T0320668

# Leukolysins and Cancer

# Contemporary Biomedicine

**Leukolysins and Cancer**
Edited by **Janet H. Ransom** and **John R. Ortaldo**, 1988

**Methods of Hybridoma Formation**
Edited by **Arie H. Bartal** and **Yashar Hirshaut**, 1987

**Monoclonal Antibodies in Cancer**
Edited by **Stewart Sell** and **Ralph A. Reisfeld**, 1985

**Calcium and Contractility:** Smooth Muscle
Edited by **A. K. Grover** and **E. E. Daniel**, 1984

**Carcinogenesis and Mutagenesis Testing**
Edited by **J. F. Douglas**, 1984

**The Human Teratomas:** Experimental and Clinical Biology
Edited by **Ivan Damjanov, Barbara B. Knowles,** and **Davor Solter**, 1983

**Human Cancer Markers**
Edited by **Stewart Sell** and **Britta Wahren**, 1982

**Cancer Markers:** Diagnostic and Developmental Significance
Edited by **Stewart Sell**, 1980

# Leukolysins and Cancer

Edited by

## Janet H. Ransom

*Bionetics Research, Inc.*
*Rockville, Maryland*

and

## John R. Ortaldo

*National Cancer Institute,*
*Frederick, Maryland*

**Humana Press · Clifton, New Jersey**

**Library of Congress Cataloging in Publication Data**

Main entry under title:

Leukolysins and Cancer.

   (Contemporary biomedicine)
   Includes bibliographies and index.
   1. Leukolysins. 2. Cancer—Immunotherapy.
I. Ransom, Janet H. II. Ortaldo, John R. III. Series.
[DNLM: 1. Cytotoxicity, Immunologic. 2. Cytotoxins—
immunology. 3. Interferons—immunology. 4. Interferons—
therapeutic use. 5. Killer Cells, Natural—immunology.
6. Lymphokines—immunology. 7. Neoplasms—
immunology. QZ 200 L652]
QR185.8.L49L48   1987      616.99'4061      87-17221
ISBN 0-89603-125-X

© 1988 The Humana Press Inc.
Crescent Manor
PO Box 2148
Clifton, NJ 07015

Printed in the United States of America

# Preface

Regulation of malignant cell growth by the immune system has been extensively studied by cancer researchers hoping to develop immuno-therapeutic approaches to cancer management. For years these studies revolved around the recognition and destruction of tumors by cytotoxic immune effector cells. Recently, however, attention has focused on the leukolysins, which are the soluble cytotoxic molecules secreted by activated leukocytes, because of their anticancer activities. The purpose of this book is to give an overview of the leukolysins, with emphasis on their ability to regulate malignant cell growth. Because this is such a new field in cancer research, there remains some confusion regarding the terminology of, and biological activity ascribed to, the different leukolysins. Therefore, we sought to present a comprehensive review of the leukolysins currently under intensive study and to compare and contrast their biological activities in an attempt to clarify the nature of these diverse biological species. This book is intended for both immunologists conducting basic research and clinical oncologists, since it reviews not only the clinical applications of the leukolysins, but presents a current update on those leukolysins that are in early developmental stages of research and could enter into clinical trials in a few years.

The introduction gives an overview of the status of research on the leukolysins. In the first section, the biological activities and biochemical characteristics of the leukolysins are presented. The lymphokines, lympho-toxin, leukoregulin, natural killer cell cytotoxic factor, and interferons and the monokines tumor necrosis factor, and macrophage cytotoxic factor are discussed. Also included are chapters on cytolysin and the mechanism of target cell destruction by pore-forming proteins that are not hormonal in action, but are relevant to the understanding of the tumoricidal activity of leukocytes. In the second section, an update of the clinical cancer therapy results using the interferons will be presented, along with information re-garding preclinical studies of two of the leukolysins that are being developed for clinical studies. There have been many literature reviews on the interferons with regard to their basic biology and clinical use. The purpose of this book is to briefly extend the available literature on the interferons, but more importantly to provide in-depth reports on the new leukolysins with potential for cancer therapy. To our knowledge, no single review has comprehensively presented all of the cytotoxic immunological hormones. Therefore, this treatise will be an invaluable aid to researchers and clinicians concerned with immunological approaches to the regulation of malignancy.

We would like to acknowledge the excellent secretarial assistance in the preparation and organization of the manuscripts by Ms. Linda Burdette and wish to thank the personnel of the Immunopharmacology Laboratory of Bionetics Research, Inc., Linda Cleveland, David Eardley, Barbara Pelle, and Douglas White, for their editorial assistance.

*Janet H. Ransom*
*John R. Ortaldo*

# CONTENTS

*Preface* ............................... v

*List of Contributors* .................... xvii

## Part 1. Biology and Biochemistry
### Introduction
#### Janet H. Ransom and John R. Ortaldo
1. The Interferons ......................... 4
2. Lymphotoxin ........................... 4
3. TNF ................................... 4
4. Natural Killer Cell Cytotoxic Factor (NKCF) ............. 6
5. Leukoregulin ........................... 6
6. Macrophage Cytotoxic Factors .......................... 6
7. Cytolysin ............................. 7
   References ........................... 7


### Cytolytic Pore-Forming Proteins
#### John Ding-E Young, Chau-Ching Liu, Lauren G. Leong, Angela Damiano, Marie A. DiNome, and Zanvil A. Cohn
1. Introduction ........................... 9
2. *Entamoeba histolytica* ....................... 10
   2.1. Contact-Dependent Cytolysis Produced by Amebae ..... 10
   2.2. Properties of the Pore-Forming Protein Isolated
        from Amebae ...................... 11
3. Cytotoxic T-Lymphocytes and NK-Like Cells ............. 20
   3.1. Nature of Cytolysis Mediated by CTLs and NK Cells .. 20
   3.2. Cytolytic Granules from Effector Cells .............. 22
   3.3. Properties of the Pore-Forming Protein Isolated from
        Granules ......................... 27

4. Eosinophils ........................................... 32
   4.1. Eosinophils Mediate Cell Killing by a Contact-
        Dependent Mechanism ............................ 32
   4.2. Eosinophil Cationic Protein as a Pore-Forming Protein .. 34
5. Complement Cascade and the Ninth Component of Complement  36
   5.1. Polymerization of C9 into Functional and Structural Ion
        Channels ........................................ 36
   5.2. Relationship Between C9 and Pore-Forming Protein
        from Lymphocytes ............................... 37
6. Conclusion ........................................... 37
   References ........................................... 39

## Cytolysin: *Its Purification, Biological Properties, and Mechanisms of Action*
### Craig W. Reynolds and Pierre Henkart

1. Introduction ......................................... 45
2. Isolation of Cytolytic Granules and Purification of Cytolysin . 46
3. Biological Properties of Cytolysin ...................... 53
4. Mechanism of Action ................................. 55
5. Summary ............................................ 60
   References ........................................... 61

## Monocyte Cytotoxic Factors
### Triggering of a Cytolytic Factor with TNF-Like Activity From Human Monocytes
### Hillel S. Koren, Karen P. McKinnon, and Allen R. Chen

1. Introduction ......................................... 67
2. Results and Discussion ............................... 72
   2.1. Role of LPS as a Critical Signal for Triggering
        Monocyte-Mediated Cytotoxicity .................. 72
   2.2. Monocyte Killing of Wehi/D Is Contact-Dependent
        and Cytolytic Factor Is TNF-Like ................. 74
   2.3. Target-Cell Selectivity and Capacity to Induce CM
        Production in Monocytes ......................... 76
   References ........................................... 81

# Antitumor Monocyte Cytotoxic Factors (MCF) Produced by Human Blood Monocytes: *Production, Characterization, and Biological Significance*
**Atsushi Uchida**

1. Introduction ........................................... 87
2. Generation of MCF ..................................... 88
   2.1. Cells Involved in MCF Production and Release ........ 88
   2.2. Optimal Conditions for MCF Generation ............. 88
   2.3. Augmentation of MCF Generation ................... 89
3. Lytic Activity of MCF ................................. 90
   3.1. Kinetics of Lysis ................................. 90
   3.2. Augmentation of MCF-Mediated Lysis by Actinomycin D  91
   3.3. Enhancement of MCF Activity by IFN ............... 91
4. Biochemical and Biophysical Characteristics of MCF ....... 92
   4.1. Temperature Stability of MCF ...................... 92
   4.2. Sensitivity of MCF to Proteolytic Enzyme ........... 93
   4.3. Effect of Protease Inhibitors on MCF Activity ........ 94
   4.4. Other Physicochemical Characteristics of MCF ....... 95
5. Biological Significance of MCF ......................... 95
   5.1. Target Cell Specificity of MCF .................... 95
   5.2. Biological Role of MCF in Human Neoplasia ......... 96
6. Conclusion ........................................... 97
   References ........................................... 97

# Antiproliferative Effects of Interferon
**Paul Aebersold**

1. Introduction ........................................... 101
2. Structure of Interferon ............................... 102
   2.1. Gene Structure ................................... 102
   2.2. Protein Structure ................................ 102
3. Interferon Receptors ................................. 103
   3.1. Types and Affinities of Receptors ................. 103
   3.2. Receptor Interactions with the Cytoskeleton ......... 105
4. Mechanisms of Action ................................. 105
   4.1. Intracellular Messengers ......................... 105
   4.2. Alterations in Gene Expression ................... 106
   4.3. Cell Cycle Progression ........................... 107

5. In Vitro Antiproliferative Effects ...................... 108
   5.1. Assays for Interferon Activity ................... 108
   5.2. Cells Inhibited by Interferon ..................... 109
   5.3. Differentiation Affected by Interferon .............. 109
   5.4. Interferon Synergisms ........................... 110
6. Structure–Function Relationships ...................... 110
7. In Vivo Tumor Biology ............................. 112
   7.1. Antibodies to Interferon ......................... 112
   7.2. Interferon-Resistant Tumors ...................... 112
   7.3. Xenografts in Nude Mice ........................ 113
   7.4. Direct vs. Indirect Effects ....................... 113
8. Conclusion ........................................ 114
   References ........................................ 115

# Natural Killer Cell Cytotoxic Factor
Human and Rodent Natural Killer Cytotoxic Factors (NKCF):
*Characterization and Their Role in the NK Lytic Mechanism*
**Susan C. Wright and Benjamin Bonavida**

1. Introduction ........................................ 121
2. Materials and Methods ............................. 122
   2.1. Production of NKCF ........................... 122
   2.2. Assay of NKCF .............................. 123
3. Results and Discussion ............................. 123
   3.1. NK Cells Produce NKCF ....................... 123
   3.2. Mechanism of NKCF Release and Its Regulation ...... 123
   3.3. Mechanism of Action of NKCF .................. 125
   3.4. Properties That Determine NK Sensitivity in a Tumor
        Cell Line ................................... 127
   3.5. Biochemical Characterization of NKCF ............. 130
   3.6. Relationship of NKCF to Other Cytotoxins ......... 130
4. Concluding Remarks ............................... 132
   References ........................................ 133

# Human Natural Killer Cytotoxic Factor (NKCF): *Relevance, Mode of Action, and Relationship to Other Cytotoxic Factors*
**John R. Ortaldo**

1. Introduction ........................................ 137

2. Results ........................................... 138
   2.1. Production of NKCF by Human LGL .............. 138
   2.2. Biochemical Characterization of Purified NKCF ...... 141
   2.3. Relationship of NKCF to Other Cytotoxic or Cytostatic
        Effectors ................................... 141
3. Discussion ....................................... 144
   References ....................................... 146

Natural Killer Cell Cytotoxic Factor
**Richard L. Deem and Stephan R. Targan**

1. Introduction ..................................... 149
2. Biology of NKCF ................................. 150
   2.1. Generation of NKCF .......................... 150
   2.2. NKCF Receptor ............................... 151
   2.3. NKCF as an Immunoregulatory Factor ........... 154
3. Biochemistry of NKCF ............................ 155
   3.1. Molecular Weights ........................... 155
   3.2. Susceptibility to Chemical Attack and pH .......... 155
   3.3. Temperature Stability ........................ 156
   3.4. Susceptibility to Enzymatic Attack ............... 156
4. Mechanism of Action of NKCF ..................... 156
   4.1. Kinetic Model for NKCF-Mediated Lysis .......... 156
   4.2. Effects of Chemical Crosslinking Agents ........... 157
   4.3. Effects of Agents That Break Disulfide Bonds ....... 158
   4.4. Effects of Inhibitors of Serine Proteases ........... 158
   4.5. Effects of Membrane Active Agents .............. 158
   4.6. Effects of Inhibitors of Receptor-Mediated Endocytosis   159
5. Future Studies ................................... 162
   References ....................................... 163

# Leukoregulin

Leukoregulin: *Biology, Biochemistry, and Mode of Action*
**Janet H. Ransom and Randall E. Merchant**

1. Introduction ..................................... 169
2. Biology of Leukoregulin .......................... 169
   2.1. Cell Source of Leukoregulin ................... 169

2.2. Bioassays ....................................... 172
2.3. Target Cell Sensitivities ......................... 173
2.4. Relationship of Leukoregulin to Other Cytotoxic
     Lymphokines .................................... 173
2.5. Leukoregulin Species Specificity ................. 178
2.6. Mechanism of Action ........................... 178
3. Physicochemical Characteristics of Leukoregulin .......... 182
   3.1. Leukoregulin Sensitivity to pH and Enzymatic Digestion  182
   3.2. Molecular Weight .............................. 182
   3.3. Isoelectric pH ................................ 183
   3.4. Stability ...................................... 186
4. Conclusions ....................................... 186
   References ........................................ 187

## Leukoregulin Mechanisms of Anticancer Action
### Charles H. Evans

1. Discovery of Leukoregulin ........................... 189
2. Assays Defining Leukoregulin Activity ................ 192
   2.1. Cytostasis—Inhibition of Cell Proliferation .......... 192
   2.2. Cytolysis—Target Cell Dissolution ................. 196
   2.3. Inhibition of Target Cell Transformation and Tumor Cell
        Outgrowth ..................................... 196
   2.4. Augmentation of Target Cell Sensitivity to Natural Killer
        Lymphocyte Cytotoxicity ....................... 198
   2.5. Destabilization of the Target Cell Membrane ......... 198
3. Preparation of Leukoregulin ......................... 202
   3.1. Cell Sources and Stimuli for Induction ............. 202
   3.2. Isolation Procedures and Retention of Biological Activity  207
4. Pathways of Leukoregulin Action .................... 208
5. Role of Leukoregulin in Homeostasis and Pathophysiology .  212
6. Therapeutic Implications and Research Directions ......... 213
   References ........................................ 214

## Lymphotoxins: *Mediators of Cellular Activation, Inflammation, and Cell Lysis That Are Immunologically Related to Macrophage Toxins and Tumor Necrosis Factors*
### Robert S. Yamamoto, Bruce J. Averbook, Mary T. Fitzgerald, Irene K. Masunaka, Sally L. Orr, and Gale A. Granger

1. Introduction ....................................... 217

2. Studies of Lymphotoxin from Normal Lymphocytes ....... 218
   2.1. Human B-Cell Lymphotoxin ..................... 219
   2.2. Human T-Cell Lymphotoxin ...................... 220
3. Immunological Relationships of LT-1, LT-2, LT-3, MCT,
   and TNF ......................................... 221
4. Effects of Lymphotoxins on Cells In Vitro .............. 222
5. Antitumor Effects of Lymphotoxins In Vivo ............. 224
6. Lymphotoxins as Inducers of Inflammation ............. 227
7. Conclusion ....................................... 229
   References ....................................... 232

## Tumor Necrosis Factors Alpha and Beta: *A Family of Biochemically Related Cytokines*
**Michael A. Palladino, Jr. and Arthur J. Ammann**

1. History of Tumor Necrosis Factors ................... 235
2. Nomenclature: In Vivo Necrosis Activities .............. 236
3. HuTNF-$\alpha$ and HuTNF-$\beta$: Biochemistry and Molecular Biology 238
   3.1. Bioassays ..................................... 238
   3.2. HuTNF-$\alpha$ and HuTNF-$\beta$ Induction Schemes ........ 238
   3.3. HuTNF-$\alpha$ ..................................... 239
   3.4. HuTNF-$\beta$ ..................................... 241
   3.5. Amino Acid Homologies ......................... 242
4. Summary ........................................ 242
   References ....................................... 243

# Part 2. Clinical Applications
# Interferons
## Clinical Aspects of Interferon Therapy in Human Cancer
**Mark S. Roth and Kenneth A. Foon**

1. Introduction ...................................... 247
2. Human Trials ..................................... 247
3. Solid Malignancies ................................ 249
   3.1. Osteosarcoma and Soft Tissue Sarcoma ............. 249
   3.2. Melanoma ..................................... 252
   3.3. Breast Cancer ................................. 253

3.4. Renal Cell Carcinoma .......................... 254
3.5. Kaposi's Sarcoma .............................. 255
3.6. Colorectal Adenocarcinoma ..................... 255
3.7. Carcinoid ..................................... 256
3.8. Lung Cancer .................................. 256
3.9. Ovarian Carcinoma ............................ 256
3.10. Bladder Carcinoma ........................... 257
3.11. Head and Neck Carcinoma ..................... 257
3.12. Cervical Cancer .............................. 257
4. Hematologic Malignancies .......................... 258
  4.1. Hairy Cell Leukemia ........................... 258
  4.2. Non-Hodgkin's Lymphoma and Hodgkin's Disease .... 258
  4.3. Cutaneous T-Cell Lymphoma ................... 259
  4.4. Chronic Lymphocytic Leukemia ................. 260
  4.5. Multiple Myeloma ............................ 260
  4.6. Chronic Myelogenous Leukemia ................ 261
  4.7. Essential Thrombocythemia ..................... 261
  4.8. Acute Leukemia .............................. 262
5. Mode of Action ................................... 262
  5.1. Oncogene Expression .......................... 263
6. Immunomodulatory Activity ......................... 264
7. Conclusion ....................................... 264
  References ......................................... 265

## Antiproliferative and Clinical Antitumor Effects of Interferons

### Joan H. Schiller and Ernest C. Borden

1. Introduction ....................................... 273
2. Direct Antiproliferative Activity of Interferons .......... 274
3. Clinical Antitumor Activity ......................... 276
  3.1. Solid Tumors ................................ 276
  3.2. Hematological Malignancies .................... 286
4. Toxicities ......................................... 293
5. Perspective ....................................... 293
  5.1. IFN and Other Lymphokines .................... 294
  5.2. IFN and Hyperthermia ........................ 294
  5.3. IFN and Cytotoxic Agents ..................... 294
6. Conclusion ....................................... 295
  References ......................................... 296

## Biologic Effects of Tumor Necrosis Factors Alpha and Beta
**Arthur J. Ammann and Michael A. Palladino, Jr.**

1. Introduction ........................................ 303
2. In Vivo Production of TNF ........................... 304
3. Effects of TNF on Tumors In Vivo ................... 305
4. Metabolic Effects of TNF In Vivo ................... 306
5. Tumor Necrosis Factor: Additional Biological Effects ..... 307
   5.1. Endotoxin Shock .............................. 307
   5.2. Inflammation ................................. 307
   5.3. Autoimmune Disease ........................... 308
   5.4. Infection .................................... 308
6. Summary ............................................ 308
   References ......................................... 309

## Leukoregulin: *Potential as a Clinical Cancer Therapeutic Agent*
**Janet H. Ransom and Linda S. Cleveland**

1. Introduction ........................................ 313
2. In Vitro Preclinical Tests ......................... 313
3. In Vivo Preclinical Tests .......................... 314
4. Conclusions ........................................ 317
   References ......................................... 317

Index ................................................. 319

# CONTRIBUTORS

PAUL AEBERSOLD · *Bionetics Research, Inc., Rockville, Maryland (Current address: Bethesda Research Laboratories, Gaithersburg, Maryland)*

ARTHUR J. AMMANN · *Department of Pharmacological Sciences, Genentech, Inc., South San Francisco, California*

BRUCE J. AVERBOOK · *Department of Molecular Biology and Biochemistry, University of California, Irvine, California*

BENJAMIN BONAVIDA · *Department of Microbiology and Immunology, School of Medicine, University of California at Los Angeles, Los Angeles, California*

ERNEST C. BORDEN · *Departments of Human Oncology and Medicine, University of Wisconsin Clinical Cancer Center, Madison, Wisconsin*

ALLEN R. CHEN · *Division of Immunology, Duke University Medical Center, Durham, North Carolina*

LINDA S. CLEVELAND · *Bionetics Research, Inc., Rockville, Maryland*

ZANVIL A. COHN · *Laboratory of Cellular Physiology, The Rockefeller University, New York, New York*

ANGELA DAMIANO · *Laboratory of Cellular Physiology, The Rockefeller University, New York, New York*

RICHARD L. DEEM · *Departments of Medicine and Microbiology and Immunology, UCLA School of Medicine, Los Angeles, California*

MARIE A. DiNOME · *Laboratory of Cellular Physiology, The Rockefeller University, New York, New York*

CHARLES H. EVANS · *Tumor Biology Section, Laboratory of Biology, National Cancer Institute, Maryland*

MARY T. FITZGERALD · *Department of Molecular Biology and Biochemistry, University of California, Irvine, California*

KENNETH A. FOON · *Department of Medicine, Division of Hematology and Oncology, University of Michigan, Ann Arbor, Michigan*

GALE A. GRANGER · *Department of Molecular Biology and Biochemistry, University of California, Irvine, California*

PIERRE HENKART · *Immunology Branch, National Cancer Institute, National Institutes of Health, Bethesda, Maryland*

HILLEL S. KOREN · *US Environmental Protection Agency, Inhalation Toxicology Division, Health Effects Research Laboratory, Research Triangle Park, North Carolina*

LAUREN G. LEONG · *Laboratory of Cellular Physiology, The Rockefeller University, New York, New York*

CHAU-CHING LIU · *Laboratory of Cellular Physiology, The Rockefeller University, New York, New York*

IRENE K. MASUNAKA · *Department of Molecular Biology and Biochemistry, University of California, Irvine, California*

KAREN P. McKINNON · *Division of Immunology, Duke University Medical Center, Durham, North Carolina*

RANDALL E. MERCHANT · *Department of Anatomy, Medical College of Virginia, Richmond, Virginia*

SALLY L. ORR · *Department of Molecular Biology and Biochemistry, University of California, Irvine, California*

JOHN R. ORTALDO · *Biological Therapeutics Branch, Biological Response Modifiers Program, Division of Cancer Treatment, National Cancer Institute, Frederick Cancer Research Facility, Frederick, Maryland*

MICHAEL A. PALLADINO, JR. · *Departments of Molecular Immunology and Pharmacological Sciences, Genentech, Inc., South San Francisco, California*

JANET H. RANSOM · *Bionetics Research, Inc., Rockville, Maryland*

CRAIG W. REYNOLDS · *Laboratory of Experimental Immunology, Division of Cancer Treatment, National Cancer Institute, National Institutes of Health, Frederick Cancer Research Facility, Frederick, Maryland*

MARK S. ROTH · *Department of Medicine, Division of Hematology and Oncology, University of Michigan, Ann Arbor, Michigan*

JOAN H. SCHILLER · *Departments of Human Oncology and Medicine, University of Wisconsin Clinical Cancer Center, Madison, Wisconsin*

STEPHAN R. TARGAN · *Wadsworth Veterans Administration Medical Center, Los Angeles, California*

ATSUSHI UCHIDA · *Department of Tumor Biology, Karolinska Institutet, Stockholm, Sweden*

SUSAN C. WRIGHT · *Department of Microbiology and Immunology, School of Medicine, University of California at Los Angeles, Los Angeles, California*

ROBERT S. YAMAMOTO · *Department of Molecular Biology and Biochemistry, University of California, Irvine, California*

JOHN DING-E YOUNG · *Laboratory of Cellular Physiology, The Rockefeller University, New York, New York*

# Part 1
# BIOLOGY AND BIOCHEMISTRY

# Introduction

JANET H. RANSOM and JOHN R. ORTALDO

The immune system has long been linked with the natural homeostatic regulation of the growth of malignant cells. Moreover, immunotherapeutic approaches have been sought to control cancer because of the inherent specificity of the immune system. The majority of these immunotherapeutic approaches has relied on specific or nonspecific activation of immune effector cells. Recently, however, interest has centered on leukolysins, the term recently adopted by the Reticuloendothelial Society to denote the soluble cytotoxic molecules secreted by activated leukocytes with anticancer activities. This specialized class of immunologic hormones is rapidly being brought to the clinic as a result of genetic engineering. A typical pattern has emerged in the clinical development of these cytotoxic molecules. Initially, a biologic "activity" is described, generally the growth inhibition or cytolysis of some type of tumor cell by the soluble product of an activated leukocyte. The "activity" is biochemically characterized and purified. Because these molecules are difficult to isolate in large quantities, only limited clinical trials have been performed with native materials. Hence, genetically engineered molecules are being used clinically. The leukolysins represent a whole new type of therapeutic agent, and much new research needs to be done to determine their best methods of use. Further, because these hormones have potent synergies with other immune effectors and chemotherapeutics, it will take time to discover the best possible combinations.

The purpose of this book is to describe biologically and biochemically the leukolysins secreted by monocytes and lymphocytes and to present the clinical data that have accumulated regarding the therapeutic effects of this new type of drug on different cancers and its side effect on patients. The only leukolysins that have undergone significant clinical testing are the interferons; therefore, we have included discussions of the preclinical trials of two other hormones, tumor necrosis factor (TNF) and leukoregulin.

3

In an effort to clarify the distinctions and interrelationships between the leukolysins discussed in this book, we have compiled a table comparing the known biologic and biochemical characteristics of each (Table 1).

## 1. The Interferons

The interferons (IFN) as a general class of leukolysins have in common the ability to induce protection against viral infection of mammalian cells. The three different types of interferons, alpha, beta, and gamma, differ in their relative abilities to augment in vivo immune responsiveness and induce tumor cell cytotoxicity. This work will concentrate on the interferons direct cytotoxic effect on tumor cells (which is primarily tumor cell cytostasis) and will not detail the interferon's stimulation of the immune system and its possible role in controlling cancer. Interferon was initially described by Isaacs and Lindeman in 1957 (1). All three types of interferons have been genetically engineered and are being evaluated in clinical trials. The interferons have their greatest success with malignancies of hematologic origin, although some solid cancers do respond. One interesting aspect of the interferon-induced clinical response is that although the direct antitumor response is one of cytostasis, complete tumor rejection does occur.

## 2. Lymphotoxin

Lymphotoxin is a term introduced in 1968 by Granger to denote the soluble product of antigen- or mitogen-stimulated lymphocytes that lyses the murine L-929 cell line (2). Lymphotoxin probably more appropriately denotes a class of molecules with similar biological characteristics, but comprised of several biochemically distinct molecular species. A lymphotoxin secreted by the human B-lymphoblastoid cell line RPMI 1788 and stimulated lymphocytes has recently been genetically engineered (3). This form of lymphotoxin has extensive amino acid sequence homology with TNF, as well as similar biological effects (4). In addition to inhibiting the murine L-929 cell line, lymphotoxin inhibits a few human tumor cell lines, but more significantly, has potent synergistic effects on numerous human tumor cell lines when combined with IFN$\gamma$, but not IFN$\alpha$ (5,6).

## 3. TNF

The discovery of TNF was unique because, unlike the other leukolysins discussed in this book, TNF was initially observed in vivo (7). Carswell

## Table 1
## Molecular and Biologic Characteristics of the Leukolysins[a]

| Parameter | Cytokine | | | | | | | |
|---|---|---|---|---|---|---|---|---|
| | TNF | Cytolysin | NKCF | Lymphotoxin | Leukoregulin | Interferon-α | Interferon-β | Interferon-γ |
| Cell sources | Monocytes, monocytic leukemias | LGL and CTL | NK cells (LGL) | T-cells, B-lymphoblastoid cell lines | T-cells, NK cells, LGL, B-lymphoblastoid cell lines | Lymphoblastoid cell lines, T-cells, LGL | Fibroblasts | T-cells, NK cells |
| Inducing agents | LPS, BCG, PMA | None | PHA, Con A, NK-sensitive target cells | PHA, antigen, PMA, SEB, thymosin α1 | PHA, antigen, NK-sensitive target cells | Virus, RNAs mitogen, PMA | Virus, RNA | Mitogen, antigen IL-2 |
| Other names | TNF-α, cachetin | Perforin | None | TNF-β | None | IFN type I, lymphoblastoid IFN | IFN type I, fibroblast IFN | IFN type II, immune IFN |
| Biologic actions | Hemorrhagic necrosis of tumors; tumor cell cytotoxicity | Pore formation, cell lysis | Lysis of NK-sensitive targets | Tumor cell lysis, tumor necrosis | Tumor cell cytolysis, tumor cell cytostasis, enhancement of target cell sensitivity to NK killing | Virus protection in cells, cytostatis of tumor and normal cells | Virus protection in cells, cytostatis of tumor and normal cells | Virus protection in cells, cytostatis of tumor and normal cells |
| Species | Human, mouse, rat, rabbits | Human, mouse, rat | Human, mouse, rat | Human, mouse, hamster, guinea pig | Human, hamster | Human, mouse, hamster, guinea pig, rat, rabbit | Human, mouse | Human, mouse, hamster, guinea pig, rat, rabbit, bovine |
| Most commonly used target cells | L-929, Wehi-164 | SRBC, YAC-1 | K562, YAC-1, U937 | L-929 | RPMI 2650, HT-29, K562 | Daudi, L-929 | Daudi, L-929 | WISH |
| mw | 19 $K_d$ 157 Amino acids | 50–60 $K_d$ | 20–40 $K_d$ | 20,000; other forms 25,000–70,000 | 25–50 $K_d$ | 20 $K_d$, 165–166 amino acids | 20 $K_d$, 166 amino acids | 18 $K_d$, 143 amino acids |
| p$I$ | 5.3 | ND | 7.5 | 5.8 | 5.4, 7.8 | | | |
| Glycosylated | No | ND | Yes | Yes | Yes | Some species | Yes | Yes |
| Genetically cloned | Yes | No, Yes | No | Yes | No | Yes, 20 different genes | Yes | Yes |
| Specific activity[b] Natural | 1 × 10⁸ | ND | ND | 4 × 10⁷ | ND | >2 × 10⁷ | >2 × 10⁷ | >2 × 10⁷ |
| Recombinant | 4 × 10⁷ | ND | ND | 2 × 10⁷ | ND | >2 × 10⁷ | >2 × 10⁷ | >2 × 10⁷ |
| Side effects in vivo | Endotoxic shock, inflammation, autoimmune disease | Unknown | Unknown | Similar to TNF | Unknown in human, nondetected in mice | Flu-like symptoms, fatigue, anosmia, somnolence, confusion, anorexia, myelosuppression, impotence, interstitial nephritis, paresthesias | | |

[a] Abbreviations: BCG, bacillus calumette guerin; CTL, cytotoxic T-lymphocytes; IFN, interferon; LGL, large granular lymphocytes; LPS, lipopolysaccharide; PHA, phytohemagglutinin; PMA, phorbol myristate acetate; SEB, staphylococcus enterotoxin B; SRBC, sheep red blood cells.

[b] Units/mg.

et al. (7), in 1976, found a factor in the serum of mice treated with endotoxin that induced the hemmorrhagic necrosis of tumors in vivo and tumor cell cytolysis in vitro. TNF has been genetically engineered (4) and was found to be identical to cachetin (8). Cachetin, also initially described as a monocyte product, was found to be the mediator in endotoxin toxicity. This presents an interesting predicament in using TNF for cancer therapy, because, although it induces tumor regression, it also has the severe side effect of inhibiting lipoprotein lipase, resulting in patient wasting, symptoms associated with endotoxic shock, inflammation, and possibly autoimmune disease. This will present many difficulties in learning the best way to utilize this effector for therapy.

## 4. Natural Killer Cell Cytotoxic Factor (NKCF)

NKCF was initially described in 1981 by Wright and Bonavida as the soluble cytotoxic factor produced during the interaction of natural killer (NK) cells with a NK-sensitive target cell that lyses NK-susceptible targets (9). The biochemistry of NKCF is very preliminary, although much work has been done on its mechanism of action and role in NK-mediated cytotoxicity (10,11). NKCF is potentially clinically interesting because it has target cell specificity similar to NK cells.

## 5. Leukoregulin

Leukoregulin, identified in 1985 by Ransom et al. (12), is one of the most recently reported leukolysins and has the ability to inhibit the growth of a wide variety of tumor cells as well as enhancing tumor cells' susceptibility to lysis mediated by NK cells. Leukoregulin, unlike most of the other cytotoxic immune hormones, has significant species restrictions. For example, human leukoregulin, although inhibiting human tumor targets, does not inhibit the growth of most mouse, guinea pig, and hamster tumor cells, and vice versa. Leukoregulin inhibits the growth of numerous freshly dissociated human carcinomas in clonogenic-type assays and has been shown to inhibit human tumor xenografts in nude mice. Therefore, when recombinant material is available, leukoregulin will be an interesting candidate for clinical trials.

## 6. Macrophage Cytotoxic Factors

In addition to the lymphokines described above, mononuclear phagocytes also secrete tumoricidal monokines. Several soluble toxic factors have been identified as macrophage products. These include lysozyme (*13*), interferon (*14*), TNF (*15*), complement (*16*), thymidine (*17*), $H_2O_2$ (*18*), proteases (*19*), and proteinaceous cytolytic molecules (*20*). TNF and interferon have been well characterized, whereas, several protein cytotoxins are currently under investigation.

## 7. Cytolysin

Cytolysin is a cytotoxic protein(s) that is contained within the cytoplasmic granules of NK cells and cytotoxic T-lymphocytes. Cytolysin probably lyses cells at the site of effector–target cell interaction in a very localized area. Cytolysin, similarly to complement, polymerizes to form a pore that is inserted into target cell membranes. Cytolysin is not target-specific and will lyse almost any membrane; therefore, its use as a therapeutic agent is unlikely. We included a discussion of its biology, however, because it is pertinent to the understanding of one soluble mechanism in the immune regulation of cancer.

## References

*1.* Isaacs, H. and Lindemann, J. *Proc. R. Soc. Lond. (Biol.).* **147**, 257–262 (1957).
*2.* Granger, G. A. and Kolb, W. P. *J. Immunol.* **101**, 111–116 (1968).
*3.* Gray, P., Aggarwal, B. B., Benton, C. V., Bringman, T. S., Henzel, W. J., Jarret, J. A., Leung, D. W., Moffat, B., Ng, P., Svedersky, L. D., Palladino, M. A., and Nedwin, G. E. *Nature* **312**, 721–724 (1984).
*4.* Pennica, D., Nedwin, G. E., Hayflick, J. S., Seeburg, P. H., Derynck, R., Palladino, M. A., Kohr, W. J., Aggarwal, B. B., and Goeddel, D. V. *Nature* **312**, 724–729 (1984).
*5.* Ransom, J. H. and Merchant, R. E., this volume.
*6.* Williams, T. W. and Bellanti, J. A. *J. Immunol.* **130**, 518–520 (1983).
*7.* Carswell, E. A., Old, L. J., Kassel, L. J., Green, S., Fiore, N., and Williamson, N. *Proc. Natl. Acad. Sci. USA* **72**, 3666–3670 (1975).
*8.* Beutler, B., Mahoney, J., Trang, N. L., Pekla, P., and Cerami, A. *J. Exp. Med.* **161**, 984–995 (1985).
*9.* Wright, S. C., and Bonavida, B. *J. Immunol.* **126**, 1516–1521 (1981).
*10.* Blanca, I., Herberman, R. B., and Ortaldo, J. R. *Natl. Immun. Cell Growth Regul.* **4**, 48–59 (1985).
*11.* Wright, S. C., Wilber, S. M., and Bonavida, B., in *Mechanisms of Cell-Mediated Cytotoxicity* vol. II (Henkart, P. and Martz, E., eds.) Plenum, New York (1985).

12. Ransom, J. H., Evans, C. H., McCabe, R. P., Pomato, N., Heinbaugh, J. A., Chin, M., and Hanna, M. G., Jr. *Cancer Res.* **45**, 851–862 (1985).
13. Osserman, E. F., Klokars, M., Halper, J., and Fishel, R. E. *Nature* **243**, 231–233 (1973).
14. Stewart, W. E., Gresser, I., Tovey, M., Bandu, M. T., and Le Goff, S. E. *Nature* **626**, 300–339 (1976).
15. Matthews, N. *Immunology* **44**, 135–142 (1981).
16. Schorlemmer, H. V. and Allison, A. C. *Immunology* **31**, 781–785 (1976).
17. Stadecker, M. J., Calderon, J., Karnovsky, M. L., and Unanue, E. R. *J. Immunol.* **119**, 1738–1743 (1977).
18. Klebanoff, S. J., in *Advances in Host Defense Mechanisms* vol. 1 (Gallin, J. I. and Fauci, A. S., eds.) Raven, New York (1982).
19. Adams, D. O. *J. Immunol.* **124**, 286–291 (1980).
20. Uchida, A., this volume.

# Cytolytic Pore-Forming Proteins

JOHN DING-E YOUNG, CHAU-CHING LIU,
LAUREN G. LEONG, ANGELA DAMIANO,
MARIE A. DINOME, and ZANVIL A. COHN

## 1. Introduction

The mechanism(s) by which professional killer cells lyse target cells remains one of the more important and exciting problems in biology today. Of particular interest to immunologists are killer cells that lyse targets efficiently by a contact-dependent process. This surface contact can be mediated by means of antibodies directed against target surface, in the case of antibody-dependent, cell-mediated cytotoxicity (ADCC) mediated by Fc receptor-bearing cells (macrophages, neutrophils, eosinophils, NK cells) or via receptors (specific and nonspecific) that recognize target surface components in the absence of antibody, as in the case of activated macrophages and cytotoxic T-lymphocytes. In both instances, it is assumed that binding of the target elicits release of the soluble mediators into the diffusion-limited intercellular space. The search for mediators of cytolysis that might explain the cell-mediated cytotoxicity, particularly that mediated by immune effector cells, has resulted in the identification of numerous mediators produced and secreted by these cells. Cytolytic proteins that exert lethal action on targets are presumed to be released into the extracellular space during effector–target cell contact. The increased interest in these effector mediators is largely the result of the feasibility of their isolation in the laboratory in high yields and their further characterization by conventional biochemical and biophysical techniques.

Several criteria have been used to implicate a mediator in cytolysis. (1) The purified or highly enriched mediator should reproduce the killing action of intact effector cells. Killing by isolated mediators should follow

9

kinetics comparable to that observed during cytolysis by intact cells. (2) The presence and release of the mediator should correlate with the expression of activation and cytolytic potential of the effector cells. In the case of macrophages, for example, only activated macrophages should produce or secrete much higher levels of the lytic mediator. (3) Attachment to the specific target should result in release of the mediator; these observations can usually be made by immunocytochemical localization studies, using antibodies directed against the mediator. Triggering of mediator release is probably also obtained with nonspecific surface-active agents, such as calcium ionophores and surface-stimulating compounds (concanavalin A, lipopolysaccharides, phorbol esters). It is important to remember that although extracellular levels of the secreted mediator may be low, these levels may become highly concentrated in the narrow intercellular contact zone between the effector and target cells. (4) Inhibitors of the mediator may or may not block whole cell killing. Negative results in such experiments may be hard to interpret, especially since the inhibitor may not have had access to the zone of contact between the effector-target. (5) Cell lines deficient in the production or secretion of the mediator may be used to further analyze the role of the mediator in cell killing.

Here, a brief summary of some of the cytolytic proteins more recently studied in our laboratory is outlined. All these proteins share a common mechanism of action, which is the formation of ion pores in the target membranes. The assembly of functional pores in target membranes resulting in disruption of electrochemical gradients and transmembrane equilibration of water, ions, and macromolecules has long been regarded as an efficient way of mediating cell lysis (*see* ref. *1* for review). In the past, membrane pore formation has been described mainly for bacterial proteins, toxins, and antibiotics (*1,2*), a topic that is beyond the scope of this brief review. Recently, a role for pore formation in protozoan parasite and immune cell-mediated cytolysis has been proposed and will be discussed in greater detail here. We suggest that all the different killer cells described here may share a common mechanism for delivery of target cell injury.

## 2. Entamoeba histolytica

### 2.1. Contact-Dependent Cytolysis Produced by Amebae

*Entamoeba histolytica* is the enteric human parasite responsible for amebiasis. This infection is characterized by an invasive enteric illness that may spread to multiple organs. In culture, this protozoan parasite is cytolytic to a variety of cell types, including neutrophils and macrophages (reviewed in ref. *3*). The mechanism(s) involved in the expression of this potent cytolysis remain unclear. Previous studies from several laboratories have shown that the cell killing mediated by ameba is dependent on its intimate contact with the target cell membrane (4–10). Following contact, the ameba may rapidly ingest the target cell (Fig. 1A). Eaton and colleagues (5) proposed earlier a surface triggering mechanism whereby lysosomal contents would be released at the site of surface contact with target cells. These observations have been substantiated by more recent cinemicroscopic and kinetic studies (9,10; see also Fig. 1B) that indicate that the cytolysis mediated by ameba may occur prior to phagocytosis, raising the possibility of an extracellular cytolytic event triggered by surface contact. In many respects, the mode of cytotoxicity mediated by ameba resembles that produced by immune cells and has been studied in our laboratory as a model system for contact-dependent cytolysis.

Cell-free extracts of *Entamoeba histolytica* have been shown to produce a cytopathic effect on cultured cells (9,11–14). This cytotoxic factor has been isolated and shown to migrate on chromatograms with an apparent $M_r$ of 25–45 kdalton (11–14). This factor has been shown to be lectin-like in that the toxicity is neutralizable by fetuin (13,14). The cytopathic effect of this factor is reversible (9) and totally inhibited by the presence of serum (9,11–14).

Previous work from this laboratory has been concerned with isolation of plasma membrane fractions and surface polypeptides from axenically grown amebae (15,16). Studies from this laboratory dealing with the endosomal pathways used by amebae have also been reported (17). Here, we briefly outline some of the more recent evidence for the involvement of a pore-forming protein (PFP) isolated from this parasite in the contact-dependent killing that closely resembles the complement system and the killer molecules isolated from immune effector cells. Our results suggest a very similar and general mechanism of killing used by all these different effector systems.

## 2.2. Properties of the Pore-Forming Protein Isolated From Amebae

### 2.2.1. Rationale and Strategy Used

Our goal was to isolate an active principle from ameba lysates that could explain the mechanism of the potent cytolysis observed with intact amebae. In particular, we needed to design functional assays that could be used to screen and enrich for this membrane lytic activity. A pore-forming protein produced by killer cells and presumably used to lyse target cells would be expected to change the transmembrane ionic balance in a dramatic way. First, at the whole cell level, PFPs should be able to lyse

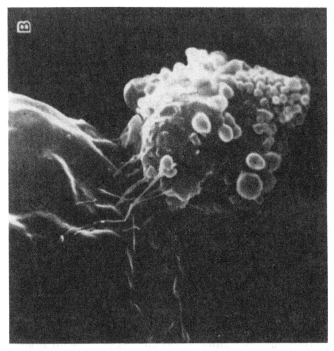

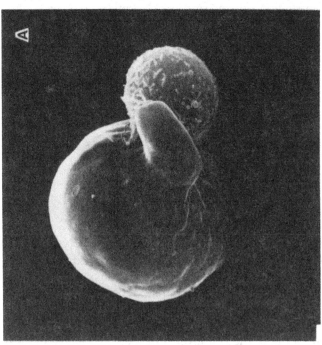

Fig. 1. Scanning micrographs of *E. histolytica* trophozoites and J774 macrophages coplated on coverslips for 10 min. (A) Initiation of phagocytosis of macrophage by ameba ($\times 970$). (B) Attachment of macrophage to ameba surface. The macrophage shows extensive membrane blebbing, a common finding at this early time point, suggesting possible extracellular cytotoxic activity mediated by the ameba ($\times 1940$) (from ref. 23).

anucleated erythrocytes and depolarize the resting membrane potential of nucleated cells. Lysis of red blood cells occurs because of the irreversible membrane permeation of electrolytes, water, and macromolecules and the lack of any significant membrane repair mechanism in those cells. Lysis of red blood cells by amebae lysates has been previously described (18). Putative PFPs can also be assayed and examined in greater details using model lipid membranes, such as lipid vesicles and planar lipid bilayers. The latter allows one to examine directly some molecular and biophysical properties associated with PFPs that would not be attained by other procedures.

## 2.2.2. Membrane Lytic Activity in Ameba Lysates

Ameba lysates depolarize dramatically the membrane potential of macrophages and lymphocytes (19) and *Fundulus* blastocells (20). Similar depolarization effects have been found with *Escherichia coli* spheroplasts (unpublished). The hemolytic activity associated with ameba lysates is unstable and rapidly decays with time when lysates are stored at 4 °C. A number of protease inhibitors have been tested and found to be ineffective in stopping the rapid loss of membrane lytic activity. Recently, the successful use of iodoacetamide has been reported (20), suggesting the possibility that sulfhydryl enzymes may be involved in this decay of lytic activity.

Ameba lysates are also active on lipid vesicles (19). Our assay consists in loading lipid vesicles with different electrolytes (19,21). In the presence of ameba membrane lytic activity, cations become more permeable through lipid vesicle membranes than anions (19). The transient asymmetric distribution of charged ions across the membrane results in the generation of transmembrane potential that can then be measured by using voltage-sensitive probes. Using this approach, it can be shown that ameba lysates make membrane permeable to $Na^+$ and $K^+$, and to a somewhat lesser degree, even to divalent ions such as $Ca^{2+}$ and $Mg^{2+}$.

As noted, the most sensitive assay for membrane lytic activity by pore formation is the high-resistance planar bilayer system (1,22,22A). Because of the high impedance of the bilayers, one can measure small conductance changes with greater time resolution than with other techniques. The bilayers are made from lipids of defined composition and can be voltage-clamped and used for direct current measurements through the use of sensitive current amplifiers. The lipid and buffer compositions are well controlled, and the clamped transmembrane potential may mimic the plasma membrane potential of living cells. The schematics of the membrane and the electrical connections of the bilayer system are outlined in Fig. 2.

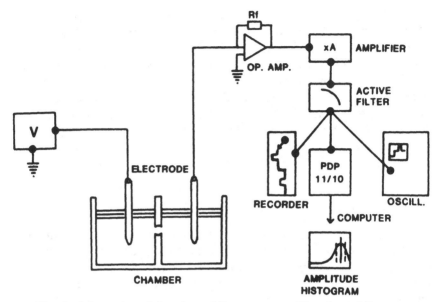

Fig. 2. Schematics of the planar bilayer system. The planar bilayer spans
the hole across the two chambers. The transmembrane voltage is clamped by a
dc battery. Current is measured via a pair of electrodes, and the signal amplified
by an operational amplifier. The output signal is shown on the oscilloscope or
chart recorder, and the data analyzed by hand or through an attached computer.

The planar bilayer gives insight into the function of individual molecules of pore formers. This technique allows the demonstration that ameba
lysates contain pore-forming proteins that rapidly increase the bilayer current (Fig. 3). The increase in current always occurs as a summation of
discrete current steps, indicative of progressive incorporation of channel
units into the bilayer. The size of each step is translated into an ion flux
of at least $10^7$ ions/channel, which is considerably higher than the rate
that would be attained by active transport or an ion carrier mechanism.

### 2.2.3. Isolation of Pore-Forming Protein from Amebae

The PFP from different strains of *Entamoeba histolytica* has been extracted with detergents (B-D-octylglucoside and SDS) and assayed as
described above (*19,20,23*). In the presence of $\beta$-D-octylglucoside, the
PFP from cell lysates may be fractionated by high-performance liquid
chromatography (HPLC), under which conditions the activity is found to
be associated with a $M_r$ of 28–30 kdalton (*19*). Interestingly, even in the
presence of high levels of B-D-octylglucoside (60 m$M$), PFP readily aggregates with time, and when rechromatographed, may assume a higher
$M_r$. Lysates fractionated by HPLC in the absence of any detergent show

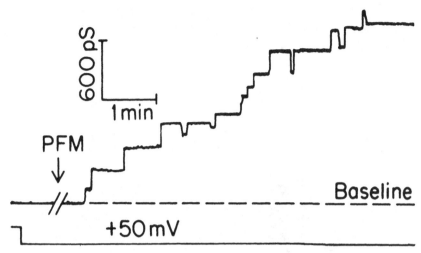

Fig. 3. Effect of ameba extracts on planar bilayer membrane conductance. The bilayer was formed in symmetrical $0.1M$ KCl solution. The voltage across the membrane was clamped at $+50$ mV. The ameba lysate was added to the positive side, followed by stirring (arrow, noise deleted). Note the increase in membrane current in steps (from ref. 19).

peaks of activity not only at the 28–30 kdalton region, but also at much higher $M_r$ values (over 200 kdalton). As noted, activity in lysates quickly decays at 4°C even in the presence of a mixture of protease inhibitors. Upon treatment with 1% SDS, the protein assumes an electrophoretic mobility of 13–15 kdalton (20,23) (Fig. 4). The 13–15 kdalton species may represent the monomeric species of PFP, whereas the larger forms may correspond to aggregates or oligomers of this monomeric species. The material extracted by SDS maintains its pore-forming activity in planar lipid bilayers (20; unpublished observations). Moreover, most of the pore-forming activity is associated with a subcellular membrane compartment that can be sedimented by high-speed centrifugation (20,23), indicating that PFP may be localized in intracellular vacuoles. We are presently deriving monospecific polyclonal antibodies for immunolocalization of this protein in amebae in order to substantiate the intriguing possibility that this protein may be packaged in lysosomal or vacuolar compartments.

PFP has also been extracted using buffers of low pH in the absence of any detergent. At low pH, PFP is in part solubilized and remains functionally active. PFP extracted at low pH and fractionated by HPLC migrates with a $M_r$ of 15 kdalton, as analyzed by SDS-polyacrylamide gel electrophoresis (Fig. 4B). The low pH extraction scheme allows for direct assay for cytotoxicity in detergent-free conditions. The planar bilayer assay may be used adequately to screen for protein preparations containing detergent,

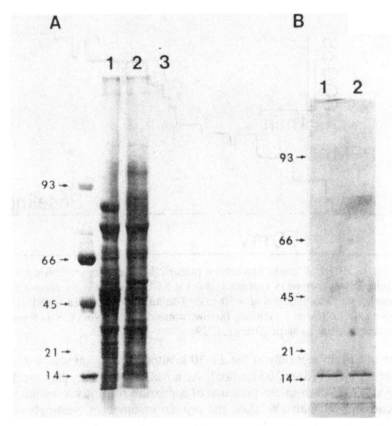

Fig. 4. Purification of the PFP from *E. histolytica*. (A) Lane 1, total post-nucleus supernatant protein, 75 μg protein. Lane 2, supernatant after centrifugation of lysate at 100,000g for 90 min, 4 °C; 75 μg protein. Lane 3, postmembrane supernatant after gel chromatography on Sephacryl S-200 and TSK-G3000 columns; fraction containing pore-forming activity was loaded on gel; 1 μg protein. (B) Lanes 1 and 2, proteins extracted from two different strains of ameba using ammonium acetate 0.2M, pH 4, followed by Sephadex G-75 and TSK-G3000 columns; the membrane active fractions were dialyzed to pH 7 and loaded on the gel; 5 μg protein each lane.

but is often laborious and time-consuming. By extracting this protein in the absence of detergent, we can now adapt a simple hemolysis microassay to screen for this protein (*24*), which may now reduce the time spent in assaying for this protein. Using the microassay, the lytic efficiency of this protein can be determined. Less than 100 ng of the enriched PFP is capable of lysing $10^8$ sheep erythrocytes suspended in 1 mL solution in less than 10 min. This lytic protein aggregates at neutral pH, as evidenced by chromatography, and loses activity rapidly at pH 7.

In view of the fact that ameba lysates contain potent proteases that appear to readily inactivate the PFP and our observation of multiple sizes for this same protein, the information gathered on the $M_r$ of this protein at the present cannot be taken as conclusive. More experiments need to be performed to elucidate the precise structure of this molecule.

## 2.2.4. Functional Properties of Ameba PFP

### 2.2.4.1. Biophysical Properties. The PFP from ameba responds remarkably to an increase in transmembrane potential. In planar bilayers containing PFP, the application of a transmembrane potential results in instantaneous current flow (Fig. 5). At voltages exceeding 30 mV, the initial current attained with the voltage pulse rapidly decays to much lower "steady-state" values with time (Fig. 5). In other words, the membrane current associated with ameba PFP increases linearly with an increase in

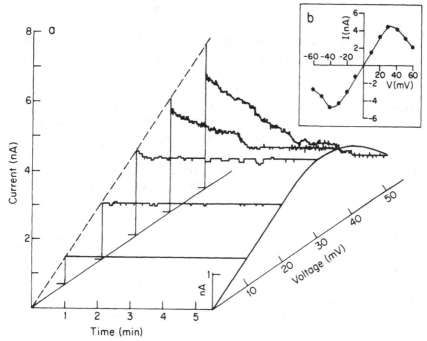

Fig. 5. The steady-state current–voltage relationship for ameba PFP. (a) Voltage steps from 0 to +60 mV at 10 mV intervals were applied to a bilayer in 0.1$M$ KCl treated with 10 µg of purified PFP. The membrane rested at 0 mV between every two pulses. The membrane current following the voltage pulse was allowed to relax for 5 min (note the time scale). The final current value was used to generate the steady-state current–voltage plot seen in the inset (b) (from ref. 23).

transmembrane potential until a sharp negative resistance region is reached (Fig. 5, inset b).

Single-channel events, corresponding to the opening and closing of individual PFP-channels, are observed when low amounts of PFP (p$M$ levels) are used (Fig. 6). Unit conductances of 67 pS (expressed in Siemens, 1 S = 1 A/1 V) are rarely observed. More often, we observe doublets with a conductance of 135 pS, hexaplets of 400 pS, and dodecaplets of 800 pS, all of which fluctuate between open and closed states in synchrony. Taken together, these results and our chromatographic observation of multiple forms of this protein suggest that PFP may oligomerize or aggregate in the membrane to form larger conducting units, in much the same way as the antibiotic alamethicin (25). Oligomerization appears not to be a requisite for functional channel formation, however, since the monomeric species forms ion channels even at very low concentrations and low temperatures (19).

The steep voltage dependence of ameba PFP mentioned above can be explained at the level of single channels. The time at which the individual channels remain open decreases with increasing voltages. Thus the transmembrane potential appears to affect directly the probability of a channel staying in the open or closed configuration.

The isolated ameba PFP confers membrane permeability to monovalent and divalent ions, in much the same way as that described for lipid vesicles.

*2.2.4.2. Secretion of PFP by Stimulated Amebae*. Amebae release constitutively low amounts of PFP into the cell medium. A significant amount of PFP can be measured in cell supernatant after only 6 h of incubation (Fig. 7a). Upon stimulation with the calcium ionophore A23187, *E. coli* LPS, and concanavalin A (con A), PFP is rapidly released by amebae (Fig. 7b). By analogy, it can be inferred that possibly other types of surface stimulation, such as cell-to-cell contact, may trigger similar and perhaps even more pronounced release of PFP into closed intercellular spaces. The relatively low amount of PFP released into the cell medium [up to 10% of total lytic activity (Fig. 7b)] may be concentrated to much higher levels in the intercellular space of cell contact, providing probably the necessary levels for cell lysis to occur.

*2.2.4.3. Cytolysis Mediated by PFP*. As described above, PFP lyses erythrocytes. Recently, the isolated PFP has also been tested against nucleated cells in standard cytotoxicity assays using [51]Cr release (unpublished observations). PFP lysed a variety of tumor cell lines, including YAC-1 and L cells.

### 2.2.5. Pore-Forming Proteins in Other Protozoan Parasites

Other protozoan parasites are known to be pathogenic and to kill by a contact-dependent mechanism. A PFP with potent hemolytic activity has

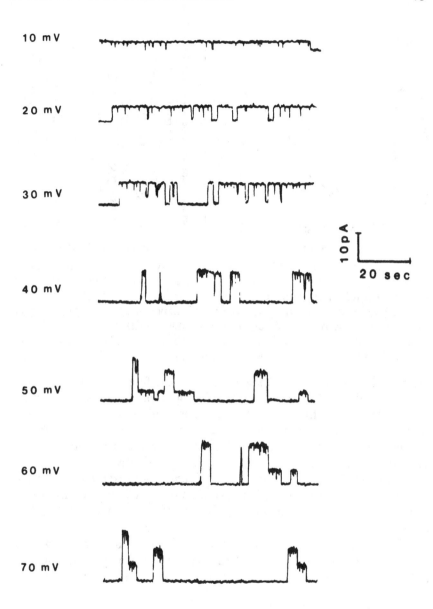

Fig. 6. Voltage-dependent conductance at the level of single channels. The membrane made in symmetrical $0.1M$ KCl was treated with 5 pg of PFP. The upward deflections represent channel openings of hexaplets at several different voltages. Note that the magnitude of current increases proportionally with an increase in voltage, whereas the opening time decreases inversely with the voltage increase. Note that at voltages over 50 mV, the unit starts to break down and smaller conductance steps may be observed to close and open synchronously.

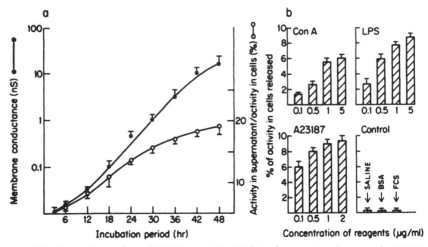

Fig. 7. (a) Secretion of PFP by viable *E. histolytica*. Amebae (strain HM1,
$2 \times 10^5$/mL) were washed three times with medium and incubated at 37 °C. At
intervals, 0.1 mL of the supernatant was tested for PFP activity in planar bilayers,
and the conductance measured after 30 min of exposure (solid bullet); activity
was also given relative to that found in cells (hollow bullet). (b) Secretion of PFP
induced by con A, *E. coli* LPS, and A23187. Saline (5%), BSA (5 mg/mL), and
FBS (5%) were used as controls (from ref. *19*).

recently been isolated from *Naegleria fowleri* and found to form functional
channels in lipid bilayers (Lowry and Young, unpublished observations).
This protein is also found to be lytic to tumor cell lines (Lowry, personal
communication). A role in cytolysis has been proposed for this membrane
lytic protein. Like the *Entamoeba* PFP, this protein assumes multiple forms,
suggesting that it undergoes a similar process of polymerization.

   We have also searched for PFPs in *Trichomonas vaginalis*, but have
not found any pore-forming activity (Young and Gorrell, unpublished observations). The protozoan *Acanthamoeba castellanii* has not been found to
produce any detectable levels of pore-forming activity.

   The closely related properties of the PFPs isolated from *Entamoeba*
and *Naegleria* support the notion that these proteins may be responsible
at least in part for the potent cytolysis mediated by these two parasites.

# 3. Cytotoxic T-Lymphocytes and NK-Like Cells

## 3.1. Nature of Cytolysis Mediated by CTLs and NK Cells

The mechanism(s) by which cytotoxic T-lymphocytes (CTL) and
natural killer (NK) cells lyse tumor cells have been extensively studied

in several laboratories over the past few years (for reviews, *see* refs. *26–31*). A permeability increase in the target membrane inflicted by effector cells via antibody–Fc receptor interaction (ADCC) was first demonstrated by Henkart and Blumenthal (*32*). The possibility of pore formation during ADCC was later substantiated by ultrastructural demonstration of target membrane-associated ring-like lesions with an internal diameter of 15 nm (*33*). These same ring structures were found to be associated with extracellular granular material released by effector cells (large granular lymphocytes), suggesting the involvement of a secretory phenomenon, by which the granular contents of effector cells are released upon contact with target cells (*34*). These studies were extended by Podack and Dennert, who demonstrated that cloned CTL (*35*) and NK cells (*36*) also assembled ring-like structures on target membranes.

Other functional studies that support a role for pore formation in lymphocyte killing include: (1) the dose–response curve of cell killing corresponds to a one-hit mechanism (*37*); (2) the release of small molecular weight markers precedes the release of cellular contents of large molecular weight (*38*); (3) inhibition of T-cell-mediated lysis employing extracellular macromolecules indicates the presence of either an osmotic or diffusion-limiting protective mechanism (*39*); (4) after initial contact, the presence of the effector cells is no longer necessary for the completion of lysis to occur since the former can leave the target cell to kill other cells (*40,41*); (5) functional sizing of the lymphocyte-mediated lesion gives estimates comparable to the size of the pores generated by complement (*42,43*).

The role of other mediators in T-cell-mediated cytolysis, such as oxygen metabolism intermediates, has also been investigated (*44*). Although $O_2$ is required for T-cell-mediated killing, reactive oxygen intermediates do not seem to play a direct role in T-lymphocyte-mediated killing (*44*). It has also been suggested that NK cell lysis may involve the action of proteases (*45–48*). Recently, it has been proposed that a soluble cytotoxic factor, NKCF, may be responsible at least in part for the cytolysis mediated by NK cells (*49–53*). It is possible that this NKCF may be related or identical to tumor necrosis factor (TNF) and lymphotoxin (LT), which has been recently cloned and expressed in *E. coli* (*54–57*). A detailed description of the potential role of TNF in killing is described elsewhere in this volume (*see* chapter by Palladino in this volume). In addition to these cytotoxic factors, multiple cytokines are known to be produced by human large granular lymphocytes (LGL), such as interleukins 1 and 2, interferons-α and -γ and B-cell growth factor (*58*). The LGLs appear to correspond morphologically and functionally to human NK cells (*59,60*).

With the advent of cloned cell lines that show high cytotoxic activity (*61–67*), it has become possible to grow large numbers of homogeneous populations of cells for biochemical analysis. Recently, work on lymphocyte and NK cell cytolysis has been extended to subcellular levels and to purified protein. Here, we outline first the cytolytic properties of cytoplasmic granules isolated from these cells and then the lytic properties of the protein responsible for the ring-like lesions produced on target cell membranes.

## 3.2. Cytolytic Granules from Effector Cells

### 3.2.1. Presence of Cytoplasmic Granules in CTL and NK Cells

The lytic apparatus of CTL and NK cells appears to be localized in the granule population of these cells. Granules isolated from cloned mouse CTL and rat LGL are cytotoxic and capable of assembling membrane lesions in the presence of $Ca^{2+}$ (68–72). All the cytotoxic T-cell lines (CTLL) and NK clones examined contain cytoplasmic granules (Fig. 8). The granules vary in size (usually ranging from 0.1 to 1 $\mu$m), but generally show a fine amorphous matrix surrounded in the periphery by electron-dense membrane-bound vesicular material (Fig. 8B).

### 3.2.2. Isolation of Cytoplasmic Granules

In order to assess which subcellular fraction is responsible for cytolysis, cloned effector cells have been subjected to fractionation and the different compartments analyzed for their lytic activity. The fractionation procedures used by several investigators who have successfully isolated granule populations from these cells have all involved centrifugation of cytoplasmic material through continuous or discontinuous gradients of Percoll (68–73) (Fig. 9A). Centrifugation through Percoll gradients allows for rapid separation of the different cytosolic compartments. The different fractions are then tested for hemolytic or pore-forming activity in planar bilayers. The granule fraction is enriched in $\beta$-glucuronidase (68,69) and other lysosomal markers (68,69), suggesting the lysosomal nature of the granules.

### 3.2.3. Functional and Structural Lesions Produced by Isolated Granules

*3.2.3.1. Structural Lesions.* The isolated granules are capable of assembling membrane lesions when incubated with target membranes at 37°C, in the presence of $Ca^{2+}$ (68–73). Tubular structures of approximately 160 Å diameter are observed (Fig. 9B–D). In addition to complete rings, partially assembled tubules are also frequently observed (Fig. 9D). Thus, isolated granules are capable of producing lesions resembling those formed by intact killer cells.

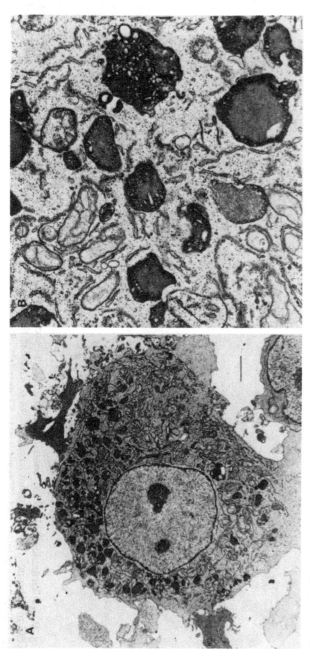

Fig. 8. (A) Morphology of Hy 3-Ag3 cell, showing numerous electron-dense granules in the cytoplasm. (B) An enlarged view of a selected region of the cytoplasm containing granules. Note the amorphous matrix of granules surrounded by the more electron-dense vesicular membranes. Scale bar corresponds to 3.5 μm in (A) and 657 nm in (B) (from ref. 73).

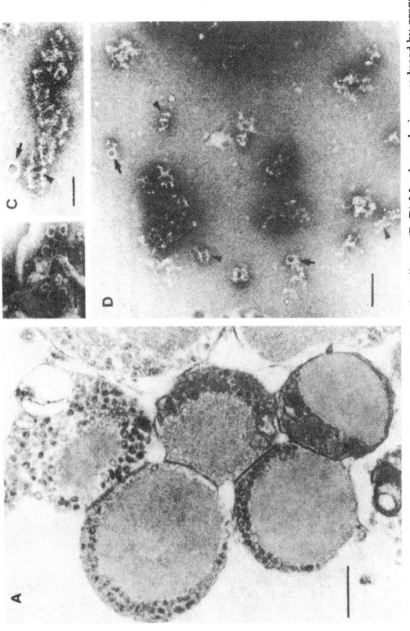

Fig. 9. (A) Granules isolated by centrifugation through Percoll gradients. (B–D) Membrane lesions produced by granules on SRBC membranes. Arrows point to top views of circular lesions. Arrowheads correspond to longitudinal views of the tubular lesions. Scale bars: (A), 270 nm; (B), 57 nm; (C), 38 nm; (D), 87 nm (from ref. 73).

*3.2.3.2. Functional Lesions.* Granules from CTLL and NK-like cells are highly hemolytic (*68–73*). The kinetics of the hemolysis can be measured simply as a decrease of turbidity of an erythrocyte suspension at 700 nm. Such kinetic studies show rapid hemolysis produced by isolated granules that is entirely $Ca^{2+}$-dependent (Fig. 10). The hemolysis can be restored in $Ca^{2+}$-free medium by addition of $Ca^{2+}$ (Fig. 10c). Similarly, hemolysis can be effectively interrupted when EGTA is added to an ongoing lysis experiment to chelate $Ca^{2+}$ to micromolar levels (Fig. 10d).

The isolated granules depolarize the membrane potential of nucleated cells (*71–73*), induce marker release and ion fluxes across membranes of lipid vesicles (*74*), and form functional channels in high-resistance planar lipid bilayers (*71–73*). Figure 11 shows a typical planar bilayer experiment, in which a membrane has been exposed to granular material from mouse CTLL. Typically, the conductance increase occurs in discrete jumps, and progresses until the membrane breaks (Fig. 11). This behavior is again indicative of incorporation of single or groups of single channels into the bilayer. Incorporation of channels into the bilayer is also dependent on the presence of $Ca^{2+}$. The sizes of the channels are heterogeneous, varying in the range of 0.4 to 6 nS/channel in $0.1M$ NaCl. It appears that the different sizes correspond to multiple forms of polymerization of the granule PFP.

Unlike ameba PFP, granule-derived channels remain permanently open at low transmembrane potentials (Fig. 12). These pores are highly resistant to changes in the electrical field, and show only a significant amount of closing at voltages that exceed 70 mV. The current–voltage relationships for these channels show a linear curve (Fig. 12, lower panel), with noise and only slight deviation from linearity (i.e., with channels closing) developing at voltages exceeding 70 mV. This behavior indicates that large, stable, and voltage-resistant channels are formed by the granule-derived material, which are attributes that would favor an active role of these channels in cytolysis.

Because of the relatively high resistance to closing, single-channel events are rare and only observed at high transmembrane potentials (*71–73*). The single channels formed by the granules are large and heterogeneous in size.

Granules that show membrane lytic activity have been isolated from a variety of cell lines. A rat tumor LGL line (corresponding possibly to rat blood NK cells) yields granule fractions with high lytic activity (*68,69*). Several mouse CTLL (*70–72*) and a mouse cell line, showing high NK-like activity (*73*), have all been successfully used to produce highly lytic granules.

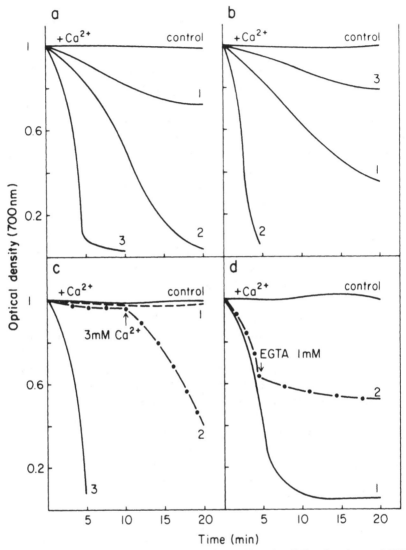

Fig. 10. Hemolytic activity associated with subcellular fractions of CTLL
A11 cells. Hemolysis of SRBC was assayed in the presence or absence of 1 m*M*
CaCl₂, as indicated. Reagents were added at time 0; for control, phosphate-
buffered saline (PBS) was added. (a) Curve 1, whole-cell, postnuclear lysate (5
μg protein/mL); curve 2, cells resuspended in 0.8% NH₄Cl, producing control
hemolysis; curve 3, granules (5 μg/mL). (b) Curve 1, granules (1 μg/mL); curve
2, granules extracted with ammonium acetate; the high-speed supernatant, dialyzed
against PBS, was added at 1 μg of protein per mL; curve 3, pellet (1 μg/mL)
from ammonium acetate extraction, followed by dialysis against PBS. (c) Curve
1, granules (5 μg/mL) added in the absence of Ca²⁺; curve 2, granules (5 μg/mL)

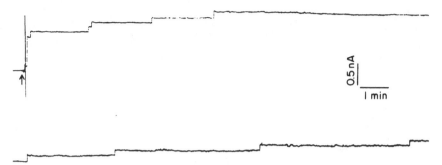

Fig. 11. Effect of granule-derived material on bilayer conductance. Planar bilayer made in buffer A and clamped at constant 30 mV was exposed to granule-proteins incubated at 37 °C for 48 h. Twenty micrograms of granule-protein mixed with 0.2% Triton X-100 was diluted into the *cis* side (400 times dilution). Note the increase of membrane current in discrete steps; current trace (top, right) is continued at the bottom (left) (from ref. *72*).

## 3.3. Properties of the Pore-Forming Protein Isolated from Granules

### 3.3.1. Isolation of Pore-Forming Proteins from Isolated Granules

The putative pore-forming protein from lymphocyte granules has received several names, even prior to its purification. Henkart and colleagues have named the putative PFP of rat LGL tumor as cytolysin (*68, 69,74*). The mouse cytotoxic T-cell and NK cell putative pore-forming monomers were termed perforin 1 and 2 by Podack and Dennert (*35,36*). Because in our hands the cytolytic protein resembles that produced by a variety of effector cell types in that they form channels in lipid bilayers, we have kept our generic terminology of pore-forming proteins (PFP) (*71*) and will refer to them as such in this review.

The PFPs from mouse cytotoxic T-cells and NK-like lymphocytes have recently been purified (*75–78*). The PFP was purified by a combination of ion exchange and molecular sieving chromatography (*76–78*). The eluted fractions from the columns are assayed for hemolytic activity using the microassay described earlier (*24*) and also for pore-forming activity in

---

← Fig. 10. (continued)

added without Ca²⁺, followed by addition of 3 m$M$ CaCl$_2$ (arrow); curve 3, control lysis with granules (5 $\mu$g/mL) in the presence of 1 m$M$ CaCl$_2$. (d) Curve 1, granules (5 $\mu$g/mL) in the presence of 1 m$M$ CaCl$_2$; curve 2, granules (5 $\mu$g/mL) followed by addition of 1 m$M$ EGTA (arrow). Under these conditions, free Ca²⁺ was brought down to micromolar levels (solid bullets) (from ref. *72*).

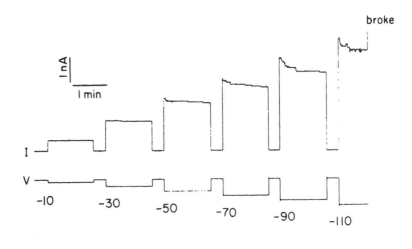

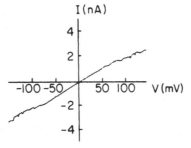

Fig. 12. Steady-state membrane current (I) as a function of membrane voltage (V). Bilayer in $0.1M$ NaCl was exposed to 15 $\mu$g of granule-protein as in Fig. 11 and allowed to sit for 30 min prior to application of voltage pulses at 20 mV increments. The membrane rested at 0 mV between every two pulses. Note the progressive decay of instantaneous current at voltage $>70$ mV. The membrane broke (as indicated) under application of $-110$ mV. (Lower panel) Current-voltage plot generated by applying a continuous voltage ramp running between $-150$ and $+150$ mV in 1 s to a bilayer treated with 15 $\mu$g of granule-protein (from ref. 72).

planar bilayers. The monomeric protein migrates with a $M_r$ of 66–68 kdalton (75) and 70–75 kdalton (76–78) under reducing conditions when analyzed by SDS-polyacrylamide gel electrophoresis (Fig. 13B). The non-reduced form has an apparent $M_r$ of 60–66 kdalton as observed by gel electrophoresis and molecular sieving chromatography (Fig. 13A). Sizing PFP by HPLC (Fig. 13A) provides an independent estimate of its apparent $M_r$ and excludes the possibility that the single band observed by SDS-PAGE could have been related to the closely comigrating bovine albumin or that the lytic activity could have been associated with some other minor species *not* identified by gel electrophoresis.

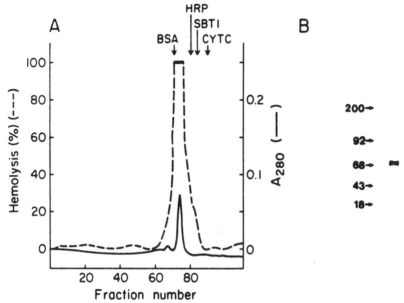

Fig. 13. Purification of PFP from cytotoxic T-lymphocytes. (A) $A_{690}$ (hemolysis) and $A_{280}$ (protein) determinations in HPLC fractions containing eluted PFP from cell granules. The injected sample was previously purified by Sephacryl S-200 and Mono Q columns. For hemolysis assay, 250 $\mu$L of SRBC suspension (at density of $5 \times 10^7$ cells/mL) was placed into each well of a 96-well plate and 2-$\mu$L aliquots from each HPLC fraction was added. Arrows delineate elution patterns of $M_r$ markers. (B) SDS-PAGE profile of peak hemolytic fraction from (A). 40-$\mu$L sample (approximately 1 $\mu$g protein) was loaded on the gel (from ref. 24).

### 3.3.2. Polymerization of the Purified Protein in the Presence of Ca²⁺

*3.3.2.1. Demonstration by Gel Electrophoresis.* The purified protein polymerizes in the presence of $Ca^{2+}$ at 37°C, resulting in the formation of a polymeric species of $M_r$ greater than 1 Mdalton that resists partial dissociation by SDS and reducing agents (Fig. 14). In the absence of $Ca^{2+}$, polymerization is not observed (77).

*3.3.2.2. Demonstration by Chromatography.* The polymerized species also migrates as multiple forms of the monomeric protein when analyzed by molecular sieving chromatography. Following incubation with $Ca^{2+}$ at 37°C and elution through Sephacry S-200 columns, most of the protein elutes in the void volume.

*3.3.2.3. Demonstration by Electron Microscopy.* The purified protein polymerizes into tubular lesions on erythrocyte membranes, as visualized by negative staining (Fig. 15). Tubular structures with a diameter averaging 160 Å are typically seen.

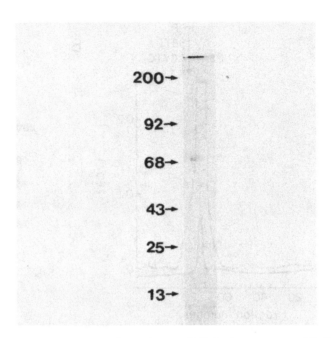

Fig. 14. Polymerization of lymphocyte PFP in the presence of $Ca^{2+}$. 10 $\mu$g PFP from TSK G3000 column was incubated at 37°C, 48 h, with 1 m$M$ $CaCl_2$, 0.1% deoxycholate, 0.5 m$M$ phenylmethylsulfonyl fluoride, and 0.1 U/mL aprotinin and applied to the gel under reducing conditions. A 4–11% gradient gel swab was used (20 cm long). An additional 3 cm of 4% gel was placed on top of the running gel to resolve high $M_r$ bands.

### 3.3.3. Functional Lesions Produced by PFP

*3.3.3.1. Effect of PFP on Cells.* The purified protein shows potent hemolytic activity directed toward erythrocytes from a number of different species. One nanogram of PFP is capable of lysing completely $10^8$ sheep red blood cells in a total volume of 200 $\mu$L (*24*). The PFP does not bind to membranes in the absence of calcium, as inferred from the following experiment: SRBCs incubated with PFP at 37°C for 15 min in the absence of calcium, washed twice, and resuspended in buffer containing 1 m$M$ $Ca^{2+}$ are not hemolyzed following subsequent incubation at 37°C (*77*).

PFP is also found to depolarize the membrane potential of a number of different cell types. Chicken embryos myoblasts, impaled with microelectrodes, rapidly depolarize following exposure to PFP (*77,78*). $Ca^{2+}$ is required for maximal depolarization activity. PFP that has been incubated at 37°C for 4 h (i.e., material that has polymerized) produces no depolarization response.

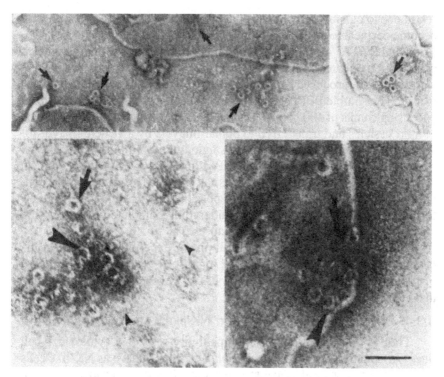

Fig. 15. Polymerization of lymphocyte PFP on erythrocyte membranes to form tubular lesions. The four panels show selected images of typical ring structures of 160 Å internal diameter (arrows) and some incompletely polymerized tubules (arrowheads). Scale bar: upper panels, 250 nm; lower panels, 85 nm (from ref. 77).

PFP inserts spontaneously into cell membranes, as measured by whole cell patch recording (76). Current steps are observed that seem to correspond to the insertion of individual channels into the cell membrane.

### 3.3.3.2. Effect on Lipid Vesicles.

The membrane perturbation effect is also observed when lipid vesicles are used as target membranes (76–78). Membranes treated with PFP become permeable to monovalent and divalent ions ($Ca^{2+}$, $Mg^{2+}$, $Ba^{2+}$, $Zn^{2+}$) and to large macromolecules like sucrose (mol wt , 342) and lucifer yellow (mol wt , 457).

### 3.3.3.3. Effect on Planar Bilayers.

PFP induces step-wise conductance increments in planar bilayers similar to those produced by solubilized granule contents (77,78). Similar voltage–current and ion selectivity ratios are obtained for the purified protein. The channels produced by PFP have large conductance steps and are relatively voltage-resistant, showing great resistance to closing by voltages under 70 mV. Bilayers treated with PFP become permeable to glucosamine (which has a Stokes diameter of 8 Å), Tris⁻, and EGTA²⁻, implying a large functional diameter for the assembled pores. Single-channel recordings obtained with the purified protein are similar to those produced by the granules. The unit steps are heterogeneous in size. The soluble PFP that inserts spontaneously into lipid bilayers produces single units of 400 pS in $0.1M$ NaCl. The protein that has polymerized in lipid vesicles and transferred to planar bilayers by a vesicle-bilayer fusion protocol produces much larger single units, in the range of 1–6 nS (Fig. 16). These results suggest that PFP may polymerize into complete and incomplete rings of multiple sizes, all of which are functionally conducting in the bilayer. It is therefore possible that PFP may produce effective membrane damage without undergoing complete polymerization to form the EM-visible tubular structures.

*3.3.3.4. Cytolytic Activity.* Preliminary experiments show that the purified protein is lytic to a variety of tumor cell types *(78)*. The amount of protein required to achieve cytolysis, however, is much higher than that required for hemolysis.

### 3.3.4. PFP Isolated from CTL and NK-like Lymphocytes

The PFP isolated from histocompatibility-restricted cytotoxic T-cell lines *(78)* and that obtained from lymphocytes that behave as NK-like cells *(77)* has a number of identical structural and functional properties. Presently, studies in our laboratory are seeking to identify similar polypeptides in human peripheral blood lymphocytes and NK cell lines.

## 4. Eosinophils

### 4.1. Eosinophils Mediate Cell Killing by a Contact-Dependent Mechanism

Eosinophils play an active role in allergic reactions and in the antibody-dependent killing of a number of helminthic parasites *(see* refs. *79–82* for review). Recently, eosinophil granule proteins have been implicated in this killing process *(79–82)*. A number of cationic proteins have been isolated and characterized from eosinophil granules of several species. A major basic protein (MBP) of 9–11 kdalton was extracted from eosinophils of several species *(83–85)*. Major eosinophil cationic proteins (ECP) with a $M_r$ of 21 kdalton have also been extracted from human eosinophil granules *(86,87)*. Other basic proteins that have been isolated from eosinophils include EP-X *(88)*, eosinophil peroxidase *(89)*, and the eosinophil-derived neurotoxin (EDN) *(90,91)*. Since all these proteins have been shown

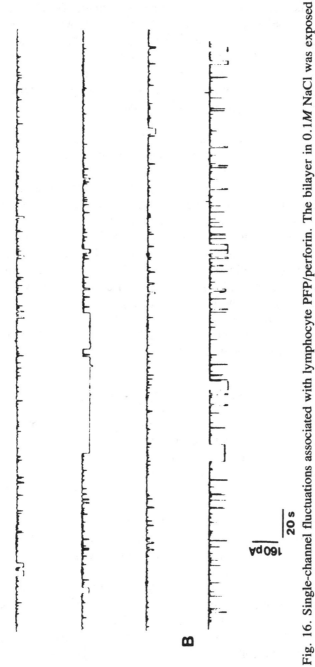

Fig. 16. Single-channel fluctuations associated with lymphocyte PFP/perforin. The bilayer in 0.1*M* NaCl was exposed to 0.5 ng/mL of purified PFP from CTLL A2. The trace shows a continuous recording from upper left to lower right, obtained 10 min after addition of protein, with bilayer clamped at +120 mV. The upward deflections represent channel openings. Note the slow channel fluctuations of 400 pS observed at this voltage. Resolution, 1 ms. (B) PPF was reconstituted into lipid vesicles and incorporated into planar bilayer. Proteoliposomes (2 μm PFP) were fused with bilayer as described in ref. 78. The current trace was obtained 15 min after perfusion of bilayer chamber with urea-free buffer. Note the 1 nS channel step (from ref. 77).

to constitute the major contents of eosinophil granules (92), their role in parasite and microbial killing has been investigated in several laboratories. MBP has been shown to damage parasites (93,94) and mammalian cells (95), but at concentrations exceeding $10^{-5}M$. At these concentrations, it is possible that surface charge interactions (because bilayer membranes are negatively charged) may result in a nonspecific permeability increase of target membranes (96,97) without the concomitant formation of ion channels.

For the human ECP, it has been shown that the purified protein damages schistosomula of the intravenous parasite *Schistosoma mansoni* at concentrations as low as $10^{-7}M$ (98). ECP also induces the classic paralytic syndrome known as the Gordon phenomenon after intrathecal injection into guinea pigs (99). ECP has been detected by radioimmunoassays in the supernatant of human degranulated granulocytes via the Fc-linked mechanism (80). Because a secretory form of ECP has been identified in eosinophil granules (100) and eosinophils kill by a contact-dependent mechanism, the extracellular release of ECP seen with cell stimulation by immunocomplexes suggests that secretion of ECP into closed intercellular spaces between the effector and target cells may play a role in cell killing. In an attempt to understand the mechanism of cell damage induced by ECP, we subjected eosinophils and their granule contents to the same rigorous treatment as that used with other effector cells (101), and our results are outlined below.

### 4.2. Eosinophil Cationic Protein as a Pore-Forming Protein

ECP can be purified from human eosinophil granules by a low-pH extraction protocol. Granules are first enriched by sucrose density gradient centrifugation of nucleus-free cell lysates. The granules are then extracted with $0.2M$ ammonium acetate, pH 4, followed by molecular sieving and ion-exchange chromatography. On SDS-PAGE, the purified protein typically migrates as a major band of 21 kdalton, associated with two closely migrating minor bands (101). The three bands show immunological cross-reactivity, suggesting a precursor relationship between the different species. ECP is extremely basic, the isoelectric point being higher than pH 11.

The isolated ECP is toxic to a number of cell types. ECP lyses sheep red blood cells, depolarizes the membrane potential of cultured nucleated cells, and induces ion flow through lipid vesicles (101). After intrathecal injection of ECP into guinea pigs, it lyses Purkinje cells (Fig. 17), consistent with the eosinophil-associated paralytic cerebellar Gordon syndrome in guinea pigs (99).

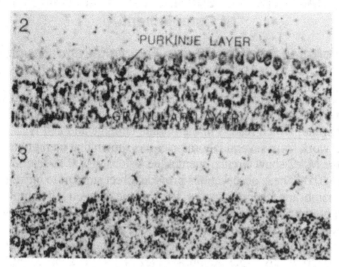

Fig. 17. Cytolysis mediated by human eosinophil cationic protein. (Panel 2) Normal Purkinje cells of a guinea pig 10 d after an intraventricular injection of 10 μL physiological saline (151 ×). (Panel 3) Seven days after an intraventricular injection of 0.3 μg of ECP. The Purkinje cells are depleted, leaving the typical cell cavities (151 ×) (from ref. *99*).

When phospholipid bilayers are exposed to lysates of human eosinophils, typical conductance steps are incorporated into the bilayers (*101*), suggesting the formation of discrete ion channels. The membrane lytic material is enriched in the granule population extracted by centrifugation of subcellular material through continuous Percoll gradients (*101*). Purified ECP forms channels that show characteristics similar to those produced by cell lysates and granule fractions.

ECP channels are very resistant to closing by high transmembrane voltages, in a way similar to the pore-forming protein from lymphocytes. Up to 100 mV, the conductance associated with ECP channels shows little or no relaxation to lower steady-state values in response to increasing voltage pulses (*101*). ECP channels appear to be stable transmembrane entities, remaining permanently open once inserted into the bilayer. Ion-selectivity experiments show that ECP channels are relatively nonselective to all the monovalent ions tested, being slightly more permeable to anions. The single-channel unit averages 120 pS in 0.1$M$ NaCl.

ECP forms channels that are indistinguishable in many ways from those formed by lymphocyte PFP (perforin). These observations suggest a similar mode of action among all these effector molecules.

## 5. Complement Cascade and the Ninth Component of Complement

### 5.1. Polymerization of C9 into Functional and Structural Ion Channels

The membrane attack complex (MAC) of complement is formed by the assembly of the five terminal components of complement in the target cell membrane, which results in membrane damage and cell lysis. Ultrastructural work from several laboratories has shown that membranes damaged by the MAC show circular membrane lesions of 100 Å internal diameter (102–105). These observations provide direct support to the doughnut or transmembrane channel model for the mechanism of complement-mediated membrane lysis first proposed by Mayer (106). The assembly of the hydrophilic precursors of complement into the lipophilic MAC involves the expression of hydrophobicity at several levels: the initial insertion of C5b-7 into target membranes (107) and the subsequent attachment of C8 and C9 leading to membrane damage (108,109).

Recently, it has been demonstrated that the ninth component of complement is largely responsible for the appearance of the tubular lesions found to be associated with the MAC (105,110,111). Purified C9 polymerizes spontaneously after prolonged incubation at 37°C to form circular polymers resembling ultrastructurally the MAC (112,113). Polymerization of monomeric C9 ($M_r$ of 70–75 kdalton) into a supramolecular transmembrane tubule ($M_r$ greater than 1 Mdalton) involves the self-association of 12–16 C9 molecules (114), which then become resistant to dissociation by SDS, reducing agents, and proteolysis.

The purified C9 can be catalyzed to polymerize at a much faster rate in the presence of heavy metals (115,116). We have recently reconstituted poly-C9 into model lipid membranes and measured directly the transmembrane current associated with poly-C9 channels (116,117). The current steps are heterogeneous in size and reveal electrical characteristics indistinguishable from those of PFP from eosinophils and lymphocytes. Monomeric C9 fails to confer any conductance change to lipid bilayers. Channel formation results only from polymerization of C9 (116,117). Poly-C9 forms stable, voltage-insensitive channels that remain permanently open at low membrane potentials (up to 100 mV), an observation that would be consistent with the expected cytolytic function associated with the MAC.

Single poly-C9 channel fluctuations show slow open–close kinetics similar to that described for the other PFPs (Fig. 18). The single-channel conductance increases proportionally with an increase in the ionic strength of the medium, indicating that water and ions are freely mobile within

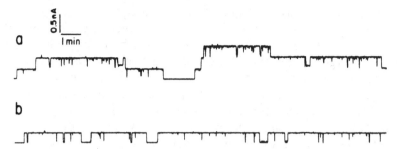

Fig. 18. Single-channel properties of poly-C9 in bilayer. (a and b) Two separate experiments with poly-C9 introduced into bilayers at ng levels. The membrane was bathed in 0.1$M$ NaCL and clamped at +120 mV (from ref. *116*).

the poly-C9 channel and supporting a water-filled tubular model for the poly-C9 structure. Poly-C9 channels are also permeable to lucifer yellow (mol. wt., 457) and sucrose (mol. wt., 342). The estimates for the minimal functional size of poly-C9 channel range from 60 to 80 Å (*116,117*), which are comparable to functional diameters of 40 Å (*43*) and 55 Å (*118*), estimated previously for the MAC.

## 5.2. Relationship Between C9 and Pore-Forming Protein from Lymphocytes

The resemblance in ultrastructural morphology and functional properties between C9 and lymphocyte PFP (perforin) has suggested to us the presence of structural domains common to both molecules. This possibility has recently been assessed by using polyclonal antibodies raised against purified C9 and lymphocyte PFP. Recent data indicate that the homology is limited to a domain that is only exposed when the two molecules are reduced (*7,119,120*).

## 6. Conclusion

It appears that a common mechanism is shared by a variety of cell types specialized in target cell killing. In the cell-mediated contact-dependent cytotoxicity, pore-forming proteins are clearly implicated at least for cytotoxic T-lymphocytes, NK cells, eosinophils, and certain protozoan parasites, such as *Entamoeba histolytica* and *Naegleria fowleri*. More work needs to be done to investigate the presence of such proteins in other cell types, such as activated macrophages and neutrophils. The strategical localization of these proteins to subcellular compartments (granules) likely to be involved in secretory phenomena suggests again an active role for these proteins during cell lysis and implies that cell killing may involve a membrane secretory phenomenon. In this model, the specificity of target cell killing is not conferred by the protein, but rather by recognition of the appropriate targets at the level of effector–target cell membrane contact. Once triggered, the killing apparatus is thought to be surprisingly similar for the various cell types: a pore-forming protein is secreted into the intercellular space, and then assembles to form structural and functional lesions in the target membrane. The cells differ mainly in how they recognize the right targets. The question of how the effector cell protects itself from injury once PFP has been released remains an exciting problem that needs to be resolved.

Pore formation may represent a general mechanism of membrane damage. In this respect, it is intriguing that the complement system (and mainly C9) may form channels that are similar in a number of ways to the channels formed by effector cells. This homology has recently been substantiated by evidence that points to immunological cross-reactivity between C9 and the lymphocyte PFP. It is possible that the highly effective mechanism of delivering membrane damage by pore formation may have remained functionally conserved during evolution. Our immediate goal is to find out the extent of structural homology that exists between these various molecules at the level of primary amino acid sequence and gene expression. It is entirely conceivable that all these proteins may have emerged from one single ancestral parent protein that diverged during evolution and became specialized later to serve the purposes of either humoral or cellular immune responses. The fact that even certain distantly related pathogenic protozoan parasites have proteins with similar function substantiates further our view that these effector molecules must play an important role during cell killing.

Other granule constituents, especially those of lymphocytes, should be analyzed for their possible role in cell killing. Efforts in our laboratory are concerted toward characterizing each one of those components and testing their function in cell killing. It is possible that the protein channel described here could actually work as a transmembrane conduit for other toxic molecules (such as proteases or nucleases) that might go through these channels and penetrate the target cell. It is easy to envision such a role for channels of the diameter described here. The permeation of a second toxic molecule from the granules of lymphocytes, for example, would be able to explain the nucleus breakdown commonly observed in target cells exposed to NK-like and cytotoxic T-cells.

In the next few years, it will be exciting to see the molecular structure of each of these proteins and their gene expression elucidated and to start thinking in terms of their in vivo therapeutic applications in tumor cell lysis.

## Acknowledgments

We thank the following researchers for sharing their advice and collaborative help during the course of this work: Drs. C. F. Nathan, E. R. Podack, P. Venge, C. G. B. Peterson, and M. A. Palladino. The excellent technical assistance of S. S. Ko during the initial part of this research is also well appreciated. This work was supported in part by grants from the Cancer Research Institute and from the Lucille P. Markey Charitable Trust to J.D.-EY. and by grants CA30198 and AI070127 from NIH to Z.A.C. J.D.-EY. is a Lucille P. Markey Scholar.

## References

1. Latorre, R. and Alvarez, O. *Physiol. Rev.* **61**, 77–150 (1981).
2. Eaker, D. and Wadstrom, T., eds., in *Natural Toxins* pp. 1–713, Pergamon, Oxford (1980).
3. Ravdin, J. I. and Guerrant, R. L. *Rev. Infect. Dis.* **4**, 1185–1207 (1982).
4. Jarumilinta, R. and Kradolfer, F. *Ann. Trop. Med. Parasitol.* **58**, 375–381 (1964).
5. Eaton, R. D. P., Meerovitch, E., and Costerton, J. W. *Trans. R. Soc. Trop. Med. Hyg.* **63**, 678–680 (1969).
6. McCaul, T. F. and Bird, R. G. *Int. J. Parasitol.* **7**, 383–388 (1977).
7. Bos, H. J. *Acta Leidensia* **47**, 23–40 (1977).
8. Knight, R., Bird, B. B., and McCaul, T. F. *Ann. Trop. Med. Parasitol.* **69**, 197–202 (1975).
9. Ravdin, J. I., Croft, B. Y., and Guerrant, R. L. *J. Exp. Med.* **152**, 377–390 (1980).
10. Ravdin, J. I. and Guerrant, R. L. *J. Clin. Invest.* **68**, 1305–1313 (1981).
11. Lushbaugh, W. B., Kairalla, A. B., Cantey, J. R., Hofbauer, A. F., and Pittman, F. E. *J. Infect. Dis.* **139**, 9–17 (1979).
12. Bos, H. J. *Exp. Parasitol.* **47**, 369–372 (1979).
13. Mattern, C. F. T., Keister, K. B., and Natovitz, P. C. *Am. J. Trop. Med. Hyg.* **29**, 26–0 (1980).
14. Kobiler, D., Mirelman, D., and Mattern, C. F. T. *Am. J. Trop. Med. Hyg.* **30**, 955–959 (1981).
15. Aley, S. B., Scott, W. A., and Cohn, Z. A. *J. Exp. Med.* **152**, 391–404 (1980).
16. Aley, S. B., Scott, W. A., and Cohn, Z. A. *Arch. Invest. Med.* **11** (suppl. 1), 41 (1979).
17. Aley, S. B., Cohn, Z. A., and Scott, W. A. *J. Exp. Med.* **160**, 724–737 (1984).
18. Lopez-Revilla, R. and Said-Fernandez, S. *Am. J. Trop. Med. Hyg.* **29**, 209–212 (1980).
19. Young, J. D. -E, Young, T. M., Lu, L. P., Unkeless, J. C., and Cohn, Z. A. *J. Exp. Med.* **156**, 1677–1690 (1982).

20. Lynch, E. C., Rosenberg, I. M., and Gitler, C. *EMBO J.* 1, 801-804 (1982).
21. Young, J. D. -E., Blake, M., Mauro, A., and Cohn, Z. A. *Proc. Natl. Acad. Sci. USA* 80, 3831-3835 (1983).
22. Montal, M. and Mueller, P. *Proc. Natl. Acad. Sci. USA* 69, 3561-3566 (1972).
22A. Young, J. D. -E., Unkeless, J. C., Young, T. M., Mauro, A., and Cohn, Z. A. *Nature* 306, 186-189 (1983).
23. Young, J. D. -E. and Cohn, Z. A. *J. Cellular Biochem.* 29, 299-308 (1985).
24. Young, J. D. -E., Leong, L. G., DiNome, M. A., and Cohn, Z. A. *Anal. Biochem.* 154, 649-654 (1986).
25. Boheim, G. *J. Membr. Biol.* 19, 277-303 (1974).
26. Berke, G. *Immunol. Rev.* 72, 5-42 (1983).
27. Martz, E. *Contemp. Top. Immunobiol.* 7, 301-361 (1977).
28. Henney, C. S. *Contemp. Top. Immunobiol.* 7, 245-272 (1977).
29. Trinchieri, G. and Perussia, B. *Lab. Invest.* 50, 489-513 (1984).
30. Herberman, R. B. *Transplantation* 34, 1-7 (1982).
31. Podack, E. R. *Immunol. Today* 6, 21-27 (1985).
32. Henkart, P. and Blumenthal, R. *Proc. Natl. Acad. Sci. USA* 72, 2789-2793 (1975).
33. Dourmashkin, R. R., Deteix, P., Simone, C. B., and Henkart, P. *Clin. Exp. Immunol.* 42, 554-560 (1980).
34. Henkart, M. P. and Henkart, P.A., in *Mechanisms of Cell-Mediated Cytotoxicity* (Clark, W. R. and Martz, E., eds.)(pp. 227-247, Plenum, New York (1982).
35. Dennert, G. and Podack, E. R. *J. Exp. Med.* 157, 1483-1495 (1983).
36. Podack, E. R. and Dennert, G. *Nature* 302, 442-445 (1983).
37. Henney, C. S. *J. Immunol.* 110, 73-84 (1973).
38. Ziegler, H. K. and Allison, A. C. *Immunol.* 115, 1500-1504 (1975).
39. Ferluga, J. and Allison, A. C. *Nature* 250, 673-675 (1974).
40. Golstein, P. and Smith, E. *Contemp. Top. Immunobiol.* 7, 273-300 (1977).
41. Koren, H. S., Ax, W., and Freund-Moelbert, E. *Eur. J. Immunol.* 3, 32-37 (1973).
42. Simone, C. B. and Henkart, P. A. *J. Immunol.* 124, 954-963 (1980).
43. Giavedoni, E. B., Chow, Y. M., and Dalmasso, A. P. *J. Immunol.* 122, 240-245 (1979).
44. Nathan, C. F., Mercer-Smith, J. A., DeSantis, N. M., and Palladino, M. A. *J. Immunol.* 129, 2164-2171 (1982).
45. Ades, E. W., Hinson, A., Chapuis-Cellier, C., and Arnaud, P. *Scand. J. Immunol.* 15, 109-113 (1982).
46. Gravagna, P., Gianazza, E., Arnaud, P., Neels, M., and Ades, E. W. *Scand. J. Immunol.* 15, 115-118 (1982).
47. Hiserodt, J. C., Britvan, L., and Targan, S. *J. Immunol.* 131, 2705-2709 (1983).
48. Hiserodt, J. C., Britvan, L., and Targan, S. *J. Immunol.* 131, 2710-2713 (1983).
49. Wright, S. C. and Bonavida, B. *J. Immunol.* 129, 433-439 (1982).

50. Wright, S. C., Weitzen, M. L., Kahle, R., Granger, G. A., and Bonavida, B. *J. Immunol.* **130**, 2479-2483 (1983).
51. Farram, E. and Targan, S. R. *J. Immunol.* *130*, 1252-1256 (1983).
52. Wright, S. C. and Bonavida, B. *Proc. Natl. Acad. Sci. USA* **80**, 1688-1692 (1983).
53. Steinhauer, E. H., Doyle, A. T., and Kadish, A. S. *J. Immunol.* **135**, 294-299 (1985).
54. Old, L. J. *Science* **230**, 630-632 (1985).
55. Mathews, N. and Watkins, J. F.*Br.J.Cancer***38**, 302-309 (1978).
56. Pennica, D., Nedwin, G. E., Hayflick, S., Seeburg, P. H., Derynck, R., Palladino, M. A., Kohr, W. J., Aggarwal, B. B., and Goeddel, D. V. *Nature* **312**, 724-729 (1984).
57. Gray, P. W., Aggarwal, B. B., Benton, C. V., Bringman, T. S., Henzel, W. J., Jarrett, J. A., Leung, D. W., Moffat, B., Ng, P., Svedersky, L. P., Palladino, M. A., and Nedwin, G. E. *Nature* **312**, 721-724 (1984).
58. Allavena, P., Scala, G., Djeu, J. Y., Procopio, A. D., Oppenheim, J. J., Herberman, R. B., and Ortaldo, J. R. *Cancer Immunol. Immunother.* **19**, 121-126, 1985.
59. Timonen, T., Saksela, E., Ranki, A., and Hayry, P. *Cell. Immunol.* **48**, 133-148 (1979).
60. Timonen, T., Ortaldo, J. R., and Herberman, R. B. *J. Exp. Med.* **153**, 569-582 (1981).
61. Gillis, S. and Smith, K. A. *Nature* **268**, 154-156 (1977).
62. Dennert, G. *Nature* **287**, 47-49 (1980).
63. Nabel, G., Bucalo, L. R., Allard, J., Wigzell, H., and Cantor, H. *J. Exp. Med.* **153**, 1582-1591 (1981).
64. Bracilae, T. J., Andrew, M. E., and Braciale, V. T. *J. Exp. Med.* **153**, 910-923 (1981).
65. Kedar, E., Ikejiri, B. L., Sredni, B., Bonavida, B., and Herberman, R. B. *Cell. Immunol.* **69**, 305-329 (1982).
66. Sugamura, K., Tanaka, Y., and Hinuma, Y. *J. Immunol.* **128**, 1749-1752 (1982).
67. Acha-Orbea, H., Groscurth, P., Lang, R., Stitz, L., and Hengartner, H. *J. Immunol.* **130**, 2952-2959 (1983).
68. Millard, P. J., Henkart, M. P., Reynolds, C. W., and Henkart, P. A. *J. Immunol.* **132**, 3197-3204 (1984).
69. Henkart, P. A., Millard, P. J., Reynolds, C. W., and Henkart, M. P. *J. Exp. Med.* **160**, 75-93 (1984).
70. Podack, E. R. and Konigsberg, P. J. *J. Exp. Med.* **160**, 695-710 (1984).
71. Young, J. D.-E, Nathan, C. F., and Cohn, Z. A. *J. Cellular Biochem.* **9A** (suppl.) 161 (1985).
72. Young, J. D.-E, Nathan, C. F., Podack, E. R., Palladino, M. A., and Cohn, Z. A. *Proc. Natl. Acad. Sci. USA* **83**, 150-154 (1986).
73. Young, J. D. -E, Hengartner, H., Podack, E. R., and Cohn, Z. A. *Cell* **44**, 849-859 (1986).

74. Blumenthal, R., Millard, P. J., Henkart, M. P., Reynolds, C. W., and Henkart, P. A. *Proc. Natl. Acad. Sci. USA* **81**, 5551-5555 (1984).
75. Masson, D. and Tschopp, J. *J. Biol. Chem.* **260**, 9069-9072 (1985).
76. Podack, E. R., Young, J. D. -E, and Cohn, A. A. *Proc. Natl. Acad. Sci. USA* **82**, 8629-8633 (1985).
77. Young, J. D. -E,R., Podack, E. R., and Cohn, Z. A. *J. Exp. Med.* **164**, 144-155 (1986).
78. Young, J. D.-E, Cohn, Z . A., and Podack,, E. R. *Science* **233**, 184-190 (1986).
79. Dessin, A. J. and David, J. R. in *Advances in Host Defense Mechanisms* vol. 1 (Gallin, J. I. and Fauci, A. S., eds.) pp. 243-268, Raven, New York 1982).
80. Venge, P., Dahl, R., Hallgren, R., and Olsson, I, in *The Eosinophil in Health and Disease* (Mahmoud, A.F.F. and Austen, K. F. eds.) pp. 131-142, Grune & Stratton, New York (1980).
81. Spry, C. J. F. *Immunol. Today* **6**, 332-335 (1985).
82. Gleich, G. J. and Loegering, D. A. *Annu. Rev. Immunol.* **2**, 429-459 (1984).
83. Gleich, G. J., Loegering, D.A., and Maldonado, J. E. *J. Exp. Med.* **137**, 1459-1741 (1973).
84. Gleich, G. J., Loegering, D. A., Kueppers, F., Bajaj, S. P., and Mann, K. G. *J. Exp. Med.* **140**, 313-332 (1974).
85. Gleich, G. J., Loegering, D. A., Mann, K. G., and Maldonado, J. E. *J. Clin. Invest.* **57**, 633-640 (1976).
86. Olsson, I. and Venge, P. *Blood* **44**, 235-246 (1974).
87. Olsson, I., Venge, P., Spitznagel, J. K., and Lehrer, R. I. *Lab. Invest.* **36**,493-500 (1977).
88. Peterson, C. G. B., and Venge, P. *Immunol.* **50**, 19-26 (1983).
89. Carlson, M. G. Ch., Peterson, C. G. B., and Venge, P. *J. Immunol.* **134**, 1875-1879 (1985).
90. Durack, D. T., Sumi, S. M., and Klebanoff, S. J. *Proc. Natl. Acad. Sci. USA* **76**, 1443-1447 (1979).
91. Durack, D. T., Ackerman, S. J., Loegering, D. A., and Gleich, G. J. *Proc. Natl. Acad. Sci. USA* **78**, 5165-5169 (1981).
92. Ackerman, S.J., Loegering, D. A., Venge, P., Olsson, I., Harley, J. B., Fauci, A. S., and Gleicyh, G. J. *J. Immunol.* **131**, 2977-2982 (1983).
93. Butterworth, A.E., Wassom, D. L., Gleich, G. J., Loegering, D. A., and David, J. R. *J. Immunol.* **122**, 221-229 (1979).
94. Wassom, D. L. and Gleich, G. J. *Am. J. Trop. Med. Hyg.***28**, 860-863 (1979).
95. Gleich, G. J., Frigas, E., Loegering, D. A., Wassom, D. L., and Steinmuller, D. *J. Immunol.* **123**, 2925-2927 (1979).
96. Montal, M. *J. Membr. Biol.* **7**, 245-266 (1972).
97. Bach, D. and Miller, I. R. *J. Membr. Biol.* **11**, 237-254 (1973).
98. McLaren, D. J., McKean, J. R., Olsson, I., Venge. P., and Kay, A. B. *Parasite Immunol.* **3**, 359-373 (1981).

99. Fredens, K., Dahl, R., and Venge, P. *J. Allergy Clin. Immunol.* **70**, 361–366 (1982).
100. Tai, P.-C., Spry, C. J. F., Peterson, C. G. B., Venge, P., and Olsson, I. *Nature* **309**, 182–184 (1984).
101. Young, J. D. E, Peterson, C. G. B., Venge, P., and Cohn, Z. A. *Nature* **321**, 613–616 (1986).
102. Humphrey, J. H. and Dourmashkin, R. R. *Adv. Immunol.* **11**, 75–115 (1969).
103. Bhakdi, S., Bjerrum, O. J., Rother, U., Knufermann, H., and Wallach, D. F. H. *Biochim. Biophys. Acta* **406**, 21–35 (1975).
104. Biesecker, G., Podack, E. R., Halverson, C. A., and Muller-Eberhard, H. J. *J. Exp. Med.* **149**, 448–458 (1979).
105. Podack, E. R., Esser, A. F., Biesecker, G., and Muller-Eberhard, H. J. *J. Exp. Med.* **151**, 301–313 (1980).
106. Mayer, M. M. *Proc. Natl. Acad. Sci. USA* **69**, 2954–2958 (1972).
107. Michaels, D. W., Abramovitz, A. S., Hammer, C. H., and Mayer, M. M. *Proc. Natl. Acad. Sci. USA* **73**, 2852–2856 (1976).
108. Hu, V. W., Esser, E. F., Podack, E. R., and Wisnieski, B. J. *J. Immunol.* **127**, 380–386 (1981).
109. Podack, E. R., Stoffel, W., Esser, A. F., and Muller-Eberhard, H. J. *Proc. Natl. Acad. Sci. USA* **78**, 4544–4548 (1981).
110. Dourmashkin, R. R. *Immunology* **35**, 205–212 (1978).
111. Podack, E. R., Tschopp, J., and Muller-Eberhard, H. J. *J. Exp. Med.* **156**, 268–282 (1982).
112. Podack, E. R. and Tschopp, J. *Proc. Natl. Acad. Sci. USA* **79**, 574–578 (1982).
113. Tschopp, J., Muller-Eberhard, H. J., and Podack, E. R. *Nature* **298**, 534–538 (1982).
114. Podack, E. R. and Tschopp, J. *Fed. Proc.* **41**, 486 (1982).
115. Tschopp, J. *Fed. Proc.* **43**, 1450 (1984).
116. Young, J. D. -E., Cohn, Z. A., and Podack, E. R., in *Perspectives in Inflammation, Neoplasia and Vascular Cell Biology* (in press).
117. Young, J. D. -E, Cohn, Z. A., and Podack, E. R. (submitted).
118. Ramm, L. E. and Mayer, M. M. *J. Immunol.* **124**, 2281–2287 (1980).
119. Liu, C. -C., Perussia, B., Cohn, Z. A., and Young, J. D. -E. *J. Exp. Med.* **164**, 2061–2076 (1986).
120. Young, J. D. -E., Liu, C. -C., Leong, L. G., and Cohn, Z. A. *J. Exp. Med.* **164**, 2077–2082 (1986).

# Cytolysin

## Its Purification, Biological Properties, and Mechanism of Action

CRAIG W. REYNOLDS and PIERRE HENKART

## 1. Introduction

The mechanism of lymphocyte cytotoxicity has been the subject of investigation for well over ten years. In spite of this intensive effort, the exact mechanism(s) involved in the destruction of target cells by lymphocytes remains controversial. Over the past few years, however, several groups have been able to demonstrate a number of common features for the cytolytic process by different lymphocyte populations, including T-cells and natural killer (NK) cells. These common features have led to the suggestion that lymphocyte-mediated cytotoxicity proceeds in a series of stages, ultimately resulting in the secretion of cytolytic molecules leading to target cell lysis. These distinct stages include: (1) the binding of effector and target cell via a specific receptor–antigen interaction, (2) a calcium- and energy-requiring rearrangement of cytoplasm and secretion of cytotoxic material into the intercellular space, (3) the interaction of the cytolytic material with target-cell membranes, leading to (4) lysis of the target cell.

Recently, an appreciable amount of experimental evidence has accumulated that is consistent with the hypothesis that the mechanism of lymphocyte cytotoxicity involves the secretion of cytolytic molecules. This evidence includes: (a) the presence of distinct cytoplasmic granules in many cytotoxic lymphocyte populations, (b) rearrangement of cytoplasmic organelles and release of granules from these cytotoxic cells following their binding to target cells (1–2), (c) decreased NK activity in Chediak-Higashi patients (3–5) and Beige (bg/bg) mice (6), genetic mutations with abnormal lysosomal granule formation, (d) the inability of agranular lymphocytes to kill following tumor cell contact (7), (e) a reduction in cytotoxic activity by strontium (8,9), which has been shown to promote leukocyte degranulation, (f) a requirement for lipid metabolism (transmethylation and phospholipase $A_2$ activity) for both secretion of lysosomal enzymes and cytotoxic activity (10,11), and (g) the inhibition of cytotoxicity by lysosomotropic amines, which interfere with lysosomal function (12). Studies have also demonstrated the release of soluble cytolytic factors from T-cells and NK cells upon incubation with target cells or lectins (see additional chapters, this volume), further suggesting that a secretory process is involved in the lysis of tumor cells by cytotoxic lymphocytes.

Given all of the above lines of evidence suggesting a secretory process and role for cytoplasmic granules in lymphocyte cytotoxicity, we have begun a study of the biochemical and functional properties of these granules from cytotoxic lymphocytes. The present manuscript will review the data from this and other studies on the nature of cytotoxic molecules from cytoplasmic granules, with special emphasis on how these molecules might be involved in the lysis of target cells by cytotoxic lymphocytes.

## 2. Isolation of Cytolytic Granules and Purification of Cytolysin

Recent evidence has clearly demonstrated that most, if not all, of the NK and antibody-dependent cell-mediated cytotoxicity (ADCC) of freshly isolated rat (13,14), mouse (15,16), and (17) human leukocytes is mediated by a distinct population of cells termed large granular lymphocytes (LGL). These cells are easily identified by the presence of azurophilic granules in the cytoplasm of Giesma-stained cells. The presence of these distinctive granules in cytotoxic lymphocytes suggests that LGL-mediated lysis of susceptible target cells may be dependent upon the secretion of cytolytic material from these cytoplasmic granules.

In order to provide direct evidence for the role of LGL granules in the lysis of tumor cells, we have purified the cytoplasmic granules from rat LGL tumors (18,19). These cells were chosen since they provide a convenient and uniform source of highly active cytolytic cells with normal NK morphology, surface markers, and cytotoxic specificity (20,21). As a first step in this project, we have developed a method for the isolation of the cytoplasmic granules from these cells (18). The purification scheme is largely dependent upon a self-formed Percoll gradient, which results in pure granules banding near the bottom of the gradient. The presence of the granules was initially detected by assays for lysosomal enzymes and EM morphology, and later by the cytolytic activity described below.

Figure 1 shows the fractionation rat LGL tumor cells on a Percoll gradient, with both the cytolytic activity and peak lysosomal enzyme activity restricted to tubes 2–6. A variety of marker enzymes was also measured on these gradients to localize other cellular components, such as plasma membrane and mitochondria, which were found to occur higher up in the gradient (*18*).

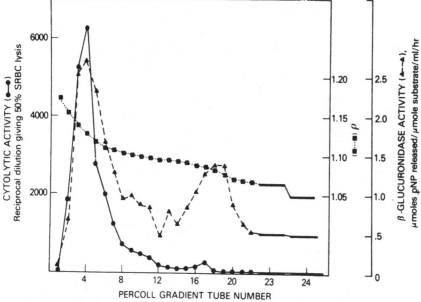

Fig. 1. Percoll gradient fractionation of LGL tumor homogenate (*see* ref. *18* for conditions). Each fraction contained 0.8 mL, except 23 and 24, which contained 2.4 mL.

Figure 2 shows that the pool of lytically active material in tubes 2–5 contains a pure population of granules that appear very similar morphologically to those in rat LGL tumors and blood LGL. The heterogeneity in granule morphology reflects that seen in the cells, and leaves open the possibility that more refined separation techniques could resolve the granules into subpopulations. No significant contamination by other cellular organelles was observed.

The cytolytic reproducibility and potency of these granule preparations is demonstrated in Fig. 3 (*19*). Virtually complete lysis (80–90%) of sheep red blood cells (SRBC) occurred at granule protein concentrations of 1 $\mu$g/mL in all preparations, with detectable lysis still observable at 20 ng/mL in some preparations. Of more than 50 LGL tumor granule preparations, all displayed cytolytic activities comparable to those shown

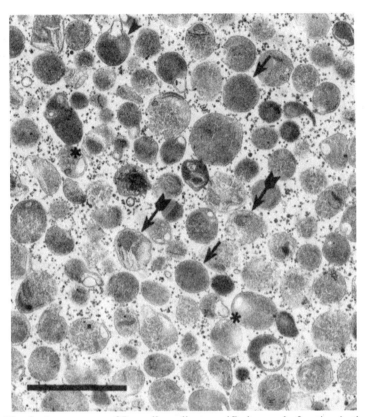

Fig. 2. Appearance of Percoll gradient-purified granule fraction in the electron microscope. Arrows and asterisks indicate different morphological forms of granules (Bar, 1 μm; from ref. *18*).

here. For comparison with the cytotoxicity of intact effector cells, an equivalent effector/target (E/T) ratio can be calculated for granule cytotoxicity. Using a granule purification yield of 1 mg protein/$10^8$ RNK tumor cells, the value of 1 μg/mL granule protein shown in Fig. 3 corresponds to an equivalent E/T ratio of 0.2 (i.e., the granule content of one effector cell could kill at least five targets). This approximation illustrates the potency of the cytolytic effect. Curves similar to those shown in Fig. 3 were also obtained when hemoglobin release was used as an indicator of lysis when sheep or human erythrocytes were used as targets (data not shown).

Analysis of the proteins in the Percoll fractions by SDS gel electrophoresis provides further evidence of the purity of our granule preparation. As shown in Fig. 4, the granules contain five major protein bands of 60, 58, 30, 28 and 27 kdalton. The purity of the granule preparation is shown by the lack of proteins found maximally in other regions of the

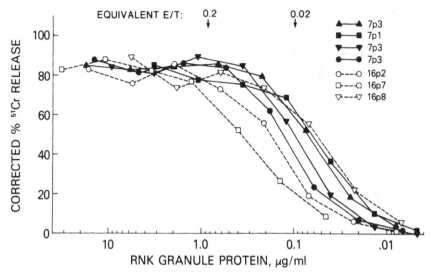

Fig. 3. Cytolytic activity of purified rat LGL tumor cytoplasmic granules on sheep erthrocytes. Titrations of seven independent preparations of purified granules are shown. These preparations are from the RNK 7 and RNK 16 tumor lines, whose in vivo passage number is indicated by the "p" (from ref. *19*).

gradient (*18*). Even with the more sensitive silver stain technique, minimal contamination by other proteins is detectable.

Analysis of the protein patterns and the enzymatic properties of the granule fractions leads to the conclusion that they are distinct from other known cytoplasmic granules such as those from mast cells and polymorphonuclear leukocytes (*19*). To further investigate the question of whether cytotoxic molecules were present in the granules from other types of cells, we next examined a series of granule preparations for cytolytic activity from a variety of cell types. The results in Table 1 demonstrate that only the LGL tumor cells and normal LGL and CTL lines contain cytoplasmic granules with cytolytic activity. Similar studies by Dennert and Podack (*22,23*) have also demonstrated the presence of cytolytic granules in various cell lines with either T-killer or NK-like activity, but not in noncytotoxic cell lines.

The lack of cytolytic activity of granule preparations from noncytotoxic lymphoid cells (Table 1) suggests that the cytolytic potential of cytoplasmic granules may be the result of a product(s) of lymphocyte differentiation specialized for the cytotoxic function. It seems unlikely that normal lysosomal enzyme activities can account for granule-mediated cytolytic activity, since most of the noncytotoxic cells in Table 1 gave granule fractions containing levels of lysosomal enzymes at least as high as those in

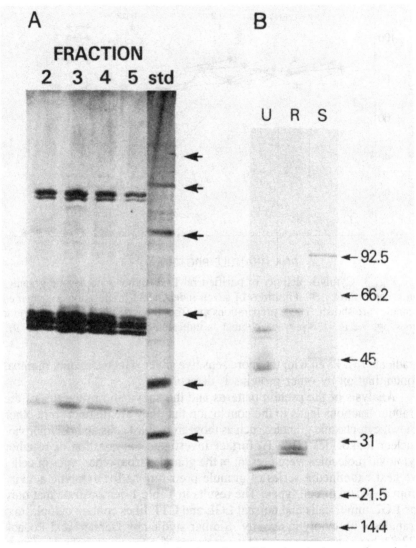

Fig. 4. SDS gel pattern of proteins from Percoll fractions in the granule region. (A) Reduced gels, silver stain, with 1 μg protein/lane. (B) Coomassie stained gels showing reduced (R) vs. unreduced (U) pattern. Molecular weights of protein standards (S) are shown for both (A) and (B) in panel (B) (from ref. *18*).

LGL tumors. The activity of such lysosomal enzymes has been suggested to be responsible for the lethal hit in NK (*24,25*) and CTL cytoxicity (*26*). We, however, favor the hypothesis that the lysosomal enzymes present in these granules are not responsible for either granule- or cell-mediated lytic activity. In this regard we would point out that lysosomal enzymes

Table 1
Cytolytic Activity of Purified Cytoplasmic Granules and Lysosomes
from Various Cells[a]

| Granules from:[b] | Granule lysosomal enzymes[c] | Maximal granule protein concentration[d], $\mu$g/mL | Maximum % SE lysis[e] | Granule lytic units per $10^8$ cells[f] |
|---|---|---|---|---|
| LGL tumor | + | 100 | 90 | 1000–4000 |
| Peripheral blood LGL | + | ND[g] | 90 | 3000 |
| Peripheral blood T-cells | + | ND[g] | 3 | < 10 |
| Spleen | + | 120 | 2 | < 10 |
| Thymus | − | 94 | 3 | < 10 |
| EL-4 (mouse) cell lymphoma | + | 500 | 4 | < 10 |
| Peripheral blood granulocytes | + | ND[g] | 2 | < 10 |
| Peritoneal macrophages | − | ND[g] | 3 | < 10 |
| Liver lysosomes[h] | + | 1 | 2 | < 10 |
| Peritoneal mast cells[h] | + | 37 | 2 | < 10 |

[a]From ref. (19).
[b]Fresh rat tissue, except EL-4.
[c]Plus sign indicates a peak of $\beta$-glucoronidase activity was observed in tubes 2–5.
[d]Final protein concentration of 1:10 dilution of mean of granule pool (tubes 2–5) of Percoll gradient.
[e]All tubes of Percoll gradients tested at final dilutions of 1:10 and 1:100.
[f]Sum of activity in all tubes of gradient divided by cell input.
[g]Insufficient number of cells available to determine protein above Percoll interference.
[h]Not prepared by the Percoll gradient technique.

in eosinophil granules (27) and mast cell granules (28) are not known to play a functional role after secretion. The calcium requirement of granule-mediated cytolytic activity also casts doubt on the role of lysosomal enzymes in this process, since known lysosomal enzymes do not show this property.

In order to better study the nature of the cytolytic molecule, experiments were done to see whether the whole granules were required for the lytic effect, or if a soluble molecule(s) within the granules were solely responsible for target cell lysis. The involvement of a protein was suggested by the temperature lability and pronase sensitivity of the cytolytic activity (see section 3). When we attempted to solubilize the lytic activity from the granules, simple membrane rupture by freezing or mild sonication failed to make the activity nonsedimentable. Nondenaturing detergents also had no effect, although their use was complicated by their own lytic effect on target cells. We found that 1–2*M* NaCl or KCl would successfully solubilize the cytolytic activity, however.

Solubilization of the active cytolytic molecule shows that the intact granule structure is not required for the lytic activity, and allows for the further purification of the active molecule(s). As a first step in this purification, we have performed gel filtration chromatography on ACA 54, as shown in Fig. 5. These data show that the active molecule behaves like a protein of 50–60 kdalton. The SDS gels of the active peak from this column show that the components of 60, 58, and 28 kdalton are still pres-

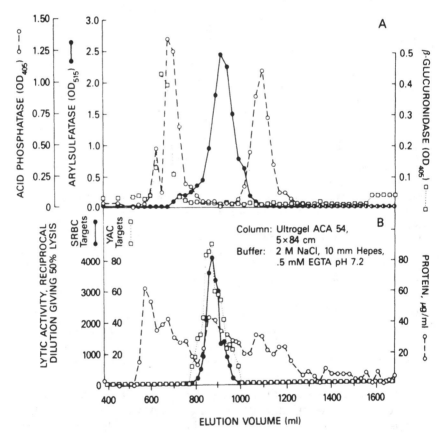

Fig. 5. Gel filtration of LGL granule cytolysin on ACA 54. LGL tumor granules were extracted with 2*M* NaCl and the extract chromatographed at 5 °C on Ultrogel ACA 54 (84 × 5 cm). (A) Enzymatic activity. (B) Cytolytic activity of column fractions.

ent; the other major granule proteins are gone, however, along with most of the lysosomal enzyme activities we have measured (data not shown).

Further detailed studies on the biochemistry of the cytolytic molecule are underway.

## 3. Biological Properties of Cytolysin

From the start of our efforts to purify LGL tumor granules, we sought to detect a lytic activity that fit into a secretory model for cytotoxicity. Like others in the past, our initial attempts did not succeed in detecting plausible levels of lytic activities in cytotoxic lymphocyte homogenates. After we did succeed, it became clear that the interesting properties of the lytic agent, which we call cytolysin, may well have prevented its earlier discovery.

As shown in Fig. 6, the major controlling variable in cytolysin activity is calcium (19). In the absence of calcium, no lytic activity can be detected on any target cell. The activity is maximal in the physiological extracellular calcium range, and although magnesium and barium cannot replace calcium, strontium will substitute at tenfold higher concentrations. We feel that this calcium dependence makes physiological sense for a lytic agent stored in the effector cell interior, where the calcium concentration is very low and its destructive power must be restrained. After exocytosis into the extracellular space where the calcium concentration is in the millimolar range, the lytic potential of the cytolysin is unleashed.

Another interesting finding with respect to divalent ions is that cytolysin activity is not stable in the presence of calcium. In order to assay cytolysin activity, our routine procedure is to dilute the granules or extract into calcium-free PBS, followed by addition of an equal volume of target cells in balanced salt solution containing calcium. If the granules are exposed to 2 m$M$ calcium prior to addition of the target cells, a time-dependent loss of activity occurs, with a half life of about 10 min at room temperature (19). One interpretation of this behavior is that an unstable intermediate is generated when calcium is added. It again seems plausible that a physiologically relevant lytic agent should have such a property, since it would clearly be a problem for a highly lethal agent to be able to diffuse and destroy "innocent bystander" cells, which does not seem to happen with NK-mediated cytoxicity (24).

One of the most striking features of the granule lytic activity is its rapid kinetics (19). As shown in Fig. 7, the lysis of red cells and nucleated cells is complete within a few minutes at room temperature and is faster

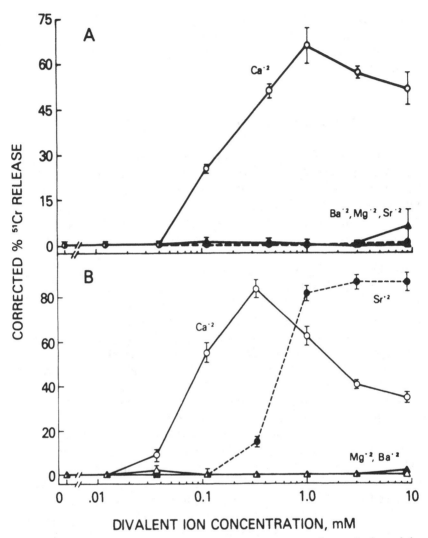

Fig. 6. Effect of divalent cations on LGL tumor granule cytolysin activity. Divalent cations were added with the (A) SRBC or (B) YAC-1 target cells (from ref. *19*).

at 37°C. This rate is in dramatic contrast to NKCF lysis, which takes hours to achieve completion. This rapid rate is compatible with a detergent type of lytic mechanism or with the creation of large membrane pores that allow for the direct egress of cytoplasmic components. It is clearly faster than the lysis of cells by complement, however, which occurs by a colloid osmotic mechanism requiring many minutes to achieve release of cytoplasmic proteins (*29*). The rate of target cell lysis during the NK cell killer-cell-

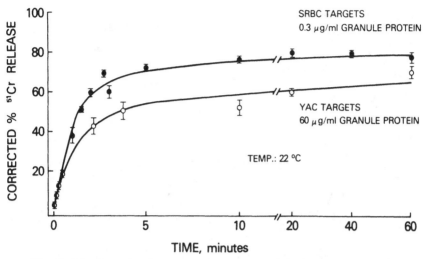

Fig. 7. Kinetics of lysis by LGL tumor granules. $^{51}$Cr-labeled target cells in BSS were mixed with an equal volume of diluted granules in PBS followed by harvesting the supernatant at the indicated time (from ref. *19*).

independent phase of lysis has recently been determined, and is close to the speed of the cytolysin-induced lysis (*30*).

As shown in Fig. 8, cytolysin from LGL tumor granules does not show a specificity identical to NK cells. In fact, the most sensitive targets we have found are red cells, which are not recognized or killed by NK cells. In general, nucleated cells are about 10–100-fold less sensitive, with some nucleated cells still less sensitive. If one considers only the lymphoid tumor cells, however, there is a general correlation of their lysability by LGL granules and NK cells. If one considers the red cell lysis by mg/mL levels of cytolysin, it can be said that the cytolysin molecule is comparable in potency to purified complement proteins such as poly-C9 and is more lytic than known hemolysins and toxins from bacteria.

## 4. Mechanism of Action

The results described so far strongly support a model of granule exocytosis during NK cytotoxicity. There is, however, little direct evidence that the cytolysin is responsible for the lethal damage to the target cell. As one approach to provide such evidence, we have raised rabbit antibodies against the purified granules (*31*). These antibodies form two precipitin bands in agar gel diffusion against salt extracts of granules and do not react with comparable extracts of granules from the noncytotoxic mouse

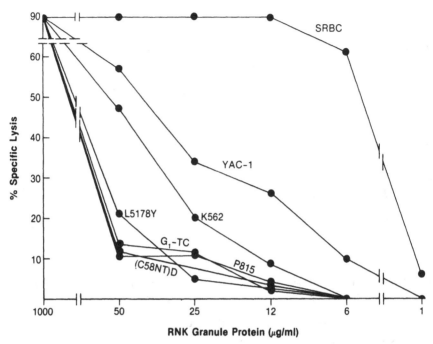

Fig. 8. Lytic activity of purified LGL tumor granules against various target cells.

tumor EL-4. On Western blots of SDS gels of granule proteins, the antibodies recognize four of the five major bands and some minor ones as well. When immunofluorescence experiments are carried out, the antibodies do not detectably stain the surface membranes of any lymphoid cells including LGL tumors or LGL. If the cells are fixed and permeabilized, however, a bright and discrete cytoplasmic staining pattern reminiscent of granules is seen in rat LGL and LGL tumors. Other lymphoid cell granules do not stain under conditions in which the LGL are brightly stained. Thus the antibodies appear to be specific for LGL granules. More importantly, $F(ab')_2$ fragments of these antibodies specifically block the lytic activity of purified rat LGL in NK and ADCC assays, in addition to the cytolysin activity (Table 2). In contrast, the antibodies do not interfere with binding of LGL to target cells (% conjugates), a result that would be expected for specific antibodies to cytoplasmic granules. We regard these experiments with antigranule antibodies as strong direct evidence for a role of granule components in NK activity. We presume that the antibodies have access to the granule cytolysin upon its release from the NK cells and prior to its effective interaction with target cell membranes. The failure of NK cells to normally lyse red cells is presumably caused by the failure of LGL to bind these cells.

Table 2
Effect of Anti-Granule Ab on Cytolysin, NK, and ADCC Activity[a]

| Treatment | % [51] Cr-release[b] | | | % Conjugates of LGL with[c] | |
| | SRBC | YAC-1 | P815 + AB | YAC-1 | P815 + AB |
| --- | --- | --- | --- | --- | --- |
| None | NT[d] | 34 ± 1 | 38 ± 3 | 18 ± 5 | 34 ± 1 |
| PBS control | 78 ± 2 | 34 ± 3 | 37 ± 3 | 20 ± 2 | 33 ± 2 |
| Anti-TNP control[e] | 81 ± 3 | 30 ± 6 | 38 ± 2 | 17 ± 4 | 26 ± 1 |
| Anti-LGL granule[e] | 1 ± 1 | 3 ± 1 | 14 ± 1 | 18 ± 5 | 35 ± 2 |

[a]From ref. (*31*).
[b]With either 10 units cytolysin (versus SRBC targets) or purified rat LGL (versus YAC-1 or P815 + Ab), E/T = 25:1.
[c]E/T = 2.1 at 37°C for 5 min.
[d]Not tested.
[e]Rabbit F(ab')$_2$ antibodies at 300 μg/mL in the assay.

To provide further insights into the nature of the interaction between cytolysin and target cells, we have studied the effects of a number of different compounds on the lysis of target cells by LGL granules (*32*). In order to compare the ability of various compounds to inhibit the cytolytic activity of LGL tumor granules, we have titrated the test compound into lysis assays with $^{51}$Cr-labeled target cells. Table 3 is a summary of the data obtained in typical inhibition experiments with SRBC and YAC-1 targets and some of these compounds. The lytic activity of granule cytolysin was inhibited by inorganic phosphate, and various monophosphoesters with 50% inhibition ($I_{50}$) values in the range of 8–20 m$M$. Choline phosphate was exceptionally potent, with an $I_{50}$ of 1.4 m$M$. In contrast to the inhibition of phosphate esters, the parent compounds, such as neutral sugars, glycerol, and choline, showed no detectable inhibition at 50 m$M$. A lysolipid bearing a short aliphatic chain (L-α-lysocaproylphosphatidylcholine) and some detergents (CHAPS) were inhibitory with $I_{50}$ values in the range of 1 m$M$. Lysolipids with longer aliphatic chains (L-α-lysopalmitoylphosphatidylcholine), phospholipids as liposomes, and related lipid compounds were also found to display potent inhibition of the hemolytic activity of LGL granule cytolysin, with $I_{50}$ values in the range of 0.2–30 μ$M$. Soluble globular proteins inhibited LGL granule cytolysin hemolytic activity with $I_{50}$ of 0.1–0.4 mg/mL. Lipoproteins were two to three orders of magnitude more potent inhibitors, with $I_{50}$ values less than 1 μg/mL. These results on the inhibition of LGL granule cytolysin by various compounds related to lipids lend support to a model of the lytic action of LGL granules in which soluble cytolysin molecules insert into membrane lipid during the course of the lytic event.

Table 3
Inhibition of LGL Granule Cytolysin[a]

| Compounds tested | $I_{50}$, m$M$[b] | |
|---|---|---|
| | SRBC | YAC-1 |
| *Phosphate compounds* | | |
| Inorganic phosphate | 12 | ND[c] |
| Organic phosphate[d] | 0.4–8 | 2–7 |
| Monophosphate esters | | |
| Glycerophosphate | 10 | >36 |
| Choline phosphate | 1.4 | ND |
| Sugar phosphate[e] | 9–21 | >50 |
| *Lipids and lipid-like compounds* | | |
| L-α-Lysocaproylphosphatidylcholine | 0.8 | ND |
| L-α-Lysopalmitoylphosphatidylcholine | $2 \times 10^{-3}$ | $>9 \times 10^{-3}$ |
| CHAPS detergent | 0.7 | ND |
| Phosphatidylcholine liposomes | $0.2 \times 10^{-3}$ | ND |
| Lipoprotein fraction of FCS | $<1 \times 10^{-3}$ | $1.5 \times 10^{-3}$ |
| *Globular proteins* | | |
| Bovine serum albumin (BSA) | 0.4 | 2.7 |
| Bovine gamma globulin (BGG) | 0.2 | 2.5 |
| Ovalbumin | 0.1 | >6 |
| *Other* | | |
| Glycerol | >50 | ND |
| Choline | >50 | ND |
| Neutral sugars[f] | >50 | >50 |

[a]From ref. (*32*).
[b]Concentration of inhibition giving 50% reduction in granule cytolysin activity.
[c]ND, not done.
[d]ATP, GTP, RNA, and DNA.
[e]Glucose-1 and glucose-6-phosphate, fructose-1 and fructose-6-phosphate and mannose-6-phosphate.
[f]Glucose, fructose, mannose, galactose, *N*-acetylglycosamine, and *N*-acetylgalactosamine all gave similar results.

The possibility that the NK lethal hit occurs via the creation of large pores in the target cell membrane is attractive to us because of a series of experiments on target cell damage induced by LGL in ADCC. In 1975 we showed that planar lipid bilayers modeling target cells were attacked so that their ionic permeability increased by several orders of magnitude. More recently, a study of resealed erythrocyte ghosts containing molecular size markers showed that ADCC induced formation of large pores, as evidenced by sieving of the released markers (*33*). When compared to complement, the LGL induced the release of larger markers, and a surprisingly large maximal pore size of 14 nm was estimated to be induced by the cytotoxic lymphocytes in these studies. Later we showed that pore-like structures with this internal diameter were visible in the red cell ghost targets after negative staining and EM (34). These structures were generally similar to those associated with complement lysis, but were larger. Similar structures were shown to be associated with cytotoxicity by cloned NK cells (35) in thin sections made of NK-target conjugates (36) and on red cell membranes exposed to LGL tumor granules in the presence of calcium (19). It should be emphasized that the appearance of these pore-like structures requires the presence of calcium, and the structures appear rapidly after its addition, correlating nicely with the lytic potential of the granules. If no target cells are present, the pore-like structures become associated with the granule membranes.

As we have shown, the appearance of pore-structures in the EM was strongly reminiscent of complement, and we felt that the cytolysin was likely to act by a similar membrane-insertion mechanism. In order to test this hypothesis, we carried out a series of experiments with liposomes, using the water soluble dye carboxyfluorescein as a marker for liposome permeability. We found that liposomes of all types make excellent targets for LGL granule cytolysin (37). A typical experiment is shown in Fig. 9, in which one can see the carboxyfluorescein release occurring over the course of few minutes. This marker release was absolutely dependent on divalent cations in the medium, with magnesium and barium being inactive and strontium being tenfold less active than calcium. These titration curves were virtually identical to the data shown in Figs. 6 and 7. Thus, the liposome permeabilization parallels the kinetics and divalent ion requirements of target-cell lysis by the cytolysin. The liposome fluidity as determined by the fatty acids of the phospholipids had only a minor effect on cytolysin activity (Fig. 9), and variation of the lipid head group had negligible effect (37).

The carboxyfluorescein techniques enabled us to show that marker release from individual liposomes was all-or-none, as predicted by a pore insertion hypothesis. The most striking evidence in favor of this hypothesis came from EM examination of the liposomes after treatment with partially purified cytolysin in the presence of calcium. Negative staining showed pore structures that appear deeply inserted into the lipid bilayer of these small unicellular liposomes (37). The liposomes that contained inserted pore structures had become permeabilized to the negative stain, whereas the other liposomes remained unstained.

These results suggest that the lytic action of granule cytolysin occurs through the insertion of the pore-forming cytolysin molecules into the target-

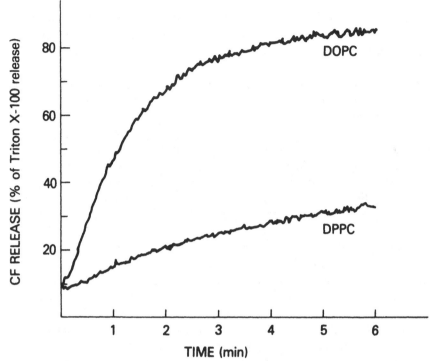

Fig. 9. Release of carboxyfluorescein from small unicellular liposomes by
partially purified LGL granules cytolysin. DOPC, dioleoyl phosphatidyl choline;
DPPC, dipalmitoyl phosphatidyl choline (from ref. *32*).

cell lipid bilayer, in a mechanism generally analogous to that of
complement.

## 5. Summary

The data summarized in the present report provides increasing evidence
that a secretory process involving cytoplasmic granules plays an important role in the mechanism of target cell lysis by cytotoxic lymphocytes.
Using biochemical techniques, it is possible to purify a single protein
molecule of 60,000 molecular weight that is responsible for most, if not
all, of the cytolytic activity of these cytoplasmic granules. This molecule,
termed cytolysin, is an extremely potent protein present only in the granules
of cytotoxic lymphocytes (NK cells and CTL), but that is able to lyse a
wide range of targets in an extremely rapid and $Ca^{2+}$-dependent manner.
When tested on liposomes, cytolysin is able to induce the release of carboxyfluorescein and the appearance of ring-like structures inserted into the mem-

brane. In addition, the lytic activity of cytolysin is inhibited by both compounds related to lipids and by antibodies made against purified granules. These data lend further support to the hypothesis that the lytic action of lymphocytes involves the release of soluble cytolysin molecules from cytoplasmic granules followed by their insertion into the target cell membrane leading to formation of complement-like pores and the eventual death of the target cell.

The evidence for involvement of granule cytolysin and other soluble factors in lymphocyte-mediated cytotoxicity (see additional chapters in this volume), raises the question of the possible relationship between these molecules. From the limited available evidence, it is hard to reconcile the major differences between cytolysin and the other cytostatic or cytotoxic factors (such as lymphotoxin, tumor necrosis factor, natural killer cytolytic factor) in their apparent molecular weights, patterns of activity against various target cells, and biological properties, and in the kinetics of their lytic effects on target cells. On the one hand, it is possible that all these agents are part of a closely related family of molecules, or may even represent different complexed or degraded forms of a single precursor protein. Alternatively, these agents may be biochemically unrelated molecules that all lead to target cell lysis, but through substantially different mechanisms of action. In fact, it remains an attractive hypothesis to think that a number of these molecules, working in concert, may normally be involved in the lysis of target cells by cytotoxic lymphocytes. The further resolution of this question will rely on our ability to purify proteins to homogeneity, and also to produce highly specific monoclonal antibodies for use in the inhibition of cell-mediated cytotoxic activity. It is hoped that these types of experiments will, in the very near future, lead to a much better understanding of the relative roles of these molecules in the mechanism of target cell lysis by cytotoxic lymphocytes.

## References

1. Henkart, M. P. and Henkart, P. A., in *Mechanisms in Cell Mediated Cytotoxicity* (Clark, W. R. and Goldstein, P., eds.) Plenum, New York (1982).
2. Carpen, O., Virtanen, I., and Saksela, E. *J. Immunol.* **128**, 2691–2697 (1982).
3. Haliotis, T., Roder, J., Klein, M., Ortaldo, J. R., Fauci, A. S., and Herberman, R. B. *J. Exp. Med.* **151**, 1039–1048 (1980).
4. Katz, P., Zaytoun, A. M., and Facui, A. S. *J. Clin. Invest.* **69**, 1231–1238 (1982).
5. Abo, T., Cooper, M. D., and Balch, C. M. *J. Clin. Invest.* **70**, 193–197 (1982).

6. Roder, J. C. and Duwe, A. K. *Nature* **278**, 451-453 (1979).
7. Itoh, K., Suzuki, R., Umezu, Y., Hanaumi, K., and Kumagai, K. *J. Immunol.* **129**, 395-400 (1982).
8. Neighbour, P. A. and Huberman, H. S. *J. Immunol.* **128**, 1236-1240 (1982).
9. Neighbour, P. A., Huberman, H. S., and Kress, Y. *Eur. J. Immunol.* **12**, 588-595 (1982).
10. Hoffman, T., Hirata, F., Bougnoux, P., Fraser, B. A., Goldfarb, R. H., Herberman, R. B., and Axelrod, J. *Proc. Natl. Acad. Sci. USA* **78**, 3839-3843 (1981).
11. Hattori, T., Hirata, F., Hoffman, T., Hizuta, A., and Herberman, R. B. *J. Immunol.* **131**, 662-665 (1983).
12. Verhoef, J. and Sharma, S. D. *J. Immunol.* **131**, 125-131 (1983).
13. Reynolds, C. W., Timonen, T., and Herberman, R. B. *J. Immunol.* **127**, 282-287 (1981).
14. Reynolds, C. W., Timonen, T. T., Holden, H. T., Hansen, C. T., and Herberman, R. B. *Eur. J. Immunol.* **12**, 577-582 (1982).
15. Luini, W., Boraschi, D., Alberti, S., Aleotti, A., and Tagliabue, A. *Immunology* **43**, 663-668 (1981).
16. Kumagai, K., Itoh, K., Suzuki, R., Hinuma, S., and Saitoh, F. *J. Immunol.* **129**, 388-394 (1982).
17. Timonen, T., Ortaldo, J. R., and Herberman, R. B. *J. Exp. Med.* **153**, 569-582 (1981).
18. Millard, P., Henkart, M. P., Reynolds, C. W., and Henkart, P. A. *J. Immunol.* **132**, 3197-3204 (1984).
19. Henkart, P. A., Millard, P. J., Reynolds, C. W., and Henkart, M. P. *J. Exp. Med.* **160**, 75-93 (1984).
20. Ward, J. M. and Reynolds, C. W. *Am. J. Pathol.* **111**, 1-10 (1983).
21. Reynolds, C. W., Bere, E. W., and Ward, J. M. *J. Immunol.* **132**, 534-540 (1984).
22. Podack, E. R. and Konigsberg, P. I. *J. Exp. Med.* **160**, 695-710 (1984).
23. Criado, M., Lindstrom, J. M., Anderson, C. G., and Dennert, G. *J. Immunol.* **135**, 4245-4251 (1985).
24. Roder, J. C., Argov, S., Klein, M., Peterson, C., Kiessling, R., Anderson, K., and Hanson, M. *Immunoogy* **40**, 107-116 (1980).
25. Zucker-Franklin, D., Grusky, G., and Yang, J-S. *Proc. Natl. Acad. Sci. USA* **80**, 6977-6981 (1983).
26. Zagury, D., in *Mechanisms of Cell-Mediated Cytotoxicity* (Clark, W. R. and Goldstein, P., eds.) Plenum, New York (1982).
27. Butterworth, A. E., Vadas, M. A., Wassom, D. L., Dessein, A., Hogan, M., Sherry, B., Gleich, G. J., and David. J. R. *J. Exp. Med.* **150**, 1456-1471 (1979).
28. Schwartz, L. B., Austen, K. F., and Wasserman, S. I. *J. Immunol.* **123**, 1445-1450 (1979).
29. Mayer, M. M. *Adv. Exp. Med. Biol.* **146**, 193-216 (1982).
30. Callewaert, D. M. and Makle, N. H., in *Mechanisms of Cytotoxicity by NK Cells* (Herberman, R. B. and Callewaert, D. M., eds.) Academic, New York (1985).

*31.* Reynolds, C. W., Reichardt, D., Henkart, M., Millard, P., and Henkart, P. (submitted for publication).
*32.* Yu, C. C., Reynolds, C. W., and Henkart, P. A. (submitted for publication).
*33.* Simone, C. B. and Henkart, P. *J. Immunol.* **124**, 954–963 (1980).
*34.* Dourmashkin, R. R., Deteix, P., Simone, C. B., and Henkart, P. A. *Clin. Exp. Immunol.* **43**, 554–650 (1980).
*35.* Podack, E. R. and Dennert, G. *Nature* (Lond.) **302**, 442–445 (1983).
*36.* Henkart, M. P. and Henkart, P. A. *Adv. Exp. Med. Biol.* **146**, 227–242 (1982).
*37.* Blumenthal, R., Millard, P. J., Henkart, M. P., Reynolds, C. W., and Henkart, P. A. *Proc. Natl. Acad. Sci. USA* **81**, 5551–5555 (1984).

# Monocyte Cytotoxic Factors

# Triggering of a Cytolytic Factor with TNF-Like Activity From Human Monocytes

HILLEL S. KOREN, KAREN P. McKINNON,
and ALLEN R. CHEN

## 1. Introduction

Mononuclear phagocytes (MNP) have been implicated in host defense mechanisms against tumors (*1*), in addition to well-established roles as scavengers (*2*), microbicidal effectors (*3*), antigen-processing and presenting cells (*4*), and secretors of immunoregulatory mediators (*5,6*). Evidence that MNPs participate in tumor surveillance has recently been extensively reviewed (*7*). Macrophage function is deficient in old age, immunosuppression, and immunodeficiencies, conditions associated with both decreased immune function and increased cancer incidence. Stimulation of macrophage function can decrease tumor incidence (*8*). Mononuclear phagocytes may also reject established tumors. Murine (*9–11*) and human (*12,13*) MNP have been observed to infiltrate tumors. Macrophages capable of lysing tumor targets have been isolated from tumors and ascitic fluid (*14–16*). Such macrophages may affect the course of disease because, in the mouse, higher macrophage tumoricidal activity is associated with regression and dormancy of certain tumors, and in humans, greater tumor infiltration is associated with fewer metastases (*17*). Furthermore, some tumors regress when injected with agents that activate macrophages (*18–20*).

Cytotoxicity against tumor cells mediated by macrophages in vitro was demonstrated first by using macrophages obtained from rodents either immunized with the homologous tumor cell line (*21*), injected with protozoa (*22*), or treated with lipopolysaccharide (LPS) (*23*). Hibbs (*24–26*) demonstrated that embryo fibroblast cytolysis was independent of H-2 compatibility and correlated instead with spontaneous transformation in vitro, and furthermore, that loss of contact inhibition and acquisition of tumorigenicity predicted susceptibility to lysis better than aneuploidy, continuous growth, or abnormal morphology. This selectivity for neoplastic cells has been confirmed repeatedly in rodent macrophage systems (e.g., 27,28). Similar selectivity has been observed for cytolysis and cytostasis by human monocytes (e.g., 29–32) and macrophages (33), even when normal and transformed targets are mixed (34). Although the selectivity of mononuclear phagocytes (MNP) for transformed targets is now well accepted, some studies indicate that this pattern is not absolute (35–37).

Alexander and Evans (23) showed that 2.5–25-$\mu$g/mL doses of lipopolysaccharide (LPS) or lipid A in vitro or in vivo render murine peritoneal macrophages cytotoxic for L5178Y lymphoma targets. By using $^{51}$Cr-release assays, Doe and Henson (38) showed that LPS-activated macrophages are not only cytostatic, but actually lyse tumor cells. Furthermore, these authors have shown that LPS acts on purified macrophages (39) via the lipid A portion of the molecule (40). The first evidence for a two-stage activation sequence for murine macrophages for tumoricidal activity was that macrophages isolated from *Mycobacterium bovis* strain BCG- or toxoplasma-infected mice are cytolytic when tested in fetal calf serum (FCS), but not in human sera unless 1–5 ng/mL LPS is added, a dose of LPS that does not activate normal macrophages for cytotoxicity (41). It was soon confirmed that murine macrophages activated in vivo by BCG infection or in vitro by macrophage-activating factor (MAF) also require triggering for cytotoxicity, but the quantity of LPS required is only on the order of 1 ng/mL (41), an amount often present as an inadvertant contaminant of media and sera (41). The synergistic effect of MAF and LPS requires MAF treatment before or contemporaneous with LPS treatment (42).

There is not a similarly well-understood activation pathway for human MNP. There have been several reports of spontaneous cytotoxicity (defined as cytotoxicity without intentional activation) against tumor cells mediated by human peripheral blood monocytes (e.g., 43), cultured monocyte-derived macrophages (44,45), and macrophages (46–48). Fresh adherence-purified monocytes have demonstrated spontaneous tumoricidal activity (49–51), even when LPS contamination is excluded (51,52). Several studies indicate that freshly isolated human monocytes are activated by various lymphokines (LK) or interferon (IFN) preparations (53–57). The potential contribution of natural killer (NK) cell contamination (58,59) poses particularly severe problems of interpretation of these studies (60), however, and the possibility of LPS contamination was seldom excluded.

As far as the killing mechanism of tumor cells by MNP is concerned, several lines of evidence in both murine (*21,23,26,31*) and human systems (*54*) indicate that binding plays an important role in target selectivity by MNP. Activation of murine macrophages and human monocyte-derived macrophages is associated with increased binding activity. Moreover, prevention of binding of activated murine macrophages by means of trypsinization or addition of a chelating agent or unlabeled target cells to the assay abolishes cytotoxicity (*61*). Contact dependence of cytotoxicity does not exclude the possibility that the mediators of cytotoxicity may be soluble. Cell contact may be required to trigger directed secretion of a cytotoxic mediator. A chemically unstable cytotoxic mediator may act only in the immediate vicinity of effector cells. Electron microscopic observations suggest that the zone of contact between an effector and a target cell may be narrow enough to limit diffusion of macromolecules in and out of the zone (*62*). Therefore, the attachment of an effector to a target cell may allow for the accumulation of a sufficiently high local concentration of a soluble mediator, or may prevent inactivation of the soluble mediator by inhibitors.

Mononuclear phagocytes secrete a large variety of molecules (*63,64*). The MNP products reported to have selective cytotoxic effects on neoplastic cells include lysozyme (*65*), IFN (*66*), $C_3A$ (*67*), thymidine (*68*), and hydrogen peroxide (*69,70*). The role of thymidine and $C_3A$ at physiologic rates of production has been disputed. Hydrogen peroxide and other reactive oxygen species, whose role in microbial defense is well established (*71*), have received the most attention.

Several observations suggest that the oxidative burst may mediate monocyte tumoricidal activity. Mammalian cells are sensitive to lysis by reactive oxygen species (*72*). Moreover, lysis by peroxide is rapid enough (*73*) to account for the kinetics of antibody-dependent cellular cytotoxicity (ADCC) and antibody-independent cytotoxicity by fresh peripheral blood monocytes (*43,74*). Mononuclear phagocytes effectively generate reactive oxygen metabolites (*75,76*). Moreover, macrophages activated for cytotoxicity by IFNγ, bacterial products such as LPS and muramyl dipeptide, and inflammatory proteases have increased levels of oxidative burst activity (*77–80*). Also, fresh blood monocytes have relatively high oxidative burst potential that declines gradually in culture (*81*), roughly in parallel with their loss of spontaneous cytotoxic potential (*55*).

Nathan and coworkers (*69,70*) have shown that lysis of neoplastic targets by activated murine macrophages stimulated by phorbol myristate acetate (PMA) depends on hydrogen peroxide production. These observations have been extended to fresh human peripheral blood monocytes stimulated by PMA (*82–85*). Although these studies demonstrate that the oxidative burst of monocyte and macrophages *can* lyse neoplastic cells, they do not establish that the oxidative burst does mediate tumor lysis under physiologic conditions. Indeed, Weinberg and Haney (*84*) found that scavengers of reactive oxygen species could not inhibit spontaneous cytolysis of HeLa target cells by unstimulated human monocytes or peritoneal macrophages. These results suggest that reactive oxygen species play no role in cytolysis unless the oxidative burst is stimulated extrinsically. It is conceivable, however, that in these experiments the scavengers of reactive oxygen intermediates inhibited monocyte/macrophage-mediated lysis, and NK contaminants accounted for at least part of the observed lytic activity. Another possibility is that hydrogen peroxide mediates lysis both with and without PMA, but without extrinsic stimulation, the effects of hydrogen peroxide are confined to a contact zone from which catalase is excluded (*85*).

An alternative approach to the problem of defining lytic mediators now appears more promising. Several groups have detected cytotoxic activity in the supernatants of activated macrophages (*86–94*) and monocytes (*95–97*).

Currie and Basham (*89*) showed that activated murine macrophages release a factor that selectively lyses malignant, but not normal, cells. Subsequently, Currie showed that the factor has arginase activity that accounts for its cytotoxicity (*98*). Although this observation has been confirmed in the mouse (*99*), it has not been extended to humans. It is also questionable whether in vivo arginine could be depleted to cytolytic levels.

Adams and coworkers have demonstrated that one cytolytic mechanism of activated murine macrophages is secretion of a cytolytic protease (*100*). They showed that: (a) activated murine macrophages secrete a neutral protease; (b) serum-free supernatants of activated macrophages lyse a spectrum of neoplastic targets; and (c) inhibitors of serine proteases inhibit lysis both by supernatants and macrophages; therefore, secretion of protease is one cytolytic mechanism of activated macrophages (*100*). They have also shown that secretion of the cytolytic protease is a property of murine macrophages that have been fully activated in vivo (*86*) or in vitro (*101*). Cytolytic protease secretion is increased by binding tumor targets or target membrane preparations (*102*).

Reidarson has described activated murine macrophage cytotoxins (MCT) of molecular weights 150 and 60 kdalton (*92*) whose activities, like cytolytic protease, are inhibited by serine protease inhibitors (*93*). MCT activity has been purified 2000- to 5000-fold (*103*). This group has isolated similar cytotoxins that can be inhibited by protease inhibitors from supernatants of a PMA-treated human monocytic leukemia cell line (*104*).

TNF is defined as the substance that causes necrosis and regression of certain tumors that is found in the sera of mice, rabbits, and rats primed with BCG and elicited with LPS (*105*). TNF activity as measured in vivo correlates with cytotoxicity to various tumor cell lines in vitro, suggesting that the same molecule mediates both in vivo and in vitro effects (*105–107*). The mode of action of TNF is not known. The slope of the dose-response curve is shallower even against cloned targets than predicted for single-hit kinetics, suggesting that TNF may act enzymatically (*108*). O-Phenanthroline, a metal chelator, blocks TNF killing by over 99%, suggesting that TNF may be a metalloenzyme. Sodium azide also chelates metals and inhibits action of TNF. Colchicine and chloroquine inhibit its effects, suggesting that TNF must be endocytosed, and lysosomal function is required for action (*109*). In addition to cytotoxicity against tumors, TNF may mediate resistance to malaria (*110,111*) and may regulate the activity of lipoprotein lipase in cultured adipocytes (*112*).

Matthews (*113*) demonstrated that human monocytes stimulated with LPS also produce a cytotoxin detected in TNF assays in vitro against L-929. Weinberg (*114*) showed that HL-60, a human promyelocytic leukemia cell line, when treated with PMA, acquires cytolytic capacity. These cells also secrete a cytotoxin, whose production is stimulated by LPS, with physicochemical and functional properties similar to those of TNF (*115*). Recently, two groups have cloned cDNA for this cytotoxin, identified as TNF as defined by cytotoxicity in vitro and tumor necrosis in vivo (*116,117*).

McKinnon et al. (*118*) and Chen et al. (*52*) have recently shown that unstimulated human monocytes can produce a cytolytic factor against actinomycin D-treated Wehi-164 (Wehi/D) targets in line with the findings of Ziegler-Heitbrock et al. (*50*). The cytolytic activity was shown by Colotta et al. (*119*) to be inhibited by serum protease inhibitors; furthermore, cytolysis by monocytes in cell-mediated assays is inhibited by macromolecular, but not micromolecular, protease inhibitors (*119*).

Hammerstrom et al. have described factors selectively cytostatic for transformed cells. These factors are produced by human monocytes cultured in vitro for 4 d, and then stimulated with LK and LPS (*97*). These factors are not cytolytic; they cause a reversible increase in cell-cycle time, inhibiting DNA synthesis earlier and more severely than protein synthesis (*120,121*).

In this chapter, we will discuss some of our recent findings as they related to major issues in the area of macrophage cytotoxicity mentioned above. The key questions that our studies addressed are as follows:

1. Is LPS an obligatory and sufficient trigger for the induction of human monocyte-mediated cytotoxicity?

2. What are some of the biological and biochemical characteristics of the monocyte-derived cytolytic factor?
3. What is the spectrum of target cells sensitive to the cytolytic factor, and what is the relationship between susceptibility to lysis and ability to trigger the production of cytolytic factor?

## 2. Results and Discussion

### 2.1. Role of LPS as a Critical Signal for Triggering Monocyte-Mediated Cytotoxicity

It has recently been shown that Wehi-164 murine sarcoma tumor cells that have been pretreated with actinomycin-D (Wehi/D) are sensitive to human monocyte-mediated killing in a 6-h $^{51}$Cr-release assay, although they remain insensitive to lysis by natural killer (NK) cells (50,51). We have made use of this target cell to investigate the role LPS plays in cytolytic reactions (52). All the tissue culture reagents and cells used in those studies were prepared under LPS-free conditions (<0.05 ng/mL LPS as detected by the Limulus amebocyte lysate assay).

Monocytes prepared and assayed under sterile conditions had significant cytolytic activity against Wehi/D targets (Fig. 1). There was considerable variation in baseline cytolytic activity among donors. Invariably, however, addition of 10 ng/mL LPS directly to the tumoricidal assay resulted in enhanced lysis ($n = 11$, $p < 0.001$, Wilcoxon two-tailed rank-sum test). The addition of polymyxin B at 10 $\mu$g/mL to the assay inhibited the most active preparations of cytotoxic monocytes, though significant levels of cytolysis persisted in all three experiments. It should be mentioned that LPS by itself does not lyse Wehi/D cells, and monocytes pulsed with LPS and washed retain enhanced cytolytic activity. Therefore, the increase in cytolysis of Wehi/D in the presence of LPS was caused by stimulation of the monocytes, not merely weakening of the target cells (52). Previous work has shown that LPS activates murine macrophages for cytostasis (122) and cytolysis (123), and that LPS stimulates cytotoxicity of human macrophages (48,124) and cultured monocyte-derived macrophages (43,125,126). Previous studies of fresh monocytes, however, revealed inconsistent and small (127) or no (84) effect of LPS. Our studies, therefore, represent the first unequivocal evidence that LPS augments tumor cytolysis by freshly isolated human monocytes. In the earlier studies, NK cells may have contributed significantly to the activity measured in these earlier studies (128), but do not lyse Wehi/D (50,51). Also, because the previous studies used long-term 48–60 h) assays, the effector cells may

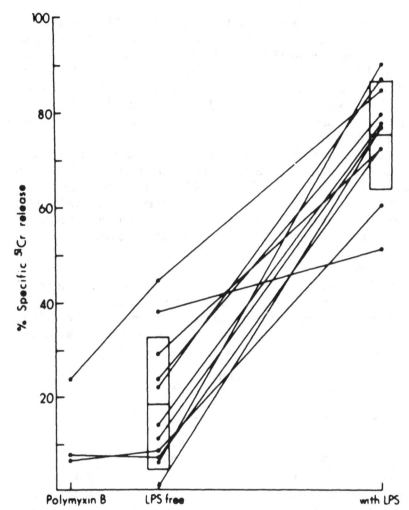

Fig. 1. Cytolytic activity of freshly isolated monocytes in 6-h $^{51}$Cr-release assays against Wehi/D. Means of triplicate determinations are plotted at E:T = 5:1. Each line connects results from samples of a single monocyte preparation tested in plain assay media (negative for endotoxin by *Limulus* amebocyte lysate gelation) or in the presence of 10 μg/mL polymyxin B or 10 ng/mL LPS. Each box represents the mean ±1 standard deviation. The increase in cytolytic activity with LPS is highly significant ($p < 0.001$, Wilcoxon two-tailed rank-sum test) (from ref. *52*).

have lost their capacity to respond to LPS as a result of maturation. In accordance with previous work (*84,127*), LPS was not absolutely required for expression of cytolytic activity, because 10 of 11 donors had significant levels of killing in the absence of LPS.

Titration of LPS added directly to the tumoricidal assay revealed a half-maximal effect at a dose of 100 pg/mL (Table 1). Because most endotoxin effects are mediated by the lipid A portion of the molecule, we tested a purified lipid A preparation in parallel with LPS. Lipid A alone was as effective as, but less potent than, intact LPS, with a half-maximal effect at a dose between 100 pg/mL and 1 ng/mL (Table 1), suggesting that the polysaccharide chains of LPS may enhance binding. Endotoxin preparations from different bacteria were equally effective, however, despite having different polysaccharide structures. All LPS preparations tested, including polysaccharide-deficient LPS of the mutant *Salmonella typhimurium* Re G30/31, had half-maximal effects at 100 pg/mL (Table 1) (*52*).

Because of the potential clinical value of a detoxified activating agent, we tested monophosphoryl lipid A in our assay. Although we confirmed that this preparation activated the *Limulus* amebocyte lysate assay, in six out of six experiments, monophosphoryl lipid A caused no increase in cytolytic activity (*52*).

The half-maximal activity of LPS observed in our study is in accordance with the sensitivity of primed murine macrophages (*129,130*), but demonstrates much greater sensitivity than has been observed with the use of cultured human monocytes (*125,126*). Unlike murine macrophages, however, fresh human monocytes did not require priming in vitro.

Table 1
Comparison of Various Endotoxin Preparations to Induce
Monocyte-Mediated Cytotoxicity[a]

| Endotoxin preparation | Capacity to induce cytotoxicity | Half-maximal effect |
|---|---|---|
| LPS *Escherichia coli* 0111:B4 | + | 100 pg/mL |
| LPS *Salmonella minnesota* WT | + | 100 pg/mL |
| LPS *Salmonella typhimurium* Re G30/C21 | + | 100 pg/mL |
| LPS *Salmonella typhimurium* WT | + | 100 pg/mL |
| LPS *Salmonella enteritidis* | + | 100 pg/mL |
| Lipid A | + | 100 pg/mL–1 ng/mL |
| Monophosphoryl lipid A | − | |

[a]Various endotoxin preparations were tested at 10 ng/mL in a 6-h cytolytic assay of fresh monocytes against Wehi/D target cells.

## 2.2. Monocyte Killing of Wehi/D Is Contact-Dependent and Cytolytic Factor Is TNF-Like

Because excess unlabeled targets did not competitively inhibit cytolysis of Wehi/D by monocytes, studies were performed to examine the possible involvement of soluble factors (52,118). Supernatants from 5-h cultures of fresh monocytes lysed Wehi/D as effectively as monocytes themselves. The kinetics of lysis by the cytolytic factor, which was termed cytolytic monokine (CM), were identical to those observed in direct cell-mediated assays (50,51). Lipopolysaccharides added to monocyte cultures increased CM titers 100- to 1000-fold, so CM titers were sufficient to account for total cell-mediated cytolysis both without LPS and at every dose of LPS tested. Taken together, these data demonstrate that monocytes lyse Wehi/D in a contact-independent manner by secretion of CM, and that the mechanism whereby LPS activates monocytes for cytolysis is to trigger secretion of CM. Cytolytic monokine was found to be filtrable, heat labile, and trypsin sensitive (Table 2). The apparent mol wt of CM by S-200 column chromatography was between 25,000 and 40,000. Experiments using actinomycin D and cycloheximide revealed that release of CM requires both transcription and translation (Table 2).

Table 2
Biochemical Characteristics of CM

| Characteristic | Procedure | Control activity, % |
|---|---|---|
| Heat stability | Boiling, 10 min | 1 |
| | 56°C, 30 min | 1 |
| Storage stability, 24 h | 37°C | 56.3 |
| | 4°C | 74.7 |
| | −20°C | 45.0 |
| Protease sensitivity | 100 U Trypsin, 90 min | 4.4 |
| Requirements for synthesis | 10 μg/mL Actinomycin D | 1 |
| | 10 μg/mL Cycloheximide | |
| Reactivity with rabbit anti-TNF antibodies | 10 TNF-neutralizing units/mL | 40.4 |

| Characteristic | Procedure | Result |
|---|---|---|
| Mol wt | Sephacryl S-200 Column | 25–40 kdalton |
| Rate of production | "Time window experiment" | Highest between 2nd and 5th |

Other investigators have described cytotoxic factors produced by human MNP stimulated by LPS (77,94,95). Because monocytes of a chronic granulomatous disease (CGD) patient produce high levels of CM (131), it is unlikely that oxygen intermediates are involved in lysis of Wehi/D. Cytolytic monokine is unlikely to be a neutral serine protease because its activity, even at high dilutions, is unaffected by 10% FCS and by a mixture of protease inhibitors known to inhibit murine cytolytic protease (*132*). In contrast, antisera to recombinant human TNF neutralize CM activity (*52*; Table 2). Together with the observation that recombinant TNF lyses Wehi/D, these data suggest that CM is antigenically and functionally similar, if not identical, to TNF. The human monocyte cytotoxin described by Matthews (*95*) is qualitatively similar to CM, except that it is harvested at 20 h, by which time CM activity has declined substantially. We also observed greater stimulation by, and sensitivity to, LPS than did Matthews, perhaps because we carefully excluded endotoxin contamination of our control monocyte preparations or perhaps because of differences in our cytotoxic assays.

## 2.3. Target-Cell Selectivity and Capacity to Induce CM Production in Monocytes

Regarding the target cell spectrum of CM, we have observed that several neoplastic targets, including K562, L-929, and CEM, were lysed by some CM preparations (Table 3). No nonneoplastic target was lysed

Table 3
Susceptibility of Targets to CM and Their Ability to Trigger CM Release

| Target | Susceptibility to lysis | Capacity to stimulate CM production |
|---|---|---|
| *Transformed targets* | | |
| A375 | − | − |
| A375/D | ± | |
| CEM | − | |
| CEM/D | − | |
| K562 | Variable | − |
| K562/D | − | |
| L-929 | Variable | |
| L-929/D | Variable | |
| Natusch | − | |
| Natusch/D | − | |
| TU5 | + | + |
| TU5/D | + + | |
| Wehi-164 | + | − |
| Wehi/D | + + | − |
| *Nontransformed targets* | | |
| Lymphocytes | − | |
| Lung | − | + |
| Lung/D | − | |
| RBC (human) | − | |
| RBC (sheep) | − | |

by CM, and not all neoplastic targets are susceptible to CM. Actinomycin D pretreatment of Wehi-164 and TU5 target cells enhanced the cytolytic effect. The observation of selectivity for a range of tumor cells supports the notion that CM may contribute to surveillance against tumor cells in vivo.

Murine macrophages cytolytic factor (*133*) and human NK cytotoxic factor (NKCF) (*134*) can be stimulated by contact of effector and target cells. In experiments performed under LPS-free conditions, we examined the possibility that some target cells may induce monocytes to secrete CM. To our surprise, enhanced CM activity was produced not by monocytes cultured with Wehi/D or K562, but by monocytes cultured with non-transformed lung cells (Fig. 2). There was no additive stimulation of CM production when monocytes were cultured with both LPS and any of the cell lines. The failure of monocyte-sensitive target cells to induce greater CM activity could have been explained by absorption of CM from the media by CM-susceptible cells. Absorption experiments performed at 4 °C (Fig. 3) or 37 °C (not shown), however, revealed no reduction of CM activity from monocyte supernatants incubated 1 h with Wehi-164, Wehi/D, TU5, TU5/D, L-929, or lung or autologous nonadherent lymphocytes. We therefore conclude that the lack of enhanced CM activity in supernatants produced by monocytes cocultured with Wehi/D was not caused by a combination of stimulation and absorption by the susceptible targets.

Further experiments done with normal lung cells showed that at ratios of 1 lung cell:100 monocytes, lung cells incubated with monocytes increased CM titers 16-fold. Similarly, TU5 and TU5/D cells at ratios of 1 TU5 cell:10 monocytes increased CM titers eightfold. This efficient stimulation suggested that the stimulation did not require cell contact. Indeed, monocytes incubated in conditioned media from 4-h cultures of TU5 or lung cells produced supernatants with high levels of CM activity, although not as high as monocytes incubated directly with TU5 cells. Interestingly, conditioned media from TU5 and lung cells activated the *Limulus* amebocyte lysate, even though the cells had been cultured in endotoxin-free media; conditioned media from Wehi-164 cells, which did not stimulate CM production, did not activate *Limulus* lysate. Stimulator cells were not contaminated with mycoplasma and still produced supernatants with stimulatory activity after being maintained in LPS-free media for months. Figure 4 shows that whereas 10 $\mu$g/mL polymyxin B reduced LPS-stimulated CM titers from 31 to 6, polymyxin B did not significantly affect CM titers stimulated by conditioned media from lung or TU5 cells. There have been several demonstrations of false-positive *Limulus* tests for endotoxin caused by similar (*135*) and unrelated (*136*) molecules. The lack of inhibition of the stimulatory effect of lung and TU5 supernatants by

polymyxin B, which binds the lipid A portion of the endotoxin molecule
(*137*), suggests that these supernatants contained a stimulatory molecule
other than LPS, the nature of which remains to be determined.

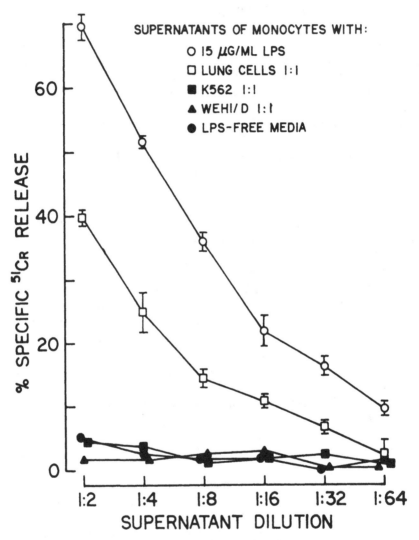

Fig. 2. Effect of coculture with various cell lines on CM production by
monocytes. Supernatants of $5 \times 10^5$ monocytes/mL incubated 5 h with $5 \times 10^5$
cultured cells/mL in endotoxin-free media. Control supernatants were from
monocytes incubated alone with or without 15 $\mu$g/mL of LPS. Cytolytic activity
was measured in 6-h assays against Wehi/D.

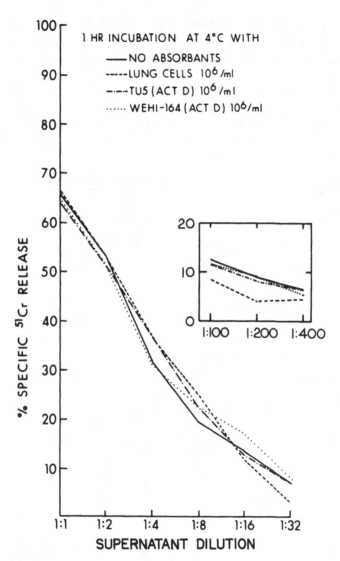

Fig. 3. Effect of CM activity against Wehi/D of absorption by target cells. Aliquots of monocyte supernatant were incubated 1 h at 4 °C alone or with 1 × $10^6$ cultured cells/mL. Inset: Aliquots of monocyte supernatant were diluted 1:50 before incubation 1 h at 4 °C alone or with 2 × $10^7$ cultured cells/mL.

Although our studies do not rule out additional cytolytic mechanisms, they provide no evidence that cytolysis of Wehi/D by monocytes is enhanced by cell contact. Therefore, although many studies have demonstrated

contact-dependent cytolysis by MNP (e.g., *28,29,138*), it is inappropriate
to extrapolate results obtained with MNP at a particular stage of maturation and activation and one target to other stages of maturation, activation,
and targets.

Conversely, the existence of a contact-independent lytic mechanism
cannot be extrapolated to all targets. Recently, Keller (*139*) also described
a contact-independent mechanism in a murine macrophage cytotoxicity
system. It should be noted that actinomycin D in our studies (data not

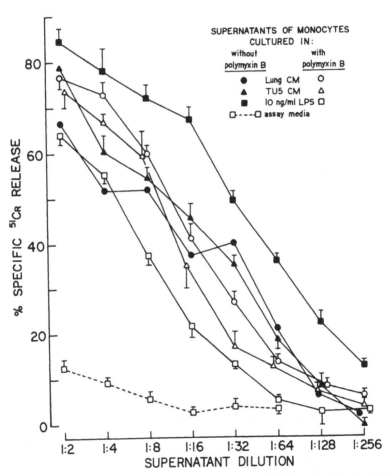

Fig. 4. Effect of polymyxin B on stimulation of CM production by LPS and
by target cell conditioned media. Aliquots of $5 \times 10^5$ monocytes/mL were incubated for 5 h, with or without 10 $\mu$g/mL polymyxin B, in target-cell-conditioned
media or fresh assay media containing 10 ng/mL LPS. Cytolytic activity in the
resulting supernatants was measured in 6-h assays against Wehi/D.

shown) was not required for cytolysis by CM: monocyte supernatants also lysed TU5 and Wehi-164 in long-term $^3$H-thymidine-release assays without drug treatment.

How CM works at the target cell level is unclear. The slope of the dose–response curve of CM is, as for TNF (*108*), shallower even against cloned targets than predicted for single-hit kinetics, suggesting that one CM molecule may kill more than one target, consistent with the hypothesis that it acts enzymatically. It is suggested that TNF may be a metalloenzyme because the metal chelator, *O*-phenanthroline, blocks TNF activity (*109*). The lack of absorption of CM activity by targets is consistent with external enzymatic action, but many other interpretations are possible. If CM binds a receptor, and is, like recombinant human TNF, effective at doses of $10^{-11}M$, the lack of absorption by $2 \times 10^7$ targets/mL of barely detectable activity indicates that fewer than 300 receptors/cell need to be occupied to effect lysis. Because actinomycin D increases the susceptibility of target cells to CM, CM most likely causes damage that can be repaired by processes requiring transcription. A lack of hemolytic activity distinguished CM from granules isolated from CTL (*140*) and NK (*141*) tumor cell lines and suggests that membrane lipids are not the primary target of CM activity.

## Acknowledgments

The research described in this article has been reviewed by the Health Effects Research Laboratory, US Environmental Protection Agency and approved for publication. Approval does not signify that the contents necessarily reflect the views and policies of the Agency nor does mention of trade names or commercial products constitute endorsement or recommendation for use.

We thank Mrs. Vickie Worrell for her excellent secretarial assistance.

## References

*1.* Hibbs, J. B., Jr., Chapman, H. A., and Weinberg, J. B. *J. Reticuloendothel. Soc.* **24**, 549 (1978).

*2.* Griffin, F. M., Jr., in *Advances in Host Defense Mechanisms* (Gallen, J. I. and A. S. Fauci, eds.) Raven, New York, (1982).

*3.* Blanden, R. V., Hapel, A. J., Doherty, P. C., and Zinkernagel, R. M., in *Immunobiology of the Macrophage* (Nelson, D. S., ed.) Academic, New York, (1976).

*4.* Thiele, D. L. and Lipsky, P. E. *J. Immunol.* **129**, 1033 (1980).

5. Rosenthal, A. S. and Unanue, E. R. *Macrophage Regulation of Immunity* Academic, New York (1980).
6. Nathan, C. F., Murray, H. W., and Cohn, Z. A. *N. Engl. J. Med.* **303**, 622 (1980).
7. Adams, D. O. and Snyderman, R. *Cancer Inst.* **62**, 1341 (1979).
8. Bast, R. C., Jr., Zbar, T. S., Borsos, T. S., and Rapp, H. J. *N. Engl. J. Med.* **290**, 1413 (1974).
9. Eccles, S. A. and Alexander, P. *Nature* **250**, 667 (1974).
10. Levy, M. H. and Wheelock, E. F. *Adv. Cancer Res.* **20**, 131 (1974).
11. Alexander, P. *Ann. Rev. Med.* **27**, 207 (1976).
12. Gauci, C. L. and Alexander, P. *Cancer Lett.* **1** 29 (1975).
13. Hayry, P. and Totterman, T. H. *Eur. J. Immunol.* **8**, 866 (1978).
14. Vose, B. M. *Cancer Immunol. Immunother.* **5**, 173 (1978).
15. Mantovani, A., Polentaratti, N., Peri, G., Shavit, Z. B., Vecchi, A., Bolis, G., and Margioni, C. *J. Natl. Cancer Inst.* **64**, 1307 (1980).
16. Haskill, S., Koren, H., Fowler, W., and Walton, L. *Br. J. Cancer* **45**, 747 (1982).
17. Lauder, I., Pherne, W., Stewart, J., and Sainsburg, R. *J. Clin. Pathol.* **30**, 563 (1977).
18. Papermaster, B. W., Holterman, O. A., Rosner, D., Klein, E., Dao, T., and Djerassi, I. *Res. Chem. Pathol. Pharmacol.* **8**, 40 (1974).
19. Snodgrass, M. J. and Hanna, M. G. *Cancer Res.* **33** 701 (1973).
20. Nelson, D. S. *Transpl. Rev.* **19**, 226 (1974).
21. Evans, R. and Alexander, P. *Nature* **22**, 620 (1970).
22. Hibbs, J. B., Jr., Lambert, L. H., Jr., and Remington, J. S. *J. Infect. Dis.* **124**, 587 (1971).
23. Alexander, P. and Evans, R. *Nature* **232**, 76 (1971).
24. Hibbs, J. B. Jr., Lambert, L. H. and Remington, J. S. *Science* **177**, 998 (1972).
25. Hibbs, J. B., Jr., Lambert, L. H. and Remington, J. S. *Proc. Soc. Exp. Biol. Med.* **139**, 1049 (1972).
26. Hibbs, J. B., Jr., Lambert, L. H., and Remington, J. S. *Nature* **235**, 48 (1972).
27. Cleveland, R. P., Meltzer, M. S., and Zbar, B. *J. Natl. Cancer Inst.* **52**, 1887 (1974).
28. Meltzer, M. S., Tucker, R. W., and Sanford, K. K. *J. Natl. Cancer Inst.* **54**, 1177 (1975).
29. Mantovani, A., Jerrells, T. R., Dean, J. H., and Herberman, R. B. *Int. J. Cancer* **23**, 18 (1979).
30. Mantovani, A., Tagliabue, A., Dean, J. H., Jerrells, T. R., and Herberman, R. B. *Int. J. Cancer* **23**, 28 (1979).
31. Hammerstrom, J. *Scand. J. Immunol.* **10**, 575 (1979).
32. Cameron, D. J. and Churchill, W. H. *J. Clin. Invest.* **63**, 977 (1979).
33. Sone, S. and Tsubura, E. *J. Immunol.* **129**, 1313 (1982).
34. Fidler, I. J. and Kleinerman, E. S. *J. Clin. Oncol.* **2**, 937 (1984).
35. Jones, J. T., McBride, W. H., and Weir, D. M. *Cell. Immunol.* **18**, 375 (1975).

36. Keller, R. *J. Natl. Cancer Inst.* **56**, 369 (1976).
37. Keller, R. *Br. J. Cancer* **37**, 732 (1978).
38. Doe, W. F. and Henson, P. M. *J. Exp. Med.* **148**, 544 (1978).
39. Doe, W. R., Yang, S. T., Morrison, D. C., Betz, S. J., and Henson, P. M. *J. Exp. Med.* **148**, 557 (1978).
40. Hibbs, J. B., Jr., Taintor, R. R., Chapman, H. A., Jr., and Weinberg, J. B. *Science* **197**, 282 (1977).
41. Weinberg, J. B., Chapman, H. A., Jr., and Hibbs, J. B., Jr. *J. Immunol.* **121**, 72 (1978).
42. Ruco, L. P. and M. S. Meltzer. *J. Immunol.* **121**, 2035 (1978).
43. Horwitz, D. A., Kight, N., Temple, A., and Allison, A. C. *Immunology* **36**, 221 (1979).
44. Rinehart, J. J., Lange, P., Gormus, B. J., and Kaplan, M. E. *Blood* **52**, 211 (1978).
45. Rinehart, J. J., Vessalla, R., Lange, P., Kaplan, M. E., and Gormus, B. J. *J. Lab. Clin. Med.* **93**, 361 (1979).
46. Balkwill, F. R. and Hogg, N. *J. Immunol.* **123**, 1451 (1979).
47. Mantovani, A., Shavit, Z. B., Peri, G., Polentarutti, N., Bordignon, C., Sessa, C., and Mangioni, C. *Clin. Exp. Immunol.* **39**, 776 (1980).
48. Sone, S., Moriguchi, S., Shimizu, E., Ogushi, F., and Tsubura, E. *Cancer Res.* **42**, 2227 (1982).
49. Golightly, M. G., Fischer, D. G., Ohlander, C., and Koren, H. S. *Blood* **61**, 390 (1983).
50. Ziegler-Heitbrock, H. W. F. and Riethmuller, G. *J. Natl. Cancer Inst.* **72**, 23 (1984).
51. Colotta, F., Peri, G., Villa, A., and Mantovani, A. *J. Immunol.* **132**, 936 (1984).
52. Chen, A. K., K. P. McKinnon, and Koren, H. S. *J. Immunol.* **135**, 3978 (1985).
53. Mantovani, A., Dean, J. H., Jerrells, T. R., and Herberman, R. B. *Int. J. Cancer* **25**, 691 (1980).
54. Herberman, R. B., Ortaldo, J. R., Mantovani, A., Hobbs, D. S., Kung, H. F., and Pestka, S. *Cell. Immunol.* **67**, 160 (1982).
55. Fischer, D. G., Golightly, M. G., and Koren, H. S. *J. Immunol.* **130**, 1220 (1983).
56. Le, Jr., Prensky, W., Yip, Y. K., Chang, Z., Hoffman, T., Stevenson, H. C., Balazs, I., Sadlik, J. R., and Vilcek, J. *J. Immunol.* **131**, 2821 (1983).
57. Dean, R. T. and Virelizier, J. L. *Clin. Exp. Immunol.* **51**, 501 (1983).
58. Chang, Z. L., Hoffman, T., Bonvini, E., Stevenson, H. C., and Herberman, R. B. *Scand. J. Immunol.* **18**, 439 (1983).
59. Chang, Z. L., Hoffman, T., Stevenson, H. C., Trinchieri, G., and Herberman, R. B. *Scand. J. Immunol.* **18**, 451 (1983).
60. Villa, A., Peri, G., Rossi, V., Delia, D., and Mantovani, A. *Cell. Immunol.* **87**, 494 (1984).
61. Marino, P. A. and Adams, D. O. *Cell Immunol.* **54**, 26 (1980).

62. Adams, D., Kao, K.-J., Farb, R., and Pizzo, S. V. *J. Immunol.* **124**, 293 (1980).
63. Nathan, C. F., Murray, H. W., and Cohn, Z. F. *N. Engl. J. Med.* **303**, 622 (1980).
64. Takemura, R. and Werb, Z. *Am. J. Physiol.* **246**, C1 (1984).
65. Osserman, E. F., Klockars, M., Halper, J., and Fishel, R. E. *Nature* **243**, 231 (1973).
66. Stewart, W. E., Gresser, I., Tovey, M., Bandu, M. T., and Le Goff, S. E., *Nature* **626**, 300 (1976).
67. Schorlemmer, H. U. and Allison, A. C. *Immunology* **31**, 781 (1976).
68. Stadecker, M. J., Calderon, J., Karnovsky, M. L., and Unanue, E. R. *J. Immunol.* **119**, 1738 (1977).
69. Nathan, C. F., Brukner, L. H., Silverstein, S. C., and Cohn, Z. A. *J. Exp. Med.* **149**, 84 (1979).
70. Nathan, C. F., Silverstein, S. C., Brukner, L. H., and Cohn, Z. A. *J. Exp. Med.* **149**, 100 (1979).
71. Klebanoff, S. J., in *Advances in Host Defense Mechanisms* vol. 1 (Gallin, J. I. and Fauci, A. S., eds.) Raven, New York, (1982).
72. Clark, R. A. and Klebanoff, S. J. *J. Exp. Med.* **141**, 1442 (1975).
73. Nathan, C. F., Brukner, L. H., Silverstein, S. C., and Cohn, Z. A. *J. Exp. Med.* **149**, 84 (1979).
74. Fischer, D. G., Hubbard, W. J., and Koren, H. S. *Cell Immunol.* **58**, 426 (1981).
75. Johnston, R. B., Jr., Lehmeyer, J. E., and Guthrie, L. A. *J. Exp. Med.* **143**, 155 (1976).
76. Nathan, C. F. and Root, R. K. *J. Exp. Med.* **146**, 1648 (1977).
77. Nathan, C. F., Murray, H. W., and Wiebe, M. E. *J. Exp. Med.* **158**, 670 (1983).
78. Lepoivre, M., Renu, J. P., Lemaire, G., and Petit, J. F. *J. Immunol.* **129**, 860 (1982).
79. Pabst, M. J., Hedegaard, H. B., and Johnston, R. B., Jr. *J. Immunol.* **128**, 123 (1982).
80. Speer, C. P., Pabst, M. J., Hedegaard, H. B., Rest, R. F., and Johnston, R. B., Jr. *J. Immunol.* **133**, 2151 (1984).
81. Nakagawara, A., Nathan, C. F., and Cohn, Z. A. *J. Clin. Invest.* **68**, 1243 (1981).
82. Weiss, S. J. and Slivka, A. *J. Clin. Invest.* **69**, 255 (1982).
83. Mavier, P. and Edgington, T. S. *J. Immunol.* **132**, 1980 (1984).
84. Weinberg, J. B. and Haney, A. F. *J. Natl. Cancer Inst.* **70**, 1005 (1983).
85. Wright, S. D. and Silverstein, S. *Cell. Biol.* **95**, 443a (1982).
86. Adams, D. O., Kao, K. J., Farb, R., and Pizzo, S. V. *J. Immunol.* **124**, 293, (1980).
87. Pincus, W. B., Spanis, C. W., and Sintex, D. E. *J. Reticuloendothel. Soc.* **9**, 552 (1971).
88. Reed, W. P. and Lucas, Z. L. *J. Immunol.* **115**, 395 (1975).
89. Currie, G. A. and Basham, C. *J. Exp. Med.* **142**, 1600 (1975).

90. Sharma, S. D., Peissens, W. F., and Middlebrook, G. *Cell. Immunol.* **49**, 379 (1980).
91. Mannel, D. N., Moore, R. N., and Mergenhagen, S. E. *Infect. Immunol.* **30**, 523 (1980).
92. Reidarson, T., Levy, W., Klostergaard, J., and Granger, G. A. *J. Natl. Cancer Inst.* **69**, 879 (1982).
93. Reidarson, T., Granger, G. A., and J. Klostergaard. *J. Natl. Cancer Inst.* **69**, 889 (1982).
94. Sone, S., Tachibana, K., Ishii, K., Ogawara, M., and Tsubura, E. *Cancer Res.* **44**, 646 (1984).
95. Matthews, N. *Immunology* **44**, 135 (1981).
96. Cameron, D. J. *J. Reticuloendothel. Soc.* **32**, 247 (1982).
97. Hammerstrom, J. *Scand. J. Immunol.* **15**, 311 (1982).
98. Currie, G. A. *Nature* **273**, 758 (1978).
99. Farram, E. and Nelson, D. S. *Cell. Immunol.* **55**, 283 (1980).
100. Adams, D. O. *J. Immunol.* **124**, 286 (1980).
101. Adams, D. O. and Marino, P. A. *J. Immunol.* **126**, 981 (1981).
102. Johnson, W. J., Whisnant, C. C., and Adams, D. O. *J. Immunol.* **127**, 1787 (1981).
103. Klostergaard, J., Reidarson, T. H., and Granger, G. A. *J. Leukocyte Biol.* **35**, 229 (1984).
104. Armstrong, C. A., Klostergaard, J., and Granger, G. A. *J. Natl. Cancer Inst.* **74**, 1 (1985).
105. Carswell, E. A., Old, L. J., Kassel, L. J., Green, S., Fiore, N., and Williamson, B. *Proc. Natl. Acad. Sci. USA* **72**, 3666 (1975).
106. Matthews, N. and Watkins, J. F. *Br. J. Cancer* **38**, 302 (1978).
107. Mannel, D. N., Meltzer, M. S., and Mergenhagen, S. E. *Infect. Immunol.* **28**, 204 (1980).
108. Ruff, M. R. and Gifford, G. E. *Infect. Immunol.* **31**, 380 (1981).
109. Ruff, M. R. and Gifford, G. E., in *Lymphokines* 2 E. (Pick, E. and Landy, M., eds.) Academic, New York, (1981).
110. Clark, I. A., Virelizier, J. L., Carswell, E. A., and Wood, P. R. *Infect. Immunol.* **31**, 1058 (1981).
111. Taverne, J., Dockrell, H. M., and Playfair, J. H. L. *Infect. Immunol.* **33**, 83 (1981).
112. Old, L. Y. *Science* **230**, 630 (1985).
113. Matthews, N. *Immunology* **44**, 135 (1981).
114. Weinberg, J. B. *Science* **213**, 655 (1981).
115. Gifford, G. E., Flick, D. A., Abdallah, N. A., and Fisch, H. *J. Natl. Cancer Inst.* **73**, 69 (1984).
116. Pennica, D., Nedwin, G. E., Hayflick, J. S., Seeburg, P. H., Derynck, R., Palladino, M. A., Kohr, W. R., Aggarwal, B. B., and D. V. Goeddel. *Nature* **312**, 724 (1984).
117. Wang, A. M., Creasey, A. A., Ladner, M. B., Lin, L. S., Strickler, J., Van Arsdell, J. N., Yamamoto, R., and Mark, D. F. *Science* **228**, 149 (1985).

118. McKinnon, K. P., Chen, A. R., Argov, S., Love, B. C., and Koren, H. S. *Immunobiology* **171**, 27–44 (1986).
119. Colotta, F., Bersani, L., Lazzarin, A., Poli, G., and Mantovani, A. *J. Immunol.* **134**, 3524 (1985).
120. Eggen, B. M., Bakke, O., and Hammerstrom, J. *Scand. J. Immunol.* **18**, 13 (1983).
121. Nissen-Meyer, J. and Seim, S. *Scand. J. Immunol.* **18**, 465 (1983).
122. Alexander, P. and Evans, R. *Nature* **232**, 76 (1971).
123. Doe, W. F. and Henson, P. M. *J. Exp. Med.* **148**, 544 (1978).
124. Peri, G., Polentarutti, N., Sessa, C., Mangioni, C., and Mantovani, A. *Int. J. Cancer* **28**, 143 (1981).
125. Hammerstrom, J. *Acta Pathol. Microbiol. Immunol. Scand.* (C) **87**, 391 (1979).
126. Cameron, D. J. and Churchill, W. H. *J. Immunol.* **124**, 708 (1980).
127. Biondi, A., Peri, G., Lorenzet, R., Fumarola, D., and Mantovani, A. *J. Reticuloendothel. Soc.* **33**, 315 (1983).
128. Chang, Z. L., Hoffman, T., Bonvini, E., Stevenson, H. C., and Herberman, R. B. *Scand. J. Immunol.* **18**, 439 (1983).
129. Russell, S. W., Doe, W. F., and McIntosh, A. T. *J. Exp. Med.* **146**, 1511 (1977).
130. Weinberg, J. B., Chapman, H. A., Jr., and Hibbs, H. B., Jr. *J. Immunol.* **121**, 72 (1978).
131. Chen, A. and Koren, H. S. *J. Immunol.* **134**, 1909 (1985).
132. Adams, D. O., Kao, K. J., Farb, R., and Pizzo, S. V. *J. Immunol.* **124**, 293 (1980).
133. Johnson, W. J., Whisnant, C. C., and Adams, D. O. *J. Immunol.* **127**, 1787 (1981).
134. Wright, S. C., Weitzer, M. L., Kahle, R., Granger, G. A., and Bonavida, B. *J. Immunol.* **130**, 2479 (1983).
135. Wildfeuer, A., Heymer, B., Schleifer, K. H., and Haferkamp, O. *Appl. Microbiol.* **28**, 867 (1974).
136. Elin, R. J. and Wolff, S. M. *J. Infect. Dis.* **128**, 349 (1973).
137. Morrison, D. C. and Jacobs, D. M. *Immunochemistry* **13**, 813 (1976).
138. Alexander, P. and Evans, R. *Nature* **232**, 76 (1971).
139. Keller, R., Keist, R., and Groscurth, P. *Int. J. Cancer* **37**, 89–95 (1986).
140. Podack, E. R. and Konigsberg, P. J. *J. Exp. Med.* **60**, 695 (1984).
141. Millard, P. J., Henkart, M. P., Reynolds, C. W., and Henkart, P. A. *J. Immunol.* **132**, 3197 (1984).

# Antitumor Monocyte Cytotoxic Factors (MCF) Produced by Human Blood Monocytes

## Production, Characterization, and Biological Significance

ATSUSHI UCHIDA

## 1. Introduction

Both lymphocytes and monocytes from the blood of normal individuals express natural cytotoxicity against a variety of tumor cells and some nonmalignant cells (for review, see ref. 1–4). There is now increasing evidence that natural killer (NK) cells and monocyte/macrophages play an important role in host defenses against tumor. For the two types of cytolytic cells, in a short-term (3–4 h) assay can be isolated from the blood of healthy killing (6) have been described. It has been shown that the monocyte population that can lyse certain tumor cells, including the NK-sensitive K562 cells, in a short-term (3–4 h) assay can be isolated from the blood of healthy donors (7,8) and of cancer patients (9–11) by adherence to plastic surfaces precoated with autologous serum.

In some experimental studies with cytotoxic macrophages, close contact between macrophages and tumor cells appears to be essential for the antitumor effect (12). In other systems, however, close contact is not prerequisite since the monocyte/macrophages release a soluble mediator. These mediators include neutral protease (13,14), arginase (15), reactive oxygen intermediates (16), the complement breakdown product C3a (17), tumor necrosis factor (TNF) (18–21), and other cytotoxic or cytostatic factors (22–26). We have recently reported that human blood monocytes can be induced to release soluble cytotoxic factors, termed monocyte cytotoxic factors (MCF), during interaction with tumor cells and suggested that this may be involved in the lytic mechanism of monocyte-mediated natural cytotoxicity (27–30). The aim of this chapter is to describe the MCF, with emphasis on generation, lytic activity, biochemical and biophysical characterization, and possible biological significance in human neoplasia.

# 2. Generation of MCF

## 2.1. Cells Involved in MCF Production and Release

Human blood monocytes obtained by adherence to autologous serum-coated plastic dishes were shown to lyse K562 cells in a 4-h $^{51}$Cr release assay, whereas little or no cytotoxicity was seen with monocytes collected from fetal calf serum (FCS)-coated dishes (7–11). Similar distinction was observed with the production of cytotoxic factors. When monocytes isolated by adherence to autologous serum-coated dishes were cocultured with K562 for 24 h in serum-free medium, the cell-free supernatants contained factors that killed K562 cells in a 48-h microcytotoxicity assay (27–30). In contrast, little or no lysis was seen with supernatants produced by coculture of monocytes from FCS-coated dishes with K562. Monocytes adhered more strongly to autologous serum-coated dishes than to FCS-coated dishes, suggesting that the adherence to autologous serum-coated dishes may activate monocytes to be highly cytotoxic.

The highly purified (>96%) adherent cell population was still contaminated with small numbers (<2%) of large granular lymphocytes (LGL). Recent evidence indicates that LGL are potent producers of natural killer cytotoxic factors (NKCF), which are released during interaction with K562 and are cytotoxic to the target cells (27–34). It is thus important to ascertain whether monocytes or NK cells are responsible for MCF production. Studies with the use of various monoclonal antibodies that were reported to recognize NK cell antigens and/or monocyte antigens have revealed that MCF production seen with the adherent cell fraction is mainly exerted by Leu-M1$^{+}$, OKM1$^{+}$, and Lue-11$^{-}$ monocytes.

## 2.2. Optimal Conditions for MCF Generation

Kinetic studies in which monocytes were incubated with K562 for time intervals varying from 3 to 48 h demonstrated that some lytic activity was detected in the supernatant as early as after 3 h of incubation (27). Maximum levels of cytotoxic activity were observed in 6-h supernatants, which were comparable to the levels obtained in supernatants, at 18, 24, and 48 h. Similar kinetics of cytotoxic factor production were reported in studies with NKCF (27,32,34) and with an antitumor cytotoxin (22).

Although supernatants from coculture of monocytes with K562 contained MCF activity, monocytes cultured alone released little or no cytotoxic factors. Resistant target cells, such as EL4 and T-blasts, failed to activate monocytes for MCF release. Blocking of monocyte binding to K562 by cytochalasin A also abrogated release of MCF in supernatants. These results may indicate the requirement of effector/target interaction for MCF production. In contrast, other cytostatic or cytotoxic factors have reportedly been released by monocytes or macrophages independently of contact with tumor cells (13–26). Lysates of monocytes produced by freezing and then thawing contained no detectable amounts of MCF activity. Similar findings were reported in other systems in which lysates of human monocytes isolated by discontinuous density gradient centrifugation are not cytotoxic to a variety of tumor cells (35). The requirement of effector/target interaction has been described for human NKCF production (29,32–34), whereas lysates of spleen cells from CBA mice were shown to contain NKCF activity (36).

Endotoxin has been implicated in the production of most cytotoxic or cytostatic factors by monocyte/macrophages (13–25). It is unlikely, however, that endotoxin plays a central role in the production of MCF since no endotoxin is detected in our system and since addition of polymixin B (10 μg/mL) does not affect the MCF production.

When monocytes were coincubated with K562 at 4 °C instead of 37 °C, the resulting supernatants contained little or no lytic activity, indicating that active cell metabolism is required for MCF production. Pretreatment of monocytes with cycloheximide, an inhibitor of protein synthesis, reduced their ability to produce MCF in response to K562. In addition, reduced generation of MCF was seen with actinomycin D-treated monocytes. The data indicate that the messenger RNA is newly synthesized in vitro. Taken together, MCF appear to be newly synthesized in vitro. Similarly, an antitumor cytotoxin was previously shown to be newly synthesized in culture of monocytes alone or with lipopolysaccharide (LPS).

## 2.3. Augmentation of MCF Generation

In vitro treatment with the streptococcal preparation OK432 or interferon (IFN)α or IFNγ has been shown to enhance natural cytotoxicity of monocytes (8–10). The OK432- or IFN-treated monocytes were found to release higher amounts of MCF in subsequent coculture with K562 (28). OK432 has a stronger enhancing effect on MCF production than IFN. There are several possible explanations for the OK432-induced enhancement of MCF generation. One possibility is that OK432-activated monocytes embark on de novo synthesis of the cytotoxic factors. This may be supported by our experiments, in which release of MCF with OK432-increased lytic activity was blocked by treating monocytes with either cycloheximide or actinomycin D. Alternatively, OK432-activated monocytes may have the same amounts of MCF, but could release greater quantities of the factors. In fact, the enhanced microfilament function has been seen with OK432-treated cells (9). Another possibility is that OK432-activated monocytes generate more lytically active forms of the cytotoxic factors than the untreated cells. The augmented production of the factors is in line with the OK432 effect with respect to the cytokines, such as IFN, interleukin 1 (IL-1), IL-2, colony stimulating factor (CSF), TNF, and NK-cell activating factor (NKAF) (37). In this regard it has been reported that release of NKCF (38) and lymphotoxin (39,40) is elevated by IFN treatment of lymphocytes.

Exposure to lymphokines of cultured human monocytes has been shown to induce the production of cytostatic protein factors (24). Similarly, tumor cytotoxic factors were released from monocytes upon stimulation with normuramyl dipeptide (25). Stimulation by OK432 alone has also induced fresh monocytes to secrete the MCF, whereas IFN alone or lymphokine alone was ineffective (28). The concurrent stimulation of monocytes with OK432 and K562 resulted in the highest level of MCF activity. Thus, it seems likely that OK432 serves as the triggering signal for monocytes like K562 and that OK432 and K562 may stimulate the different membrane moieties of monocytes. Alternatively, phagocytized OK432 could somehow activate the MCF release mechanism.

## 3. Lytic Activity of MCF

### 3.1. Kinetics of Lysis

For determination of kinetics of MCF-mediated lysis, K562 cells were incubated with MCF-containing medium for varying time intervals at 37 °C, and thereafter the viability of target cells was estimated by the trypan blue dye exclusion test (27). The lysis of target cells by MCF occurred slowly, requiring a period of incubation of 48 h or more, although some cytotoxicity was detectable at 18 h. No killing was seen with the target cells when incubated with MCF at 4 °C. NKCF-mediated lysis shows similar kinetics (27,31,33,34). In contrast, studies on the kinetics of absorption have revealed that most MCF activity could be removed from supernatants when they are incubated with K562 for 2 h at 37 °C (30). This binding also occurred at 4 °C, excluding the possible inactivation of MCF by tumor cells. In addition, after 2-h incubation of target cells with MCF, the target cells could be washed and lysis proceed with kinetics similar to that observed when they are incubated in the continued presence of MCF. Collective data indicate that by contrast with the rapid killing of intact monocytes

(2–4 h), MCF require a longer period of time (48–60 h) to produce lysis. Optimal binding can occur within 2 h, however, and this exposure is sufficient to cause subsequent lysis of target cells.

### 3.2. Augmentation of MCF-Mediated Lysis of Actinomycin D

It has been demonstrated that treatment with actinomycin D induces the resistant tumor cells to become sensitive or enhances the target cell susceptibility to lysis by cytokines (23,41,42). In fact, the lytic activity of most cytotoxic factors has been assayed in the presence of actinomycin D, cycloheximide, or mitomycin C (13–24). Pretreatment of K562 with actinomycin D or addition of the drug to cytotoxicity assays has rendered the targets more susceptible to lysis by MCF (29,30). This enhancement occurred at the concentration of actinomycin D, which alone was not toxic to the target cells. Thus, the optimal lysis by MCF has routinely been observed in an 18-h $^{51}$Cr release assay. The biological activity of TNF, lymphotoxin, and antitumor cytotoxin on L-929 has also been detected in an 18-h assay in the presence of the drugs (18–21). More rapid killing (within 6 h) by human monocyte-derived cytotoxic factors has been seen with actinomycin D-treated Wehi-164 (26). Previous studies suggested that the modification of lipid and fatty acid composition of target cells by actinomycin D or adriamycin may have profound effects on physical properties of the cells, especially membrane fluidity, permeability, or thickness, which could be responsible for the drug-induced alteration of target cell susceptibility to humoral immune attack (42). The enhanced susceptibility of actinomycin D-treated target cells to MCF is unlikely to be derived from an increase in the ability of the target cells to absorb the cytotoxic factor, but may rather result from an increase in sensitivity to the damage done by the factor (29).

### 3.3. Enhancement of MCF Activity by IFN

The addition of IFN to supernatants containing NKCF enhances their lytic activity (30,38,39). Furthermore, anti-IFNα antibodies block or neutralize the lysis by NKCF-containing medium (39). These data indicate that IFN is involved in the modulation of the lytic activity of preformed NKCF. Also, the biologic activity of lymphotoxin (43,44) and monocyte cytotoxic factors has been augmented by the presence of IFN in the assay. The addition of IFNα or IFNγ to MCF induced a synergistic enhancement of cytotoxicity (Table 1; 30). The dose of IFN required for this augmentation alone was not toxic to the target cells. The mechanism by which IFN enhances the lytic activity of MCF is unclear. It is not attributable to an increase in the number of receptors for the cytotoxic factors, since

Table 1
Enhancement of MCF Activity by IFN and Actinomycin D[a]

| Experiment | Addition of | Cytotoxicity, % |
|---|---|---|
| 1 | None | 5 |
| | IFN | 10[b] |
| | Actinomycin D | 22[b] |
| | IFN + Actinomycin D | 33[b] |
| 2 | None | 10 |
| | Anti-IFN | 8 |
| | Actinomycin D | 27[b] |
| | Actinomycin D + Anti-IFN | 25[b] |

[a]MCF-containing supernatants were produced by 24-h coculture of monocytes ($5 \times 10^6$) with K562 cells ($5 \times 10^4$) in 1 mL serum-free Iscove's modified Dulbeco's medium supplemented with 0.1% bovine serum albumin. They were then tested for lysis of K562 target cells in a 18-h $^{51}$Cr release assay in the presence of IFN$\alpha$ (human recombinant; 1000 U/mL), actinomycin D (1 $\mu$g/mL), or anti-IFN$\alpha$ antibody.
[b]Value is significantly different from that of "None" by Student's $t$-test ($p < 0.05$).

the binding capacity of target cells was not elevated by IFN. By contrast with actinomycin D, IFN pretreatment of target cells was ineffective in increasing their sensitivity to MCF. Lysis of target cells that had been pretreated with MCF, washed, and cultured in the absence of MCF as not enhanced by the addition of IFN to the assay. Conceivably, IFN may interact directly with a putative lytic molecule of MCF. Addition of IFN to the MCF assay in the presence of actinomycin D resulted in a further increase in levels of cytotoxicity. The presence of increasing doses of IFN alone or actinomycin D alone failed to augment the lytic activity of MCF to the level obtained in the presence of both agents. Anti-IFN$\alpha$ antibodies, but not anti-IFN$\gamma$ antibodies, were shown to inactivate NKCF activity (39). The lytic activity of MCF, however, was not neutralized by anti-IFN$\alpha$ antiserum, indicating that MCF may be distinct from NKCF. The anti-IFN antibodies also did not interfere with the actinomycin D-induced enhancement of target susceptibility to MCF. Collectively, it seems likely that the mechanism responsible for the syngersistic enhancing effect of IFN on MCF differs from that of actinomycin D. It is of note that IFN does not induce MCF-resistant target cells to become sensitive to lysis.

# 4. Biochemical and Biophysical Characteristics of MCF

## 4.1. Temperature Stability of MCF

MCF produced in serum-free conditions were generally stable when they were maintained at low temperatures (4°C for 7 d or −20°C for 2 mo). MCF were also stable at 56 °C for 60 min. In contrast, at higher temperatures the biological activity of MCF was labile. There was a partial loss of the lytic activity at 70 °C for 30 min and a complete loss at 100 °C for 5 min. Conceivably, the MCF may consist of more than one lytic factor with differing temperature stability. Similar temperature stability has been observed with NKCF (32). In contrast, tumor cytotoxic factors from human LPS-activated monocytes that kill adherent target cells in a 72-h assay were shown to be resistant to heating at 70 °C (25).

## 4.2. Sensitivity of MCF to Proteolytic Enzyme

For ascertaining the protein nature of MCF, supernatants containing MCF were generated in serum-free medium, treated with various proteolytic enzymes, and then tested for lysis of K562. The treatment of MCF with trypsin prior to a cytotoxicity assay resulted in a reduction of the lytic effect (Table 2). Also, the biological activity of MCF was inactivated by pretreatment with chymotrypsin. MCF activity was also abrogated by proteinase K. The same preparation of MCF was resistant to inactivation by papain and neuraminidase, however. Thus, the MCF appears to be a protein in nature. Similar patterns of enzyme sensitivity have previously been reported in studies with NKCF (33).

Table 2
Effect of Enzymes on MCF Activity[a]

| Enzyme treatment | Inhibition of MCF activity, % |
|---|---|
| Trypsin, 1 mg/mL | 60[b] |
| Chymotrypsin, 1 mg/mL | 52[b] |
| Papain, 2.5 U/mL | 4 |
| Proteinase K, 200 $\mu$g/mL | 73[b] |
| Neuraminidase | 8 |

[a]MCF produced in serum-free medium were preincubated for 60 min at 37 °C with enzymes shown.
[b]Value is significant ($p < 0.05$).

Recent evidence indicates that treatment of target cells with trypsin elevates the target susceptibility to NKCF (45). This augmentation was seen at the dose of trypsin that alone was not toxic to the target cells. This enzyme-enhancing effect was restricted to trypsin. These authors have postulated that a tryptic protease released by large granular lymphocytes (LGL) is a central and critical element.

## 4.3. Effect of Protease Inhibitors on MCF Activity

It has previously been reported that human monocytes and peritoneal macrophages are able to secrete TNF (18–21). TNF appears to play a major antitumor role in classical long-term cytotoxicity assays of monocyte/ macrophages. The biological activity of TNF has been reported to not be inhibited by protease inhibitors (19). Other antitumor factors produced by LPS-activated monocytes are also insensitive to antiprotease treatment (25). Similarly, no cytostatic protease has been produced by activated human monocytes (24,46). In contrast, cytotoxic factors that are produced spontaneously in short-term (4–5 h) cultures of human monocytes have been found to be sensitive to a series of protease inhibitors (26).

The possible involvement of protease in the lytic activity of MCF was examined by the use of antiproteases. The protease inhibitors tested included chloromethyl ketone derivatives of tosyl amino acids TLCK ($N$-$\alpha$-tosyl-L-lysine chloromethyl ketone) and TPCK (L-1-tosylamide-L-phenylethyl chloromethyl ketone), actinomyces product chymostatin, the serine-protease synthetic substrate TAME ($N$-$\alpha$-p-tosyl-L-arginine methyl ester), the macromolecular protease inhibitors $\alpha$-1-antitrypsin, and soybean trypsin inhibitor (SBTI). Treatment of MCF-containing supernatants with these protease inhibitors had little or no inhibitory effects on the lysis by MCF (Table 3). Thus, protease may not be involved in the biological activity of MCF. NKCF show similar insensitivity to antiprotease treatment (45).

Table 3
Physicochemical Characterization of MCF

| Treatment | Inhibition of MCF activity, % |
|---|---|
| TLCK, 0.1 m$M$ | 16 |
| TPCK, 0.1 m$M$ | 8 |
| Chymostatin, 1 mg/mL | 17 |
| TAME, 1 m$M$ | 0 |
| $\alpha$-1-Antitrypsin, 1 mg/mL | 0 |
| SBTI, 1 mg/mL | 0 |
| Catalase, 4000 U/mL | 0 |
| Superoxide dismutase, 500 U/mL | 0 |
| pH 2 | 90 |
| Arginine 2 mg/mL | 0 |

Other investigators, however, have reported that NKCF activity is inhibitable by a series of protease inhibitors (Bonavida, B., personal communication).

## 4.4. Other Physicochemical Characteristics of MCF

Reactive oxygen intermediates, such as superoxide and hydrogen peroxide, have been implicated in cytotoxicity of macrophages (16). Addition of catalase (which reduces $H_2O_2$ to $O_2$ and $H_2O$) or superoxide dismutase (which converts $O_2^-$ to $H_2O_2$) to MCF-containing medium had no inhibitory effect on MCF (Table 4), however. Thus, MCF-mediated lysis may be independent of reactive oxygen intermediates.

The lytic activity of MCF was destroyed by exposure to pH 2. Similar acid sensitivity has been observed with other monocyte-derived cytotoxic factors (26) and with a cytotoxin produced by phorbol myristate acetate-treated human promyelocytes (47). In contrast, a tumor cytotoxic factor produced by LPS-stimulated monocytes was shown to be resistant to acid pH treatment (25), distinguishing the factor from MCF.

Supplementation of MCF-containing medium with arginine during the lytic assay against K562 failed to prevent the biological action of MCF. Thus the MCF is unlikely to be arginase.

Table 4
Lysis of Autologous Tumor by Cytotoxic Factors Produced by
Blood Monocytes and Tumor-Associated Macrophages[a]

| Source of cytotoxic factors | Cytotoxicity, % |
|---|---|
| Monocytes | 0 |
| Monocytes + autologous tumor | 6 |
| Monocytes + OK432 | 21[b] |
| Tumor-associated macrophages | 18[b] |
| Tumor-associated macrophages + OK432 | 39[b] |

[a]Supernatants were produced by 24-h culture of blood monocytes or tumor-associated macrophages with or without autologous tumor cells or OK 432. They were then tested for lysis of autologous fresh tumor cells in a 18-h $^{51}$Cr release assay in the presence of actinomycin D. Tumor-associated macrophages contained 3% tumor cells.
[b]Value is statistically significant ($p < 0.05$).

# 5. Biological Significance of MCF

## 5.1. Target Cell Specificity of MCF

The MCFs produced by human monocytes are cytolytic to a variety of tumor cell lines, including K562, MOLT-4, U937, L-929, and Wehi-164, when target cells are pretreated with actinomycin D and tested in a 18-h Cr release assay (27–30). The MCF also has the biological effect on freshly isolated human tumor cells. No lytic activity has been seen with NK-resistant target cells, such as Raji, EL-4, YAC-1, and L1210, and with nonmalignant cells, i.e., T-cells, B-cells, T-blasts, and mesothelial cells. A minor proportion of bone marrow cells, however, are sensitive to MCF. Thus, the spectrum of cytotoxicity mediated by MCF appears to be similar to that of NKCF produced by human LGL (29–33). The target cell specificity of MCF seems to be determined mainly by binding of target cell receptors. This evidence is derived from our absorption experiments in which the lytic activity of MCF was removed from supernatants by incubation with MCF-sensitive target cells, but not with MCF-resistant target cells. The possibility that target cells with intrinsic resistance to a putative lytic molecule of MCF exist, however, still remains.

The L-929 cell line is highly sensitive to most cytotoxic or cytostatic factors. In fact, the biological activity of TNF (18–21), monocyte cytotoxin (22), lymphotoxin (40,43), NKCF (33), and leukoregulin (48) has been assayed against L-929. In contrast, the K562 cell line, which is highly sensitive to NK cell-mediated lysis, is killed only by NKCF and MCF (27–30,34,45), although leukoregulin (48) and cultured monocyte-derived cytostatic protein factors (23,24,47) can inhibit the growth of K562. It has recently been reported that recombinant human TNF is cytolytic to U937 cells and that anti-TNF antiserum blocks the lysis of U937 by NKCF (49). Moreover, NKCF-mediated lysis of K562 was shown to be inhibited by anti-TNF antibodies, and TNF was found to lyse K562 (50). My recent experiments have revealed, however, that K562s are resistant to lysis by recombinant human TNF, and that anti-TNF antibodies failed to inhibit lysis of K562 by NKCF (manuscript in preparation). Further biochemical and physiochemical investigations will be required to settle the possible relationship between MCF and TNF.

### 5.2. Biological Role of MCF in Human Neoplasia

An important issue that should be addressed is whether the MCF has biological significance. If MCF plays a role in host defenses against tumor, one would expect that MCF is produced in vivo and lyses autologous tumor cells. I have quite recently reported that MCF-containing media produced by coculture of monocytes with K562 lyse autologous as well as allogenic freshly isolated tumor cells in vitro (51,52). The contact between blood monocytes and K562 cells, however, cannot be expected to occur in vivo in cancer patients. In contrast, interaction of monocyte/macrophages with autologous tumor cells has been observed at the site of tumor growth. In this respect it should be noted that tumor-associated macrophages can be induced to release MCF-like cytotoxic factors during coculture with autologous tumor cells (Table 4; 51). The factor is cytolytic to autologous and allogenic fresh tumor cells as well as tumor cell lines. Although it seems unlikely that circulating MCF-like cytotoxic factors would be effective in controlling a large tumor mass, the locally produced cytotoxic factors might inhibit the growth of small tumors or a few tumor cells in vivo.

In vitro activation of blood monocytes and tumor-associated macrophages with OK432 has been found to produce MCF-like cytotoxic factors with strong lytic activity against autologous fresh tumor cells (51). Systemic and local treatment with OK432 has been reported to be effective in prolongation of survival time in cancer patients, in whom activation of monocyte/macrophages has been observed (53). Conceivably, the OK432-activated, tumor-associated macrophages might produce in vivo MCF-like cytotoxic factors at the site of tumor growth, which could be one mechanism of the antitumor activity of OK432. In vivo treatment with OK432 has recently been reported to induce TNF (37). The possible relationship between MCF-like factors produced by OK432 and TNF is currently unclear. Preliminary experiments have revealed that fresh human tumor cells are relatively resistant to lysis by human TNF.

## 6. Conclusion

The monocyte cytotoxic factor (MCF), a protein monokine, possesses direct cytotoxic activity for a wide variety of tumor cell lines and fresh human tumor cells. MCFs are produced by human blood monocytes during interaction with tumor cells. The production of MCF can be enhanced by OK432 and IFN. Antitumor activity of MCF is augmented by the concurrent presence of IFN. The MCF appears to be distinct from other antitumor cytotoxic factors by the criteria of temperature stability, enzyme sensitivity, antiprotease effects, acid sensitivity, and target cell specificity. The possible relation of MCF to TNF and NKCF still remains. It is of note that tumor-associated macrophages of cancer patients can produce MCF-like cytotoxic factors upon interaction with autologous tumor cells, and that the factor is cytolytic to autologous as well as allogenic fresh tumor cells. Although the mechanism by which MCF kill tumor cells is not understood, the factor might have a biological role in human neoplasia.

## References

1. Herberman, R. B., ed. *NK Cells and Other Natural Effector Cells* Academic, New York (1982).
2. Hoshino, T., Koren, H. S., and Uchida, A., ed. *Natural Killer Activity and Its Regulation* Excerpta Medica, Amsterdam (1984).
3. Hibbs, J. B., Jr., Chapman, H. A., Jr., and Weinberg, J. B. *J. Reticuloentothel. Soc.* **24**, 549–570 (1978).

4. Adams, D. O. and Snyderman, R. D. *J. Natl. Cancer Inst.* **62**, 1341–1348 (1979).
5. Kay, H. D. and Horowitz, D. A. *J. Clin. Invest.* **66**, 847–857 (1980).
6. Burns, G. F., Triglica, T., Bartlett, P. F., and Mackay, I. R. *Proc. Natl. Acad. Sci. USA* **80**, 7606–7610 (1983).
7. Fischer, D. G., Hubbard, W. J., and Koren, H. S. *Cell. Immunol.* **58**, 426–435 (1981).
8. Fischer, D. G., Golightly, M. G., and Koren, H. S. *J. Immunol.* **130**, 1220–1225 (1983).
9. Uchida, A., Yanagawa, E., and Micksche, M., in *Clinical and Experimental Studies in Immunotherapy* (Hoshino, T. and Uchida, A., eds.) Excerpta Medica, Amsterdam (1984).
10. Yanagawa, E., Uchida, A., Kokoschka, E. M., and Micksche, M. *Cancer Immunol. Immunother.* **16**, 131–136 (1984).
11. Yanagawa, E., Uchida, A., Moore, M., and Micksche, M. *Cancer Immunol. Immunother.* **19**, 163–167 (1985).
12. Hibbs, J. B. Jr. *Science* **184**, 468–471 (1974).
13. Adams, D. O., Kao, K.-J., Farb, R., and Pizzo, S. V. *J. Immunol.* **124**, 293–300 (1980).
14. Reidarson, T. H., Granger, G. A., and Klostergaard, J. *J. Natl. Cancer Inst.* **69**, 889–894 (1982).
15. Currie, G. A. *Nature* **273**, 758–759 (1978).
16. Nathan, C. F., Silverstein, S. C., Brukner, L. H., and Cohn, Z. A. *J. Exp. Med.* **149**, 100–113 (1979).
17. Fergula, J., Schorlemmer, H. U., Baptista, L. C., and Allison, A. C. *Clin. Exp. Immunol.* **31**, 512–517 (1978).
18. Carswell et al. *Proc. Natl. Acad. Sci. USA* **72**, 3666–3670 (1975).
19. Ruff, M. R. and Gifford, G. E. in *Lymphokines* vol. 2 (Pick, E., ed.) Academic, New York (1981).
20. Matthews, N. *Br. J. Cancer* **38**, 310–317 (1978).
21. Mannel, D. N., Moore, R. N., and Mergenhagen, S. E. *Infect. Immunol.* **30**, 523–530 (1980).
22. Matthews, N. *Immunology* **44**, 135–142 (1981).
23. Eggen, B. M., Bakke, O., and Hammerstrom, J. *Scand. J. Immunol.* **18**, 13–20 (1983).
24. Kindahl-Andersen, O. and Nissen-Meyer, J. *Cell. Immunol.* **89**, 365–375 (1984).
25. Sone, S., Lopez-Berenstein, G., and Fidler, I. J. *J. Natl. Cancer Inst.* **74**, 583–590 (1985).
26. Bersani, L., Colotta, F., Chezzi, P., and Mantovani, A. *Immunol. Lett.*, in press.
27. Uchida, A. and Yanagawa, E. *Immunol. Lett.* **8**, 311–316 (1984).
28. Uchida, A. and Klein, E. *Immunol. Lett.* **10**, 177–181 (1985).
29. Uchida, A. and Klein, E. *Int. J. Cancer* **35**, 691–699 (1985).
30. Uchida, A., Vanky, F., and Klein, E. *J. Natl. Cancer Inst.* **79**, 849–857 (1985).

31. Wright, S. C., Weitzen, M. L., Kehle, P., Grander, G. A., and Bonavida, B. *J. Immunol.* **130**, 2479-2483 (1983).
32. Farram, E. and Targan, S. R. *J. Immunol.* **130**, 1252-1256 (1983).
33. Hiserodt, J. C., Britvan, L., and Targan, S. R. *J. Immunol.* **131**, 2705-2709 (1983).
34. Blanca, I. R., Ortaldo, J. R., and Herberman, R. B., in *Natural Killer Activity and Its Regulation* (Hoshino, T., Koren, H. S., and Uchida, A., eds.) Excerpta Medica, Amsterdam (1984).
35. Weinberg, J. B. and Haney, A. F. *J. Natl. Cancer Inst.* **70**, 1005-1100 (1083).
36. Wright, S. C. and Bonavida, B. *J. Immunol.* **130**, 2960-2964 (1983).
37. Ishida, N., Hoshino, T., and Uchida, A., ed., *A Streptococcal Preparation OK432 as a Biological Response Modifier* Excerpta Medica, Tokyo (1983).
38. Wright, S. C. and Bonavida, B. *J. Immunol.* **130**, 2965-2968 (1984).
39. Steinhauser, E. H., Doyle, A. T., and Kadish, A. S. *J. Immunol.* **135**, 294-299 (1985).
40. Svedersky, L. P., Nedwin, G. E., Goeddel, D. V., and Palladino, M. A. *J. Immunol.* **134**, 1604-1608 (1985).
41. Reed, W. P. and Lucas, Z. L. *J. Immunol.* **115**, 395-404 (1975).
42. Schlager, S. I. and Ohanian, S. H. *J. Immunol.* **124**, 626-634 (1980).
43. Williams, T. W. and Bellanti, J. A. *J. Immunol.* **130**, 518-520 (1983).
44. Stone-Wolff, D. S. et al. *J. Exp. Med.* **159**, 828-843 (1984).
45. Ortaldo, J. R., Blanca, I., and Herberman, R. B. in *Mechanisms of Cell-Mediated Cytotoxicity* vol. II (Henkart, P. and Marz, E., eds.) Plenum, New York (1985).
46. Nissen-Meyer, J. and Kildahl-Andersen, O. *Scand. J. Immunol.* **20**, 317-325 (1984).
47. Gifford, G. E., Flick, D. A., AbdAllah, N. A., and Fish, H. *J. Natl. Cancer. Inst.* **73**, 69-73 (1984).
48. Ransom, J. H. et al. *Cancer Res.* **45**, 851-862 (1985).
49. Degliantoni, G. et al. *J. Exp. med.* **162**, 1512-1530 (1985).
50. Svedersky, L. P. et al. *Fed. Proc.* **44**, 589 (1985).
51. Uchida, A. in *Proc. 14th International Chemotherapy Congress* (in press).
52. Uchida, A. *Biochemica et Biophysica Acta* (in press).
53. Hoshino, T. and Uchida, A., eds., *Clinical and Experimental Studies in Immunotherapy* Excerpta Medica, Amsterdam (1984).

# Antiproliferative Effects of Interferon

## PAUL AEBERSOLD

## 1. Introduction

Interferon (IFN) was originally described as a product of virus-infected cells that conveyed virus-resistance to other cells (*1*). It was subsequently noted that IFN also inhibited the growth of cultured cells (*2*). IFNs produced by different methods were found to have distinct biological, biochemical, or antigenic properties: virus-induced, acid-stable IFN from leukocytes was termed IFNα; virus-induced, acid-stable IFN from fibroblasts was termed IFNβ; and mitogen-induced, acid-labile IFN from T-cells was termed IFNγ (*3*).

Because of its antiproliferative effects on cultured tumor cells, IFN has been developed commercially for treatment of human malignancies. IFNα, IFNβ, and particularly IFNγ, however, modulate a number of immune responses that may influence tumor growth. Such in vivo effects have been termed indirect to distinguish them from the direct effects of IFN on cells in culture. IFN modulation of immune responses has been reviewed elsewhere (*4,5*).

This chapter will discuss the structure of IFN, its interaction with cellular receptors, and the biochemical events so triggered that inhibit cellular growth. It will be noted that the biological effects of IFN are not a simple consequence of receptor binding, and that their nature may be determined by the affected cells. Finally, this chapter will consider animal tumor models in which direct versus indirect effects of IFN have been compared.

# 2. Structure of Interferon

## 2.1. Gene Structure

DNA sequences coding for IFNα, IFNβ, and IFNγ have been cloned (6–8). The primary structures of IFNα, IFNβ, and IFNγ have been deduced from the recombinant gene sequences (9). IFNα is actually the product of a family of 16–20 closely related genes (10) that do not contain introns (11). The genes are located on chromosome 9 (12), and two that have been characterized are flanked by sequences that are highly repetitive in the human genome (13). That humans and other species have multiple IFNα genes may or may not be biologically significant. Biological significance could result from the genes being induced differently or the gene products having different biological activities.

IFNβ appears to be the product of a single gene (10) that is homologous to IFNα (14) and likewise contains no introns. IFNα and IFNβ also have homologous 5'-flanking regions.

IFNγ and its 5'-flanking region are structurally distinct from IFNα and IFNβ and their 5'-flanking regions. IFNγ appears to be the product of a single gene that contains three introns. The first intron contains a repetitive DNA sequence (15).

## 2.2. Protein Structure

IFNα proteins contain 165 (IFNαA) or 166 amino acids, including four cysteines involved in disulfide bonds (16). The IFNα family has two subgroups based on amino acid groupings (17) and on monoclonal antibody specificity (18). Native IFNα species are generally not glycosylated, but two of the IFNα family contain N-glycosylation signal sequences, and some species of IFNα from natural sources are glycosylated (19).

IFNβ as a mature protein contains 166 amino acids, but only three cysteines. The cysteine not involved in a disulfide bond, at position 17, can be changed without altering the biological activity (20). IFNβ is naturally glycosylated, but the recombinant protein without glycosylation retains a high specific activity. Natural IFNβ is more hydrophobic than IFNα (21), and recombinant IFNβ is hydrophobic to the point of being insoluble in physiological saline.

Tertiary structure for IFNα (and thus IFNβ by homology and biological activity) has been modeled by computer (22). The proposed structure contains four roughly parallel regions of α-helix. A histidine residue appears to be critical for activity of IFNβ (23); so it is possible (24) that the active site is in the vicinity of amino acids 106–143, which are in close proximity to the antiparallel stretch of amino acids 27–57. The regions of greatest conservation between IFNα and IFNβ are amino acids 37–48 and 105–119. An active site in this region, opposite the dispensable cysteine at position 17 and glycosylation at position 80, would account for the lack of biologically active IFN fragments (25)—two noncontiguous amino acid sequences combine to form the active site.

IFNγ protein contains 143 amino acids in its native state, but 146 amino acids in the recombinant form produced in *Escherichia coli*. Native IFNγ lacks the first three amino acids, Cys-Tyr-Cys, whose cysteines are the only ones in the sequence (25). There are two N-glycosylation signal sequences, and molecular weight heterogeneity is caused by glycosylation at only one or both of the sites (26).

There are indications that IFNβ and IFNγ may in their native states form dimers and tetramers, respectively (27). IFNα apparently is monomeric. These observations based on radiation inactivation are in accord with observations of molecular weight on sizing columns (28).

## 3. Interferon Receptors

### 3.1. Types and Affinities of Receptors

IFN can induce antiviral protection in cells by binding to the cell surface—IFN bound to sepharose beads is active, but not internalized (29). Conversely, microinjected IFNβ does not induce an antiviral state in HeLa cells (30). Binding of $^{125}$I-labeled IFNαA to Daudi cells indicates the existence of 5000 high-affinity receptors per cell. The biochemistry of interferon receptors has been reviewed elsewhere (31). Competition for binding between various IFN species and iodinated IFNαA suggests that IFNα and IFNβ bind to a common receptor, to which IFNγ does not bind (32). IFNβ may also bind to the IFNγ receptors (33). Competition for binding among IFNα subspecies suggests that the specific antiviral activity of any particular IFNα correlates with its binding affinity (34). Further, the degree of receptor saturation correlates with growth inhibition of L1210 cells by murine IFNα and IFNβ and human IFNα1, even though the specific activity of human IFNα1 on mouse cells is orders of magnitude lower than the specific activity of murine IFN on mouse cells. In these systems, the biological responses are triggered by the same degree of receptor saturation regardless of the affinity of the particular IFN for the receptor.

IFNα bound to receptors is internalized by endocytosis (35). At 4 °C, binding of IFNα to cells is slow, but unaffected by metabolic events. Binding of IFNα2 to bovine cells at this temperature follows simple kinetics expected for single species of ligand and high-affinity receptor. Binding to human cells, however, follows complex kinetics suggestive of cooperative interaction among receptors (*36*). IFNα2 activates an antiviral state in bovine cells, but has no adverse effect on their growth (*37*), indicating either that the biological effects of IFN are determined by the target cells or that some biological effects are triggered by IFN subsequent to receptor binding.

At 37°C, binding of IFNα to its receptors on Daudi cells follows a complex time course. Further, the initial binding affinity appears less than the steady-state binding affinity. Analysis of the kinetics of binding suggests that IFNα first binds to receptors and subsequently transfers to an activation complex on the cell membrane (*38*). Alternatively, however, internalization of IFNα might account for the apparent increase in steady-state binding. Whichever the case, the amount of IFNα bound at steady state in this system correlates with the rate at which growth is inhibited (*38*). With an IFN-resistant Daudi line, the number of binding sites is reduced, and the high-affinity interaction is lost (*39*). Another study of IFNα binding to IFN-resistant cells also demonstrated fewer binding sites than on the parental IFN-sensitive cells. The binding sites were functional because an antiviral state could be induced in the IFN-resistant cells (*40*).

Human IFNγ is internalized and degraded by fibroblasts (*41*). Binding of $^{125}$I-labeled IFNγ to Daudi and HeLa cells indicates the presence of 13,000 and 5000 high-affinity receptors per cell, respectively, with dissociation constants in the range of $5 \times 10^{-10}M$. Analysis of the kinetics of binding shows the receptors to be of a single class (*42*). Neither IFNα nor IFNβ could displace binding of labeled IFNγ. Further, IFNγ did not induce 2',5'-oligoadenylate synthetase in Daudi cells, but did in HeLa cells.

Binding of $^{125}$I-labeled recombinant IFNγ produced in mammalian cells to human monocytes differs from binding to nonhematopoietic cells (*43*). Acid-inactivated IFNγ competes for binding to WISH cells, but not to monocytes, which suggests that receptors on monocytes are different from those on nonhematopoietic cells. Biological effects of IFNγ on monocytes also differ from those on nonhematopoietic cells in that IFNγ does not induce an antiviral state in monocytes. Kinetics of binding to the monocytes suggests negative cooperation among receptors or multiple species of receptors; another binding study with recombinant IFNγ produced in bacteria, however, showed a single class of high-affinity receptors on monocytes (*44*). Since IFNγ produced in mammalian cells is glycosylated, perhaps glycosylation affects binding to some extent. This second study also demonstrated the presence of intracellular receptors by permeabilizing cells with digitonin, and showed that activation of tumoricidal activity takes at least 4 h exposure to IFNγ.

## 3.2. Receptor Interactions with the Cytoskeleton

Various lines of evidence point to cytoskeletal involvement in cellular responses to IFN. First, the binding of [125]I-labeled IFNα2 to human primary breast carcinoma BT20 cells at 4 °C is altered by the addition of colchicine, indicating that interaction of IFN receptors with the tubulin network affects their binding affinity (36). Second, the shape of dose–response curves vary according to the density of primate receptors on the surface of mouse–monkey hybrid cells, suggesting that cooperation among primate receptors is hindered by the presence of more abundant murine receptors (45). Third, IFN inhibits cap formation by lectins whose capping is enhanced by colchicine, but not by those whose capping is unaffected by colchicine (46), and conversely lectins inhibit the antiviral effects of IFN (47). Fourth, colchicine and other cytoskeleton-disrupting drugs inhibit IFN activity (48). And fifth, restoration of the cytoskeleton in transformed cells with sodium butyrate leads to increased sensitivity to IFN (49).

IFN receptors on fibroblasts are located between microvilli (50). Diphtheria toxin receptors, on the other hand, are located primarily on microvilli. Treatment of fibroblasts with IFNβ for only 15 min diminished the number of diphtheria toxin receptors and altered their distribution. Whether IFN receptors change their distribution upon binding to IFN was not reported in that study, so evidence for aggregation of IFN receptors remains largely circumstantial. With epidermal growth factor, clustering of receptors has been shown to be necessary for complete triggering of biological responses (51).

# 4. Mechanisms of Action

## 4.1. Intracellular Messengers

Upon binding to cellular receptors, IFN activates a number of genes involved in the establishment of antiviral or antiproliferative states. The method of signal transmission from cell surface to nucleus is, however, not certain. There is interesting evidence that suggests that internalized IFNγ activates macrophages. Specifically, mouse or human IFNγ encapsulated in liposomes with muramyl dipeptide activates both mouse and human macrophages, even though free IFNγ with muramyl dipeptide is species specific (52). Pronase treatment of the macrophages abolishes their response to free IFNγ, but not to encapsulated IFNγ, so apparently internalized IFNγ or its degradation fragments are able to activate macrophages.

IFN treatment of cells does result in altered intracellular concentrations of cyclic AMP and cyclic GMP, but the alterations do not appear to correlate with the establishment of biological effects (*53,54*). In particular, cyclic AMP inhibits growth in some cells, but stimulates growth in others, and cyclic GMP does not increase when calcium is limited, but the biological effects of IFN are nevertheless induced. Treatment of cells with IFN leads to changes in membrane potential and ion fluxes (*55*), but it is uncertain whether they are causes or effects of IFN action. It has been reported that IFN–receptor complexes from Daudi cells exhibit intrinsic protein kinase activity (*56*), so perhaps the IFN receptor functions in a fashion analogous to a number of other hormone receptors.

## 4.2. Alterations in Gene Expression

IFN induces synthesis of proteins not found in untreated cells. All IFNs induce a common set of proteins, and IFNγ enhances synthesis of an additional set not affected by IFNα or IFNβ (*57*). Of the common set of induced proteins, the two best characterized are activated by double-stranded RNA to inhibit protein synthesis (*58*). One, 2′,5′-oligoadenylate synthetase, produces linked adenylate residues (*59*) that activate an endonuclease (*60*) to degrade mRNA. The other, a protein phosphokinase (*61*), inactivates protein synthesis initiation factor 2 (*62*). These induced proteins would not be expected to inhibit cellular growth under normal circumstances since they require double-stranded RNA for activation. In fact, both proteins are induced by IFN in a cell line whose growth is not inhibited by IFN (*63*). Since 12 new proteins are induced by all IFNs, however, some of them may not need activation by viral signals and may therefore be involved with growth regulation. The significance of 12 additional proteins induced by IFNγ in fibroblasts is not clear—in cells of the immune system, it would be expected that proteins uniquely induced by IFNγ would lead to immune regulation unaffected by IFNα or IFNβ.

The activities of some enzymes involved in cell proliferation are altered by IFN treatment. Induction of ornithine decarboxylase activity is inhibited by IFN, but its role in polyamine synthesis is not likely to inhibit DNA synthesis since polyamines are not limiting for short-term DNA synthesis (*64*). Interestingly, IFN may affect the synthesis of ornithine decarboxylase by inhibiting both transcription and translation of its mRNA.

Prostaglandins may mediate some IFN effects, since they are increased by IFN treatment of cells (*65*). When an essential enzyme in the prostaglandin synthesis pathway, fatty acid cyclooxygenase, is inhibited, IFN is unable to induce an antiviral state (*66*). In cells selected for resistance to IFN, fatty acid cyclooxygenase was found lacking entirely (67). The role of the enzyme in mediating IFN effects is uncertain, however, because when the enzyme is inhibited, prostaglandins are not able to overcome its inhibition.

Since growth is enhanced by a number of protooncogenes, growth inhibition by IFN could involve modulation of protooncogene expression. Daudi cells, which have reciprocal chromosomal translocations that involve c-*myc* (68), are extremely sensitive to IFN$\alpha$ and IFN$\beta$. When Daudi cells are treated with IFN$\beta$, the c-*myc* concentration decreases rapidly (69), such that the effect cannot be explained by a slower accumulation of cells in $G_0$. In cells less sensitive to IFN, c-*myc* concentration appears unaffected by IFN treatment. Further, a line of IFN-resistant Daudi cells, which responds to IFN with synthesis of 2',5'-oligoadenylate synthetase, but whose cell cycle distribution is not altered, has lost the IFN-mediated downregulation of c-*myc* (70). Another system in which c-*myc* transcription has been studied is the $G_0$ to S transition of Balb/C 3T3 cells. IFN inhibits the increase of c-*myc* stimulated by platelet-derived growth factor in those cells (71). Part of the inhibition is dependent on synthesis of new proteins, so IFN-induced proteins apparently down-regulate c-*myc* transcription. However interesting the connection between c-*myc*, IFN, and growth inhibition, down-regulation of c-*myc* may not be sufficient for growth inhibition. When Swiss 3T3 cells are stimulated to grow with up to three factors, the response can be inhibited by IFN; but when five factors are used, IFN no longer inhibits growth (72). If c-*myc* concentration is down-regulated in both cases, then other factors are capable of growth stimulation in its absence.

Mouse 3T3 cells transfected with human c-Ha-*ras*1 gene activated by an upstream promoter acquire a transformed phenotype, growing past confluence in vitro. Murine IFN$\beta$ induced phenotypic reversion to contact inhibition in a clonal line of such transformed cells. The c-Ha-*ras*1 DNA was still present in the cells, but corresponding mRNA and protein were significantly reduced (73). When the revertant cells were grown in the absence of IFN$\beta$, however, they retained their normal phenotype, but c-Ha-*ras*1 gene products increased. Incidentally, IFN$\beta$ could not induce phenotypic reversion in a clonal line transformed with the mutated EJ/T24 *ras* gene from bladder carcinoma cells (74). Effects of IFN on these and other oncogene expression have been reviewed elsewhere (75).

## 4.3. Cell Cycle Progression

Manifestations of growth inhibition by IFN vary somewhat according to the particular cells. Melanoma cells (76), 3T3 fibroblasts (77), and

$P_3HR$-1 lymphoblasts (78) accumulate in $G_0$ when treated with IFN. Fibroblasts and breast epithelial cells show prolongation of all phases of the cell cycle during IFN treatment (79). Various other cells are affected by prolongation of $G_1$, S, $G_2$, or mitosis (80).

In general, IFN exhibits cytostatic rather than cytotoxic effects on cells. With long treatment times, however, some tumor cells are lysed (81). Fibroblasts, on the other hand, survive quite well during prolonged treatment, probably because they have not lost growth-regulatory mechanisms. The basis for cytotoxicity on some tumor cells is not certain, but may be related to a loss of coordination between DNA synthesis and other events necessary for cell division. Specifically, Daudi cells synthesize DNA at about the same rate whether treated with IFN or not, yet the doubling time is prolonged by IFN treatment (82). Measurements of DNA synthesis must take into account that IFN inhibits thymidine kinase activity (83).

# 5. In Vitro Antiproliferative Effects

## 5.1. Assays for Interferon Activity

IFNs are quantitated by antiviral activity. The cytopathic effect of virus infection of cultured cells can be seen visually through a microscope or measured by viable dye uptake after overnight incubation (84). With availability of monoclonal antibodies to specific IFN classes, more rapid (4 h) radioimmunoassays can be used. To detect low levels of IFN, reduction of virus yield can be quantitated by plaque assays or immunoassays, since virus yield is reduced at IFN levels that do not protect cells from destruction.

Antiproliferative assays require about 3 d. Titers are defined as reciprocals of IFN dilutions at which treated cultures have 50% as many viable cells (85) or incorporate 50% as much $^3$H-thymidine as control cultures. Clearly, the antiproliferative titer of an IFN preparation depends on the test cells—Daudi cells, for example, are sensitive to IFN$\alpha$ and IFN$\beta$, but rather insensitive to IFN$\gamma$ (86), whereas the reverse is true on a number of other cells (87). For antiproliferative assays of IFN$\alpha$ or IFN$\beta$ using Daudi cells, a more convenient endpoint for growth inhibition is change in color of the medium (88).

A different type of antiproliferative assay measures tumor stem cell colony formation in soft agar (89). This assay has been used to rate the efficacy of different IFNs on a variety of tumors (90), of which less than half were significantly inhibited.

## 5.2. Cells Inhibited by Interferon

Although IFNs inhibit growth of a variety of cells, whether or not a particular cell type will be sensitive to any IFN class is impossible to predict. In general, tumor cell growth is inhibited more by IFN than normal cell growth; but some tumor cells are resistant to IFN (91), whereas some normal cells are sensitive (92). IFN resistance is apparently induced by exposure of tumor cells to IFN—Luria-Delbruck fluctuation analysis of the acquisition of IFN resistance indicates it is not a randomly acquired trait. In the same study, normal fibroblasts did not acquire IFN resistance (93). The resistant tumor cell clones reverted to IFN sensitivity in the absence of IFN.

Whether growth of particular cells is inhibited by IFN appears to depend on how various cells respond to the same signal. Bovine MDBK cells, which are activated to an antiviral state by human IFNα species, are not growth-inhibited by those same species, whereas Daudi cells are growth-inhibited by IFNα. Clearly, then, binding of IFN to cellular receptors cannot account for observed differences in biological responses.

## 5.3. Differentiation Affected by Interferon

IFN affects some pathways of cellular differentiation, and to some extent its antitumor activity may be caused by differentiation of tumor cells. When mouse fibroblasts are transformed by murine sarcoma virus, they acquire a capability to grow in soft agar. If these transformed cells are subsequently cultured for a number of passages in low concentrations of IFN, they lose their spindle shape, recover contact inhibition in monolayer growth, and no longer grow in soft agar (94). Their growth in monolayers is not inhibited by IFN, so their inability to grow in soft agar apparently is caused by an IFN-induced alteration in phenotype, perhaps cytoskeletal changes.

IFN exerts either inhibitory or inductive effects on differentiation pathways such as myogenesis, melanogenesis, granulopoiesis and macrophage, erythroid, and adipocyte differentiation (95). With Friend erythroleukemia cells, low levels of IFN enhance differentiation induced by dimethylsulfoxide, whereas high levels inhibit. When cells were selected for the ability to grow in IFN, they were found to be resistant to the enhancing effect of low levels of IFN on induced differentiation, but not to the inhibitory effect of high levels (96). The resistant cells were not activated to an antiviral state even by high levels of IFN, which suggests that this particular mechanism for inhibition of induced differentiation is not similar to mechanisms for antiviral and antiproliferative activities.

IFN and inducers of differentiation are synergistic in inhibiting growth and inducing differentiation of some tumor cells (97,98). Such synergisms are, of course, of potential clinical relevance.

### 5.4. Interferon Synergisms

Since IFNγ differs from IFNα and IFNβ in receptor binding and induction of specific proteins, its antiproliferative mechanism may also differ. Antiproliferative effects of IFNs on HT-294T melanoma cells have been evaluated singly and in combination, and potentiation occurred with combinations of IFNγ and either IFNα or IFNβ. Combinations of IFNα and IFNβ did not potentiate antiproliferative activity (99). These observations suggest that the mechanisms do in fact differ, and the consequent synergy may be of utility in antiviral or antitumor therapy.

## 6. Structure–Function Relationships

Since members of the IFNα family differ in specific activity, hybrid molecules have been constructed and evaluated for resulting specific activity. Neither the $NH_2$-proximal nor the COOH-proximal half of the IFNα molecule was found to determine the specific activity. Based on ratios of activities of IFNα species and hybrids thereof on various cell types, a two-idiotype interaction of IFNα with its receptor was proposed (100). As discussed earlier, the active site may consist of portions of the two halves of the IFNα molecule in close proximity in the tertiary structure.

Further study of IFNα species and IFNα/α hybrids revealed that the ratio of antiviral to antiproliferative activity varied among the molecular species. Thus it was speculated that individual IFNs can activate different biological responses to different degrees, perhaps via different IFNα receptors (101). Antiviral and antiproliferative activities were assessed on different cells, however, so any comparison of activities must be made with caution (102). Varying ratios of biological responses could be caused by differences in cellular responses. Speculation that molecular domains could be independently responsible for specific properties of IFN encouraged construction of numerous IFN analogs—one particular hybrid of IFNα and IFNβ was claimed to exhibit antiproliferative activity without any antiviral activity whatsoever (9,103). That hybrid, however, appears to have neither antiviral nor antiproliferative activity (104).

In another study, IFNαB, C, and F showed greater antiproliferative activity than IFNαA, D, and hybrids AD and DA, whereas the rankings reversed for antiviral protection (105). These comparisons were made on the same cells. The IFNαB, C, and F preparations were only about 0.1% pure, however, whereas the IFNαA, D, and hybrids were electrophoretically homogeneous, i.e., greater than 95% pure. Whether extracts of bacterial cells containing plasmids lacking IFN gene sequences had any effect on biological activity of pure preparations was not reported. Since purified IFNαA, D, and hybrids have quite different specific activities and yet appeared to have the same antiviral-to-antiproliferative ratios of activities, it would seem premature to compare ratios of activities of impure preparations with those of pure ones. IFNαC is actually considered in the same IFNα subgroup as IFNαA and IFNαD. Further, purified IFNαA, D, and hybrids had the same ranking of antiviral activity on K562 cells for either herpes simplex virus type 2 or encephalomyocarditis virus, yet in an earlier study the ranking of impure preparations of these IFNs on Vero cells was different for herpes simplex virus type 1 or vesicular stomatitis virus (*106*).

Another report in accord with speculation that the IFN receptor is a complex site that contains several independent triggers is one that shows IFNαJ unable to boost natural killer cell activity (*107*). Unfortunately no appropriate virus infection of large granular lymphocytes has been found to evaluate the antiviral activity of IFNαJ on these cells (*108*). IFNαJ inhibits boosting of natural killer cell activity by other IFNα species, so it would appear that IFNαJ binds to the receptors on these cells without activating a biological response. Thus IFNαJ could act as a competitive antagonist. Unless IFNαJ can be demonstrated to activate some biological responses in natural killer cells without boosting their lytic activities, the only conclusion is that large granular lymphocytes do not respond to IFNαJ. This conclusion does not necessarily suggest that one domain of IFNα activates antiviral responses whereas another boosts natural killer cell activity. It could equally suggest that the receptor on these cells is different from receptors on cells activated to an antiviral state by IFNαJ.

As mentioned earlier, acid-treated IFNγ competed for binding on WISH cells with [125]I-labeled IFNγ, even though 95% of its antiviral activity was destroyed (*43*). Further, the acid-treated IFNγ induced HLA-DR expression on WISH cells as effectively as untreated IFNγ. This suggests that acid-treated IFNγ binds as a competitive antagonist for inducing antiviral effects, but that some other postbinding mechanism is responsible for induction of HLA-DR expression.

Monoclonal antibodies to murine IFNγ have indicated possible separation of function according to molecular domain. Two antibodies inhibited antiviral activity and macrophage activation, whereas a different two antibodies also blocked antiviral activity, but enhanced macrophage activation (*109*). That study recognized the need to, but did not, assess antiviral activation in macrophages so that the same cells could be used to measure both activities. The antibodies that enhanced IFNγ activation of macrophages also enhanced binding, suggesting that perhaps interaction of antibodies with Fc receptors is involved.

There is evidence to suggest that degree of receptor occupancy correlates with biological response (44), regardless of the specific activity of the IFN in question (34). Correlation between receptor occupancy and biological response, however, does not imply a single activation mechanism —there could be activation following the binding of IFN to its receptors, activation caused by receptor aggregation, or activation by internalized IFN. Thus initial binding could activate an antiviral state (which cannot be reversed by removal of IFN), whereas subsequent events could activate growth inhibitory mechanisms (which can be reversed by removal of IFN) (110). It is entirely conceivable that one domain of IFN initiates certain responses by binding to receptors and that another domain activates different biological responses subsequent to that binding. If so, the different domains could independently activate different biological responses. At this time there is tempting evidence for postulating such a mechanism, but insufficient evidence for defining what it might be.

## 7. In Vivo Tumor Biology

### 7.1. Antibodies to Interferon

A number of animal tumor models have been used to investigate the role of IFN in tumor/host relationships. The effect of endogenous IFN on tumor establishment or growth has been demonstrated by administration of neutralizing antibodies to IFN. Such treatment of nude mice led to more invasive and metastatic growth of human tumors (111), which are themselves quite insensitive to direct effects of mouse IFN. Those observations suggest an indirect effect of IFN in restricting tumor growth, perhaps on natural killer cells, since nude mice are deficient in T-cell immunity. A subsequent report on the transplantability of murine tumors in normal mice again showed that anti-IFN antibodies enhanced tumor growth. The antibodies even enhanced the growth of tumors whose cells are resistant to direct in vitro effects of IFN, again suggesting the importance of indirect mechanisms (112).

### 7.2. Interferon-Resistant Tumors

The effect of exogenous IFN in mediating tumor rejection is of clinical interest. Several animal studies have used IFN-sensitive and IFN-resistant lines of the same tumor cells. Growth of Friend leukemia cells in peritoneal cavities of mice was inhibited by IFN treatment whether the cells were sensitive or resistant (*113*). Growth of IFN-sensitive and IFN-resistant L1210 cells in peritoneal cavities was similarly inhibited (*114*). More recently, a similar study was done with lines of murine meth A fibrosarcoma cells, with the same result. This later study also assessed growth of these lines in cell-impermeable diffusion chambers placed in peritoneal cavities. Growth of IFN-sensitive, but not of IFN-resistant, cells was suppressed by IFN, indicating that direct effects play some role. The IFN-treated mice had enhanced numbers of macrophages in their peritoneal cavities, however, and these were highly suppressive of in vitro growth of the IFN-resistant cells (*115*). All of these studies emphasize the importance of indirect effects of IFN on tumor growth.

### 7.3. Xenografts in Nude Mice

Human tumors grown in nude mice provide another system for comparing direct versus indirect effects of IFN. Human IFN does not activate murine natural killer cells or induce $2',5'$-oligoadenylate synthetase in murine spleen cells, yet it strongly inhibits growth of, while stimulating $2',5'$-oligoadenylate synthetase in, human tumors in nude mice (*37,116*). These observations suggest that direct effects of IFN can have in vivo benefit. With murine tumors and murine IFN, however, the therapeutic effect was much less in Balb/C nu/nu mice than in Balb/C wild type mice (*117*). This latter observation suggests that T-cell immunity is the predominant antitumor mechanism triggered by IFN.

### 7.4. Direct vs. Indirect Effects

It has been known for some time that repeated administration of IFN has antitumor effects in animal models (*118,119*). These effects were hypothesized to be caused by direct cytotoxicity on the tumor cells or by indirect activation of macrophages or alteration of tumor cell surfaces. As discussed in the preceding paragraphs, there is much evidence to suggest that IFN restricts tumor growth by indirect modulation of immune functions. There is also evidence that IFN can have direct antiproliferative effects on tumors, but these effects are not found to predominate.

What IFN does to enhance immunity against tumors is not fully understood. Enhancement of natural killer activity has been considered a probable mechanism, yet a recent study showed that depletion of natural killer cells in vivo did not lessen efficacy of IFN against Moloney sarcoma virus-transformed cells in mice (*120*). That study also showed, however, that activation of natural killer cells by IFN can play some role in tumor rejection. Macrophages activated by IFN may abrogate tumor growth to some extent, as mentioned above. Tumor-specific cytotoxic cells also appear to be involved in IFN-mediated tumor rejection, since mice whose tumor growth was completely suppressed by IFN were refractory to that tumor but not others (*117*). There have been indications from in vitro studies that IFN inhibits the generation of suppressor cells (*121*), but the IFN effect on suppressor cells in vitro depends on experimental conditions (*122*) and needs to be studied in an animal tumor model. It is reasonable to suggest that IFN activates a number of indirect mechanisms that work in concert to inhibit tumor growth.

## 8. Conclusion

Both native and recombinant IFNs are undergoing clinical trials for treatment of human malignancies. So far, IFNs have been found to compare favorably with single chemotherapeutic agents for certain malignancies (*123*). Since it is difficult in clinical trials to evaluate relative contributions of direct versus indirect effects, the bases for clinical tumor regressions are uncertain. Even though animal studies have demonstrated that indirect effects play a substantial role in tumor regression, the relationship of animal host to transplantable tumor may be substantially different from that of cancer patient to spontaneous neoplasm. If particular IFNs are found to be effective against specific tumor types, perhaps the responsible mechanisms will become more apparent.

Recombinant IFNs in clinical trials are of necessity purified to homogeneity. Recombinant IFN$\beta$ and IFn$\gamma$ are not glycosylated, so they might differ from the native molecules in pharmacokinetics or antigenicity. One recombinant IFN$\beta$ in clinical trials has an amino acid substitution, but there have been no reports of clinical evaluation of other modified IFNs. Since IFN hybrids or other analogs elicit the same biological responses as naturally occurring IFNs, clinical use of such analogs might only increase the production of anti-IFN antibodies. Thus a cautious approach should be taken toward clinical use of modified IFNs.

There are still many unanswered questions about the IFN system and its role in tumor biology. Early observations of antiproliferative effects of IFN may have stimulated interest in its therapeutic potential against cancer, but indirect effects of IFN on the immune system may prove to be its strong point. Tumor cells notoriously evolve drug resistance and, at least in vitro, IFN-resistance as well. The real clinical benefit of IFN may thus be via its indirect effects on the immune system that tumor cells cannot evade.

# References

1. Isaacs, A. and Lindenman, J. *Proc. R. Soc. Lond.* **147**, 258–267 (1957).
2. Paucker, K. et al. *Virology* **17**, 324–334 (1962).
3. Stewart, W. et al. *Nature* **286**, 110 (1980).
4. Vilcek, J. and De Maeyer, E., eds. *Interferon* vol. 2, Elsevier, Amsterdam (1984).
5. Gresser, I., in *Progress in Immunology IV* (Fougereau, M. and Dausset, J., eds.) Academic, New York (1980).
6. Nagata, S. et al. *Nature* **284**, 316–320 (1980).
7. Taniguchi, T. et al. *Gene* **10**, 11–15 (1980).
8. Gray, P. W. et al. *Nature* **295**, 503–508 (1982).
9. Stebbing, N., in *Mechanisms of Interferon Actions* (Pfeffer, L. M., ed.) CRC Press, Cleveland (1985).
10. Goeddel, D. V. et al. *Nature* **290**, 20–26 (1981).
11. Nagata, S. et al. *Nature* **287**, 401–408 (1980).
12. Owerbach, D. et al. *Proc. Natl. Acad. Sci. USA* **78**, 3123–3127 (1981).
13. Ullrich, A. et al. *J. Mol. Biol.* **156**, 467–486 (1982).
14. Taniguchi, T. et al. *Nature* **285**, 547–549 (1980).
15. Gray, P. W. and Goeddel, D. V. *Nature* **298**, 859–863 (1982).
16. Wetzel, R. et al. *J. Interferon Res.* **1**, 381–390 (1981).
17. Weissman, C., in *Interferon* vol. 3 (Gresser, I., ed.) Academic, London (1981).
18. Imai, M. et al. *J. Immunol.* **128**, 2824–2825 (1982).
19. Labdon, J. *Arch. Biochem. Biophys.* **232**, 422–426 (1984).
20. Mark, D. et al. *Proc. Natl. Acad. Sci. USA* **81**, 5662–5666 (1984).
21. Sulkowski, E. et al. *Ann. NY Acad. Sci.* **350**, 339–346 (1980).
22. Sternberg, M. and Cohen, F. *Int. J. Biol. Macromol.* **4**, 137–144 (1982).
23. McGray, J. and Weil, R. *Proc. Natl. Acad. Sci. USA* **79**, 4829–4833 (1982).
24. Sulkowski, E., personal communication.
25. Arnheiter, H. et al. *Nature* **294**, 278–280 (1981).
26. Rinderkneckt et al. *J. Biol. Chem.* **259**, 6790–6797 (1984).
27. Pestka, S. et al. *J. Biol. Chem.* **258**, 9706–9709 (1983).
28. Yip, Y. et al. *Proc. Natl. Acad. Sci. USA* **78**, 1601–1605 (1981).
29. Ankel, H. et al. *Proc. Natl. Acad. Sci. USA* **70**, 2360–2363 (1973).
30. Huez, G. et al. *Biochem. Biophys. Res. Comm.* **110**, 155–160 (1983).
31. Zoon, K. and Arnheiter, H. *Pharmacol. Ther.* **24**, 259–278 (1984).
32. Branca, A. and Baglioni, C. *Nature* **294**, 768–770 (1981).
33. Anderson, P. et al. *J. Biol. Chem.* **257**, 11301–11304 (1982).
34. Aguet, M. et al. *Virology* **132**, 211–216 (1984).
35. Zoon, K. et al. *Virology* **130**, 195–203 (1983).
36. Taylor-Papadimitriou, J. and Shearer, M. *J. Interferon Res.* **4**, 553–559 (1984).
37. Taylor-Papadimitriou, J. et al. *J. Interferon Res.* **2**, 479–491 (1982).
38. Mogensen, K. and Bandu, M.-T. *Eur. J. Biochem.* **134**, 355–364 (1983).
39. Hannigan, G. et al. *J. Biol. Chem.* **259**, 9456–9460 (1984).

*40.* Fuse, A. et al. *Gann* **75**, 379–384 (1984).
*41.* Anderson, P. et al. *J. Biol. Chem.* **258**, 6497–6502 (1983).
*42.* Littman, S. et al. *J. Biol. Chem.* **260**, 1191–1195 (1985).
*43.* Orchansky, P. et al. *J. Immunol.* **136**, 169–173 (1986).
*44.* Celada, A. et al. *J. Clin. Invest.* **76**, 2196–2205 (1985).
*45.* Chany, C. *Biomedicine* **24**, 148–157 (1976).
*46.* Matsuyama, M. *Exp. Cell Res.* **124**, 253–259 (1979).
*47.* Besancon, F. Doctoral Thesis, Universite Paris-Sud, Centre d'Orsay (1977).
*48.* Bourgeade, M. and Chany, C. *Proc. Soc. Exp. Biol. Med.* **153**, 501–504 (1976).
*49.* Bourgeade, M. and Chany, C. *Int. J. Cancer* **24**, 314–318 (1979).
*50.* Kushnaryov, V. et al. *Infect. Immun.* **36**, 811–821 (1982).
*51.* Schreiber, A. et al. *J. Biol. Chem.* **258**, 846–853 (1983).
*52.* Fidler, I. et al. *J. Immunol.* **135**, 4289–4296 (1985).
*53.* Tovey, M. et al. *Proc. Natl. Acad. Sci. USA* **76**, 3890–3893 (1979).
*54.* Tovey, M. and Rochette-Egly, C. *Virology* **115**, 272–281 (1981).
*55.* Grollmann, E. et al. *Cancer Res.* **38**, 4172–4185 (1978).
*56.* Eid, P. and Mogensen, K., in *The Biology of the Interferon System* (Kirchner, H. and Schellekens, H., eds.) Elsevier, Amsterdam (1984).
*57.* Weil, J. et al. *Nature* **301**, 437–439 (1983).
*58.* Kerr, I. et al. *Nature* **250**, 57–59 (1974).
*59.* Kerr, I. and Brown, R. *Proc. Natl. Acad. Sci. USA* **75**, 256–260 (1978).
*60.* Clemens, M. and Williams, B. *Cell* **13**, 565–572 (1978).
*61.* Roberts, W. et al. *Nature* **264**, 477–480 (1976).
*62.* Zilberstein, A. et al. *Proc. Natl. Acad. Sci. USA* **75**, 4734–4738 (1978).
*63.* Vandenbussche, P. et al. *Virology* **111**, 11–22 (1981).
*64.* Sreevalsan, T. et al. *J. Cell. Phys.* **104**, 1–9 (1980).
*65.* Yaron, M. et al. *Nature* **267**, 457–459 (1977).
*66.* Pottathil, R. et al. *Proc. Natl. Acad. Sci. USA* **77**, 5437–5440 (1980).
*67.* Chandrabose, K. et al. *Science* **212**, 329–331 (1981).
*68.* Dalla-Favera, R. et al. *Proc. Natl. Acad. Sci. USA* **79**, 7824–7827 (1982).
*69.* Jonak, G. and Knight, E. *Proc. Natl. Acad. Sci. USA* **81**, 1747–1750 (1984).
*70.* Einat, M. et al. *Nature* **313**, 597–600 (1985).
*71.* Einat, M. et al. *Proc. Natl. Acad. Sci. USA* **82**, 7608–7612 (1985).
*72.* Taylor-Papadimitriou, J. et al. *J. Interferon Res.* **1**, 401–409 (1981).
*73.* Samid, D. et al. *Biochem. Biophys. Res. Commun.* **119**, 21–28 (1984).
*74.* Samid, D. et al. *Biochem. Biophys. Res. Commun.* **126**, 509–516 (1985).
*75.* Friedman, R. *J. Exp. Pathol.* **2**, 223–228 (1986).
*76.* Creasey, A. et al. *Proc. Natl. Acad. Sci. USA* **77**, 1471–1475 (1980).
*77.* Sokawa, Y. et al. *Nature* **268**, 236–238 (1977).
*78.* Leanderson, T. and Lundgren, E. *J. Interferon Res.* **2**, 21–29 (1982).
*79.* Balkwill, F. et al. *Int. J. Cancer* **22**, 258–265 (1978).
*80.* Clemens, M. and McNurlan, M. *Biochem. J.* **226**, 345–360 (1985).
*81.* Ito, M. and Buffett, R. *J. Natl. Cancer Inst.* **66**, 819–825 (1981).
*82.* Gewert, D. et al. *Eur. J. Biochem.* **139**, 619–625 (1984).
*83.* Gewert, D. et al. *Eur. J. Biochem.* **116**, 487–492 (1981).

84. Familletti, P. et al. *Meth. Enzymol.* **78**, 387–393 (1981).
85. Evinger, M. and Pestka, S. *Meth. Enzymol.* **79**, 362–368 (1981).
86. Tomita, Y. et al. *Int. J. Cancer* **30**, 161–165 (1982).
87. Blalock, J. et al. *Cell. Immunol.* **49**, 390–394 (1980).
88. Aebersold, P. and Sample, S. *Meth. Enzymol.* **119**, 579–582 (1986).
89. Salmon, S. et al. *N. Engl. J. Med.* **298**, 1321–1327 (1978).
90. Schiller, J. and Borden, E., this volume.
91. Adams, A. et al. *J. Gen. Virol.* **28**, 207–217 (1975).
92. Balkwill, F. et al. *Int. J. Cancer* **22**, 258–265 (1978).
93. Lin, S. et al. *Nature* **297**, 417–419 (1982).
94. Chany, C. and Vignal, M. *C. R. Acad. Sci.* **267**, 1798–1800 (1968).
95. Fisher, P. and Grant, S. *Pharmac. Ther.* **27**, 143–166 (1985).
96. Affabris, E. et al. *Virology* **120**, 441–452 (1982).
97. Fisher, P. et al. *J. Interferon Res.* **5**, 11–22 (1984).
98. Grant, S. et al. *Biochem. Biophys. Res. Commun.* **130**, 379–388 (1985).
99. Czarniecki, C. et al. *J. Virology* **49**, 490–496 (1984).
100. Streuli, M. et al. *Proc. Natl. Acad. Sci. USA* **78**, 2848–2852 (1981).
101. Rehberg, E. et al. *J. Biol. Chem.* **257**, 11497–11502 (1982).
102. Evinger, M. et al. *Arch. Biochem. Biophys.* **210**, 319–329 (1981).
103. Mark, D. and Creasey, A. International Patent Publication WO 83/02461 (1983).
104. Aebersold, P., unpublished observation.
105. Fish, E. et al. *Biochem. Biophys. Res. Commun.* **112**, 537–546 (1983).
106. Weck, P. et al. *Nucleic Acids Res.* **9**, 6153–6166 (1981).
107. Ortaldo, J. et al. *Proc. Natl. Acad. Sci. USA* **81**, 4926–4929 (1984).
108. Ortaldo, J., personal communication.
109. Schreiber, R. et al. *J. Immunol.* **134**, 1609–1618 (1985).
110. Dahl, H. *J. Interferon Res.* **3**, 387–393 (1983).
111. Reid, L. et al. *Proc. Natl. Acad. Sci. USA* **78**, 1171–1175 (1981).
112. Gresser, I. et al. *J. Exp. Med.* **158**, 2095–2107 (1983).
113. Belardelli, F. et al. *Int. J. Cancer* **30**, 821–825 (1982).
114. Lee, S. et al. *Cancer Res.* **43**, 4172–4175 (1983).
115. Uno, K. et al. *Cancer Res.* **45**, 1320–1327 (1985).
116. Balkwill, F. et al. *Int. J. Cancer* **30**, 231–235 (1982).
117. Kataoka, T. et al. *Cancer Res.* **45**, 3548–3553 (1985).
118. Gresser, I. and Bourali, C. *Nature* **223**, 844–846 (1969).
119. Gresser, I. and Bourali, C. *J. Natl. Cancer Inst.* **45**, 365–376 (1970).
120. Fresa, K. and Murasco, D. *Cancer Res.* **46**, 81–88 (1986).
121. Belardelli, F. et al. *Int. J. Cancer* **30**, 813–820 (1982).
122. Aebersold, P. et al. *J. Biol. Resp. Modif.* **4**, 251–257 (1985).
123. Schiller, J. and Borden, E., this volume.

# Natural Killer Cell Cytotoxic Factor

# Human and Rodent Natural Killer Cytotoxic Factors (NKCF)

## Characterization and Their Role in the NK Lytic Mechanism

SUSAN C. WRIGHT and BENJAMIN BONAVIDA

## 1. Introduction

Natural killer (NK) cells are a subpopulation of lymphocytes with the capacity to lyse certain types of tumor cells in an NK cell-mediated cytotoxicity (CMC) reaction. Since these cells exist in the absence of any known immunization process, they are thought to function in the first line of defense against newly arising tumors and infections. For these reasons, the understanding of the NK lytic mechanism, as well as its regulation, has been a strong interest in basic cancer research.

Previous studies on the mechanism of NK CMC led to the dissection of the NK lytic pathway into a series of discreet events. Initially, the NK cell recognizes and binds to the target cells through the interaction of receptors on the NK cells that are specific for the putative NK target structure (1). This is followed by the programming-for-lysis stage of the reaction, which occurs while the effector cell is in contact with the target. In the final lymphocyte-independent stage of the reaction, the target cell is programmed irreversibly to die, even in the absence of the effector cell.

The actual mechanism of cell death is not well understood. Earlier studies demonstrated that the addition of various agents known to inhibit the secretory process will inhibit the NK CMC reaction (2,3). Thus, the stimulus-secretion model was proposed for the NK lytic mechanism, although there was no direct evidence for the postulated soluble lytic mediator. Subsequent work in this laboratory focused on examining this question

using techniques optimized for the detection of weak lytic activity in the
supernatants of NK CMC reactions. We found that these supernatants contained lytic activity specific for NK-sensitive target cells in an 18–24-h
assay. Natural killer cytotoxic factors (NKCF) were then functionally defined as lymphokines produced by NK cells that are selectively cytotoxic
to NK-sensitive tumor cells. Subsequent studies revealed that the functional characteristics of NKCF correlate well with some of the known
features of the NK system. This led us to propose a model consisting of
five sequential steps for the NK lytic mechanism in which NKCFs function as the lytic mediators (4,5). According to this model (Fig. 1), following
the initial recognition/binding event, the target cell delivers a signal to
activate the NKCF release mechanism. This may occur through the interaction of membrane determinants distinct from those involved in the initial binding event, since it is known that binding alone is not sufficient
to induce release of NKCF. The effector cell then releases NKCF in close
proximity to the target cell. These factors then bind to binding sites on
the target cell membrane and mediate cell lysis. It is known that NKCF
binding alone is not sufficient to lead to lysis, and thus subsequent events
such as pore formation, endocytosis, or enzymatic activity may be essential. This review will summarize our studies on the characterization of
NKCF as well as the experimental data supporting their role in the NK
CMC reaction as proposed in our model.

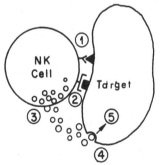

1  Effector cell recognizes and binds target

2  Target cell stimulates release of NKCF

3  Effector cell releases NKCF

4  NKCF bind to target cell

5  NKCF lyse target cell

Fig. 1. Five-step model for the mechanism of NK CMC in which NKCF
functions as the lytic mediators.

## 2. Materials and Methods

### 2.1. Production of NKCF

NKCF is routinely produced by culturing effector cells at $5 \times 10^6$/mL
in RPMI 1640 without serum for 20–24 h. In the human system, the effector cells are plastic nonadherent PBL, whereas for mice and rats, plastic

nonadherent spleen cells are employed. Effector cells are cocultured either with Con A (2.5–10.0 $\mu$g/mL) or stimulator cells at a 50:1 effector:stimulator ratio. Routinely, stimulator cells in the human system are the human NK-sensitive U937, whereas YAC-1 stimulators are used in the rodent system. All cell lines used in this study were routinely tested for mycoplasma according to Chen's technique (6) and were found to be mycoplasma free. After the overnight incubation, the cell-free supernatant was harvested and tested for NKCF activity. In some experiments PBLs were activated with recombinant IFN$\alpha$ (donated by M. Brunda of Hoffman LaRoche) prior to use as effector cells for NKCF production.

## 2.2. Assay of NKCF

The human and rodent NKCF assays are similar except that U937 was the human target, whereas YAC-1 is used to test rodent NKCF. Supernatants containing NKCF are tested at various dilutions in an 18–20 h $^{51}$Cr release assay with appropriate targets.

# 3. Results and Discussion

## 3.1. NK Cells Produce NKCF

In order to determine what cell type releases NKCF, various subpopulations were tested for their ability to produce NKCF in response to stimulation with NK-sensitive tumor stimulator cells. In the murine system, NKCF was produced by spleen cells, but not by thymocytes, and did not require the presence of mature T-cells or adherent cells (7). NKCF production did require the presence of asialo-GM1 positive cells, however, a marker known to be relatively specific for murine NK cells (8,9).

Similar to the rodent system, human NKCF production did not require the presence of adherent cells. Furthermore, NKCF-producing cells coenriched with NK cells upon fractionation of PBL by Percoll density gradient centrifugation (10). It also has been shown that human NK cells purified by selection of Fc receptor-positive LGL can produce NKCF (11).

Therefore, the available data from the murine and human systems are consistent with the NK effector cell-producing NKCF.

## 3.2. Mechanism of NKCF Release and Its Regulation

### 3.2.1. Agents That Can Stimulate Release of NKCF

Both human and rodent NKCF production can be stimulated by lectins such as Con A or PHA or by various types of tumor cell lines both

NK-sensitive and -resistant (*12*). At present, it is not known whether the activating signals induced by lectin are the same as those provided by tumor cell stimulation. We do know that binding of effector cell to the tumor cell alone is not sufficient to induce release of NKCF, however. This is based on the observation that interferon (IFN) treatment of initially NK-sensitive target cells decreases their ability to stimulate release of NKCF, although they are still able to form conjugates and are fully sensitive to lysis by NKCF (*5*). This suggests that the stimulation of NKCF release occurs through the interaction of membrane determinants in addition to and distinct from those involved in the initial binding event. Furthermore, a block in a target cell's capacity to stimulate release of NKCF could account for their IFN-induced NK resistance as originally described by Trinchieri et al. (*13*).

We have recently obtained evidence that release of NKCF can be stimulated by the combined action of phorbol myristate acetate and calcium ionophores, but not by either alone (*14*). This suggests that activation of protein kinase C is involved in the release of NKCF. Whether this is the same pathway by which tumor cells stimulate release of NKCF is not yet clear.

### 3.2.2. Evidence for the Involvement of Proteolytic Enzymes

A number of reports from other laboratories presented evidence that proteolytic enzymes are involved in the NK lytic mechanism (*3,15–19*). This was based on the observation that certain antiproteases could inhibit NK CMC, apparently by blocking some postbinding step in the pathway, since they did not affect conjugate formation. According to our model, these inhibitors could be acting on the NKCF release mechanism or else on target cell lysis by NKCF. These possibilities were tested using agents shown previously to inhibit NK CMC to determine their effect in both NKCF production and the NKCF assay (*20*). It was found that certain agents known to inhibit serine-dependent proteases and/or sulfhydryl-dependent enzymes could inhibit production of NKCF by NK cells stimulated with target cells. The same agents had no effect on target cell lysis by NKCF, however. The relevant enzymes may be associated with the effector cell surface or they may be intracellular, since the low-molecular-weight inhibitors could presumably pass through the cell membrane. It is possible that the putative enzyme(s) is involved in the NKCF release mechanism, or it may process NKCF precursors into lytically active forms. Thus, inhibition of production of lytically active NKCF could account for the observed inhibition of NK CMC by protease inhibitors.

### 3.2.3. Evidence for the Involvement of K⁺ Channels

Another recent study examined the role of $K^+$ influx in the NK lytic mechanism (*21*). Using the patch clamp technique, it was demonstrated that a voltage-dependent $K^+$ channel exists in human NK cells. Furthermore, it was found that $K^+$ channel blockers could inhibit binding of effector to target cells, as well as target cell lysis by preformed conjugates. Further analysis in the NKCF system revealed that $K^+$ channel blockers did not inhibit target cell lysis by NKCF, but they did inhibit production of NKCF in response to stimulation with U937 or Con A. These findings suggest that NK CMC requires functional effector cell $K^+$ channels in order to release lytically active NKCF.

### 3.2.4. Augmentation of NKCF Production by IFN or IL-2

In the murine system, NKCF production is augmented by pretreatment of effector cells with IFN or IFN inducers. This augmentation is dependent upon protein synthesis during the IFN pretreatment period (22). In the human system, NKCF production is also augmented by pretreatment with purified recombinant IFNα or β, as well as recombinant IL-2 (interleukin-2) (unpublished observations). These findings may account at least in part for the augmentation of NK CMC by either IFN or IL-2 reported by other investigators (13,23,24).

## 3.3. Mechanism of Action of NKCF

### 3.3.1. Kinetics of NKCF Binding and Lysis

Target cell lysis by NKCF can be divided into two stages: binding of NKCF to the target cell membrane and postbinding events. The overall kinetics of lysis by NKCF (20 h) is quite protracted compared to the kinetics of NK CMC (4 h). This is due mainly because of the kinetics of postbinding events, since NKCFs bind to the target cell quite rapidly. Target cells incubated in NKCF for only 1–2 h and then washed lysed in a subsequent 20-h incubation in the absence of NKCF (submitted for publication). The reasons for the prolonged kinetics of the post-NKCF binding events as opposed to the kinetics of NK CMC are not yet clear. It is possible that NKCFs released into the supernatant become partially inactivated or else are too diluted to mediate rapid target cell lysis. Another possibility is that there may be a specialized NKCF delivery mechanism operating when NK effector cells are in direct contact with the target, thus facilitating rapid target cell lysis.

We have recently found that the kinetics of lysis by NKCF can be augmented by addition of protein synthesis inhibitors (unpublished observations). Thus, U937 or MOLT-4 target cells incubated with NKCF in the presence of cycloheximide will lyse in only 4 h (unpublished observations). At present, it is not clear whether cycloheximide inhibits a repair mechanism or acts in some other capacity to increase the rate of lysis.

### 3.3.2. Evidence for NKCF Binding Sites

Several lines of evidence indicate that NKCFs interact with binding sites on the target cell membrane. NKCF activity can be absorbed from supernatants to different extents by different types of tumor cell lines (7). Absorption, as well as target cell lysis by NKCF, can be prevented by the addition of the same monosaccharides (25,26) shown previously to inhibit NK CMC in the human (27) or murine (28) systems. Thus, it is possible that carbohydrate determinants expressed on either NKCF molecules or target cell binding sites are essential for their interaction leading to target cell lysis in the NK CMC reaction. Results reported from another laboratory (29) support the alternate hypothesis that the relevant carbohydrate determinants are expressed on the binding site since tunicamycin-treated cells become relatively resistant to lysis by either NKCF or NK cells.

Further evidence for the role of NKCF binding sites in the NK lytic mechanism is derived from studies using enzyme-treated target cells. It was recently found that papain-treated target cells become relatively resistant to lysis by NKCF, as well as NK cells, although they could still form conjugates (30). Papain-treated targets were still lysed in an antibody-dependent cellular cytotoxicity reaction, indicating some specificity for the NK reaction. Papain-treated target cells were unable to absorb NKCF as well as normal targets, suggesting that the decrease in NK sensitivity was the result of destruction of NKCF binding sites. These results suggest that expression of protein-containing structures on the target cell destinct from the recognition structure required for conjugate formation is necessary for NK sensitivity.

The hypothesis that expression of NKCF binding sites is essential for target cell NK sensitivity was also tested by developing NKCF-resistant variants derived from YAC-1 or U937. It was found that the prolonged culture of either YAC-1 (4) or U937 (31) resulted in the development of NK-resistant variants. These variants could still form conjugates and stimulate release of NKCF; they were resistant to lysis by NKCF, however, thus accounting for their NK resistance. NKCF resistance may be caused, at least in part, by a deficiency of NKCF binding sites since the variants did not absorb NKCF as well as the parental cell lines. These findings indicate that the NKCF binding site is distinct from those membrane determinants involved in the first two steps of the lytic reaction, i.e., binding and stimulation of release of NKCF.

### 3.3.3. Post-NKCF Binding Events

Although it is readily apparent that NKCF interaction with target cell binding sites is necessary to lead to lysis, NKCF binding alone is not sufficient to lyse the cell. This stems from the observation that YAC-1 cells rendered NK resistant by passage in vivo are resistant to lysis by NKCF even though they can absorb NKCF as well as normal YAC-1 (unpublished observations). Thus, events subsequent to binding of NKCF to the target cell membrane are essential to bring about cell lysis. The nature of these post-NKCF binding events is currently under investigation. We have not been able to obtain any evidence for the involvement of proteolytic activity, since various types of antiproteases were found not to affect target cell lysis by NKCF (20). We also have evidence that NKCF will lyse target cells at 37°C, but not at 25°C. One possibility is that NKCF may lyse the target by forming pores in the membrane analagous to the complement system. Alternatively, receptor-bound NKCF may undergo endocytosis and mediate toxic effects at some intracellular site.

We have also observed some dramatic morphological changes in target cells incubated with NKCF using time-lapse cinematography. Within 1–2 h after exposure to NKCF, the target cells tend to clump up. Next follows a period of membrane blebbing and zeiosis that just precedes cell death. Zeiosis has been associated with DNA fragmentation as the ultimate cause of cell death in certain systems including target cell lysis by cytotoxic T-cells (32). Thus, it is possible that NKCF may initiate a sequence of target cell events resulting in DNA fragmentation and ultimately cell death.

### 3.4. Properties That Determine NK Sensitivity in a Tumor Cell Line

Throughout our studies on NKCF we have employed a number of different NK-resistant variants as tools to analyze the mechanism of NK CMC. In addition, the development of NK-resistant variants from initially NK-sensitive cell lines using different selection procedures has allowed us to delineate a number of properties that determine NK sensitivity. The characteristics of these variants is summarized in Table 1. Both U937 and YAC-1 have been employed as parental cells for the various types of selection procedures. The first two variants (YAC-IFN and YAC-pap) are not variants in the true sense since they were generated by brief (18 and 1 h, respectively) treatments to modify the parental line. In contrast, the other variants required the prolonged growth (at least 3 wk in the case of YAC-R, U9NR, and U9TR) under the specific selection conditions. All of these variants are relatively or completely NK resistant with the exception of U9TR. The implications of this observation concerning the relationship of TNF and NKCF and their role in the NK lytic mechanism will be further discussed in the final section. The NK resistance of these variants is not irreversible, with the possible exception of U9NR. YAC-IFN, YAC-

Table 1
Characteristics of Variant Cell Lines

| | | | Variant cell line | | | |
|---|---|---|---|---|---|---|
| Characteristics[a] | YAC-IFN | YAC-pap or U937-pap | YAC-R | U9NR | U9TR | YAC-asc |
| Parental cell line | YAC-1 | YAC-1 or U937 | YAC-1 | U937 | U937 | YAC-1 |
| Selection process | IFN treatment for 18 h | Papain treatment for 1 h | Growth in NKCF | Growth in NKCF | Growth in TNF | In vivo passage |
| Sensitive to NK CMC | +/- | +/- | - | - | +++ | - |
| Forms conjugates | +++ | +++ | +++ | +++ | +++ | +++ |
| Stimulates release of NKCF | +/- | +++ | +++ | +++ | +++ | - |
| Absorbs NKCF | ? | +/- | +/- | +/- | ? | +++ |
| Lysed by NKCF | +++ | +/- | - | - | - | - |

[a]The listed characteristics are evaluated for each of the variants with respect to the parental cell line, which is strongly positive (+ + +) for all the characteristics. A negative result (−) indicates the variant is completely defective for a given characteristic, whereas a borderline result (+/−) indicates a significant decrease in the expression of that characteristic compared to the normal parent.

pap, and U937-pap all regain full NK sensitivity within days following their treatment. YAC-R regains partial NK sensitivity after 3 wk of culture in the absence of NKCF. Although the selection process was the same, the NK-resistant phenotype of U9NR appears to be much more stable than YAC-R. U9NRs have been cultured in the absence of NKCF for as long as 41 d without any increase of NK sensitivity. A study is currently underway to determine if U9NR's NK resistance will remain stable after even longer periods of culture without NKCF. YAC-1 cells rendered NK resistant by in vivo passage regain NK sensitivity after 3 wk of in vitro culture, in agreement with previous results (33).

All the variants still express the NK target structure since they can still form conjugates with effector cells. This is in contrast to many of the variants developed in other laboratories, which appear to be NK resistant because they are not recognized and bound by the effector cell (34–36).

All of the variants can stimulate release of NKCF except YAC-IFN and YAC-asc. We have attributed the NK resistance of YAC-IFN specifically to this defect since it is still sensitive to lysis by NKCF. In contrast, YAC-asc exhibits a block at two distinct points in the NK lytic pathway. Not only are they defective in stimulating release of NKCF, but they are also inherently resistant to lysis by these factors, even though they express NKCF binding sites. It is possible that exposure to IFN in vivo induced the stimulation defect in YAC-asc. One recent report has correlated the NK resistance of YAC-IFN and YAC-asc to an increase in H-2 expression (37). Thus, it is possible that the lack of H-2 antigens on a target cell is somehow involved in activating the NK cell to release NKCF.

The remaining NK-resistant variants all exhibit the same defect—a deficiency of NKCF binding sites. Whether this is the only block in NK CMC for U9NR is currently under investigation. Since NKCF binding alone is not sufficient to lyse the target, as demonstrated by YAC-asc, it is possible that some postbinding event may also be blocked in U9NR and YAC-R.

We are also investigating what components of NKCF are responsible for induction of NK resistance using semipurified material. Currently available data suggest that IFN that may be present in supernatants containing NKCF is not responsible for inducing resistance in YAC-R and U9NR. This is based on the observation that U9NR and YAC-R can still stimulate release of NKCF, in contrast to YAC-IFN. In addition, IFN assays of a number of representative samples of human (unpublished observations) and murine (22) NKCF revealed either no IFN or else IFN concentrations much lower than that required to induce NK resistance.

The results of experiments with U9TR indicate that selection with purified recombinant human TNF is not sufficient to induce NK resistance.

U9TR cells were resistant to lysis by either TNF or NKCF, however. The possibility that there may be some similarities in the mechanisms of target cell lysis by these factors is currently under investigation.

In summary, our studies with the different types of variants revealed that target cell sensitivity to lysis by NK cells is governed by several factors. For a target cell to be NK-sensitive, it must exhibit the following properties: (1) the target cell's ability to be recognized and bound by relevant receptors and adhesion structures on the NK cell membrane, (2) the ability of the target cell to trigger the NK cell and activate the NKCF release mechanism, (3) the expression of NKCF binding sites on the target cell membrane, and (4) the inherent sensitivity of the target cell to lysis by membrane-bound NKCF.

Clearly, the ability to identify each of these properties for every new target tested allow for the precise dissection of the block(s) responsible for target cell resistance to NK cells. Thus, NK-resistant tumor cells or virally infected cells may exhibit different escape mechanisms and thus require different manipulations to render them NK sensitive.

### 3.5. Biochemical Characterization of NKCF

A number of studies have examined the biochemical characteristics of both human and rodent NKCF (38). NKCF activity is unstable at 63 °C, in 8M urea, or at pH 2. These factors are sensitive to trypsin, suggesting that NKCFs are composed at least in part of protein. NKCF activity is eliminated by reduction and alkylation, suggesting that intact disulfide bonds are essential for lytic activity. Mild oxidation with sodium periodate inactivates NKCF, suggesting that carbohydrate determinants are essential for lytic activity. Human, murine, and rat NKCF all migrate in a single broad peak exhibiting an apparent molecular weight of 15,000–40,000 by HPLC gel filtration (38). This molecular weight range roughly corresponds to that reported by other investigators for human NKCF (11,29). Although we could not resolve separate peaks by gel filtration, preliminary evidence using different fractionation techniques suggests that NKCF is composed of more than one type of cytotoxic molecule. On-going efforts to purify NKCF should help to resolve this issue.

### 3.6. Relationship of NKCF to Other Cytotoxins

Since the cytotoxic components of NKCF have not yet been purified to homogeneity, it is not clear how these factors relate to other cytotoxic molecules. It is possible, however, to make a functional comparison between supernatants containing NKCF and other cytotoxins that have been implicated as mediators of various types of CMC reactions.

Recently, cytolysins or perforins have been implicated as mediators of NK CMC reactions (39,40). These factors have been isolated from the granules of various types of cell lines and are proposed to lyse targets by forming pores in the membrane. Their functional characteristics are quite different from NKCF in that they lyse targets much more rapidly (i.e., within minutes), and this process will occur at room temperature. Although NK-sensitive targets are more sensitive to lysis by these pore-forming molecules, a wide variety of NK-resistant targets are also lysed. For these reasons, we believe NKCF to be different from cytolysins/perforins. We cannot, however, rule out the possibility that they may be related in some way.

Lymphotoxin (LT) is another type of cytotoxic factor derived from activated lymphoid cells that was originally described as cytostatic or cytotoxic to tumor cells (41,42). More recently, LT has been implicated as the mediator of various types of CMC reactions, including cytotoxic T-cell-mediated lysis (43–45), lectin-dependent cellular cytotoxicity (46), antibody-dependent cellular cytotoxicity (ADCC) (47), as well as NK CMC (48–50). Various LT forms have been described ranging in molecular weight from 12,000 to 200,000, as determined by gel filtration (51), which somewhat complicates their comparison to NKCF. Recently the α-form of LT has been biochemically purified (52,53), however, which led to the isolation of the LT gene and engineering its expression in *Escherichia coli* (54). Recently, we undertook a functional comparison between human NKCF and purified recombinant human LT (donated by Genentech). We found the target cell specificity of LT to be quite different from that of NKCF, and, furthermore, antibodies against LT did not inhibit NKCF. Therefore, we conclude that NKCF is different from recombinant LT (manuscript in preparation). The relationship, however, of the various forms of LT described previously in the literature to either NKCF or the recombinant LT is still not clear.

Tumor necrosis factor (TNF) is another type of cyotoxic mediator originally described by Carswell et al. (55). Unlike NKCF, TNF is produced primarily by monocytes and macrophages (56,57) and has been implicated as a mediator of adherent cell-mediated cytotoxicity reactions (58,59). Recently TNF has been biochemically purified (60), and its gene has been expressed in *E. coli* (61–63). Purified recombinant human TNF (donated by Genentech) was used to compare its functional characteristics with NKCF (manuscript in preparation). TNF was found to exhibit a similar target cell specificity as NKCF. Furthermore, antibodies directed against TNF mediated partial to complete inhibition of lysis of U937 target cells by NKCF. This suggested that NKCF was the same as or antigenically similar to TNF. If the two factors are identical, and if our model for the

NK lytic mechanism is correct, then it might be expected that anti-TNF would inhibit NK CMC. When we tested this hypothesis, it was found that anti-TNF caused partial inhibition of NK CMC in approximately half the experiments. The interpretation of this result is further complicated by the possibility that any mediators delivered to the target cell while it is in close contact with the effector cell may not be readily accessible to exogenous antibodies. To further analyze the possible role of TNF in the NK lytic mechanism, we developed variants by the prolonged culture of U937 in the presence of TNF. Variants selected by TNF (U9TR) were then functionally compared to variants selected by growth in NKCF (U9NR). It was found that both variants were resistant to lysis by either TNF or NKCF. U9NR was resistant to lysis by NK cells, however, whereas U9TR was still sensitive (31). Since TNF could not induce NK resistance, this suggests that TNF alone is not sufficient to mediate NK activity in a CMC reaction. It follows that the component of NKCF responsible for the induction of NK resistance in U9NR is not TNF. We are currently testing semipurified fractions of NKCF in an attempt to isolate the component that induces NK resistance.

In conclusion, it is possible that NK CMC is mediated by a mixture of cytotoxic factors that are all components of NKCF. Further biochemical analysis of NKCF should help to clarify their relationship to other cytotoxins as well as their role in the NK lytic mechanism.

## 4. Concluding Remarks

This brief description of the role of NKCF in the mechanism of NK CMC provides the basis for analyzing the possible role of soluble cytotoxic mediators in other types of cytolytic systems. The chain of events proposed for the NK lytic mechanism depicted in Fig. 1 may prove to be analogous to other types of CMC reactions. Obviously, the molecular nature of the various steps proposed in this model is not yet understood, and new probes are needed to approach their structures.

It has also become clear that the studies described above have important clinical and practical applications. For example, it should be possible to elucidate the mechanism of defective NK activity or target cell resistance in various disease states. This may lead to the introduction of new modalities to correct some of the known deficiencies. It is not unreasonable to suggest clinical modalities that can either enhance susceptibility of tumor cells to lysis by NK cells or NKCF or treatments that can restore functional NK activity where it is defective. Our laboratory is currently examining some of these potential applications.

## Acknowledgments

Supported by grant CA-35791 and in part by grant CA-37199 (S.C.W.) awarded by the National Cancer Institute. We also thank Doctor M. Brunda (Hoffman La Roche) for donating recombinant IFN and IL-2 and Doctor B. Aggarwal (Genentech, Inc.) for the recombinant TNF and LT and for his contribution in some of the studies.

## References

*1.* Roder, J. C., Rosen, A., Fenyo, E. M., and Troy, F. A. *Proc. Natl. Acad. Sci. USA* **76**, 1405–1409 (1984).
2. Roder, J. C., Argov, S., Klein, M., Peterson, C., Kiessling, R., Anderson, K., and Hansson, M. *Immunology* **40**, 107–116 (1980).
*3.* Quan, P., Ishizaka, T., and Bloom, B. R. *J. Immunol.* **128**, 1786–1791 (1982).
*4.* Wright, S. C. and Bonavida, B. *Proc. Natl. Acad. Sci. USA* **80**, 1688–1692 (1983).
*5.* Wright, S. C. and Bonavida, B. *J. Immunol.* **130**, 2965–2968 (1983).
*6.* Chen, T. P. *Exp. Cell. Res.* **104**, 255–262 (1977).
*7.* Wright, S. C. and Bonavida, B. *J. Immunol.* **129** 433–439 (1982).
*8.* Kasai, M., Iwamori, M., Nagai, Y., Okumora, K., and Tadar, T. *Eur. J. Immunol.* **10**, 175–180 (1980).
*9.* Young, W. W., Hakomori, S., Durdik, J. M., and Henney, C. S. *J. Immunol.* **124**, 199–201 (1983).
*10.* Wright, S. C., Weitzen, M. L., Kahle, R., Granger, G. A., and Bonavida, B. *J. Immunol.* **130**, 2479–2483 (1983).
*11.* Degliantoni, G., Murphy, m., Kobayashi, M., Francis, M. K., Perussia, B., and Trinchieri, G. *J. Exp. Med.* **162**, 1512–1530 (1985).
*12.* Wright, S. C. and Bonavida, B. *J. Immunol.* **133**, 3415–3423 (1984).
*13.* Trinchieri, G. and Santoli, D. *J. Exp. Med.* **147**, 1314–1333 (1978).
*14.* Graves, S. C., Bramhall, J., Wright, S. C., and Bonavida, B. (submitted for publication).
*15.* Roder, J. C., Kiessling, R., Biberfeld, P., and Anderson, B. *J. Immunol.* **121**, 2509–251k7 (1978).
*16.* Hudig, D., Haverty, T., Fulcher, C., Redelman, D., and Mendelsohn, J. *J. Immunol.* **126**, 1569–1574 (1981).
*17.* Hudig, D., Redelman, D., and Minning, L., in *NK Cells and Other Natural Effector Cells* (Herberman, R. B., ed.) Academia, New York (1982).
*18.* Goldfarb, R. H., Timonen, T. T., and Herberman, R. B., in *NK Cells and Other Natural Effector Cells* (Herberman, R. B., ed.) Academic, New York (1982).

19. Lavie, G., in *NK Cells and Other Natural Effector Cells* (Herberman, R. B., ed.) Academic, New York (1982).
20. Wright, S. C. and Bonavida, B., in *Natural Killer Activity and Its Regulation* (Hoshino, T., ed.) Excerpta Medicine, Amsterdam (1984).
21. Sidell, N., Schlichter, L. C., Wright, S. C., Hagiwara, S., and Golub, S. H. (submitted for publication).
22. Wright, S. C. and Bonavida, B. *J. Immunol.* **130**, 2960–2964 (1983).
23. Gidlund, M., Oin, A., Wigzel, H., Senik, A., and Gresser, I. *Nature* **273**, 759–761 (1978).
24. Henney, C. S., Kuribayashi, K., Kan, D. E., and Gillis, S. *Nature* **291**, 335–338 (1981).
25. Wright, S. C. and Bonavida, B. *J. Immunol.* **126**, 1516–1521 (1981).
26. Wright, S. C., Wilbur, S. M., and Bonavida, B., in *Mechanisms of Cell-Mediated Cytotoxicity II* (Henkart, P., and Martz, E., eds.) Plenum, New York (1985).
27. Forbes, J. T., Bretthauer, R. K., and Oeltmann, T. N. *Proc. Natl. Acad. Sci. USA* **78**, 5797–5801 (1981).
28. Stutman, O., Dien, P., Wisun, R. E., and Lattine, E. C. *Proc. Natl. Acad. Sci. USA* **77**, 2895–2898 (1980).
29. Blanca, I., Herbermann, R. B., and Ortaldo, J. *Natl. Immun. Cell Growth Reg.* **4**, 48–59 (1985).
30. Wright, S. C., Kane, K., Clark, W. R., and Bonavida, B. (submitted for publication).
31. Wright, S. C. and Bonavida, B. *Natl. Immun. Cell Growth Reg.* **4**, 287 (1985).
32. Cohen, J. J., Dake, R. C., Chervenak, R., Sellins, K. S., and Olsen, L., in *Mechanisms of Cell-Mediated Cytotoxicity II* (Henkart, P. and Martz, E., eds.) Plenum, New York (1985).
33. Becker, S., Kiessling, R., Lee, N., and Klein, G. *J. Natl. Cancer Inst.* **61**, 1495–1498 (1978).
34. Durdik, J. M., Beck, B. N., Clark, E. A., and Henney, C. S. *J. Immunol.* **125**, 683–688 (1980).
35. Gronberg, A., Kiessling, R., Eriksson, E., and Hansson, M. *J. Immunol.* **127**, 1734–0739 (1981).
36. MacDougall, S. L., Shustik, C., and Sullivan, A. K. *Cell Immunol.* **76**, 39–48 (1983).
37. Piontek, G. E., Taniguchi, K., Ljunggren, H., Gronberg, A., Kiessling, R., Klein, G., and Karre, K. *J. Immunol.* **135**, 4281–4288 (1985).
38. Wright, S. C., Wilbur, S. M., and Bonavida, B. *Natl. Immun. Cell Growth Reg.* **4**, 202–220 (1985).
39. Podack, E. R. and Dennert, G. *Nature* **302**, 442–445 (1983).
40. Millard, P. J., Henkart, M. P., Reynolds, C. W., and Henkart, P. A. *J. Immunol.* **132**, 3197–3204 (1984).
41. Williams, T. M. and Granger, G. A. *Nature* **219**, 1076–1077 (1968).
42. Ruddle, N. H. and Waksman, B. H. *J. Exp. Med.* **128**, 1267–1278 (1968).
43. Walker, S. M. and Lucas, Z. J. *Transpl. Proc.* **5**, 137–140 (1973).
44. Ware, C. F. and Granger, G. A. *J. Immunol.* **126**, 1934–1940 (1981).

45. Schmid, D. S., Powell, M. B., Mahoneyand, K. A., and Ruddle, N. H. *Cell. Immunol.* **93**, 68–82 (1985).
46. Sawada, J. I. and Oparoa, T. *Transplantation* **26**, 319–324 (1978).
47. Kondo, L. L., Rosenaw, W., and Wara, D. W. *J. Immunol.* **126**, 1131–1133 (1981).
48. Granger, G. A., Weitzen, M. L., Devlin, J. J., Innis, E., and Yamamoto, R. S., in *Human Lymphokines: The Biological Immune Response Modifiers* (Kahn, A. and Hill, N., eds.) Academic, New York (1982).
49. Weitzen, M. L., Yamamoto, R. S., and Granger, G. A. *Cell. Immunol.* **77**, 31–41 (1983).
50. Weitzen, M. L., Innis, E., Yamamoto, R. S., and Granger, G. A. *Cell. Immunol.* **77**, 42–57.
51. Granger, G. A., Yamamoto, R. S., Fair, D. S., and Hiserodt, J. C. *Cell. Immunol.* **38**, 388–401 (1978).
52. Aggarwal, B. B., Moffat, B., and Harkins, R. H. *J. Biol. Chem.* **259** 686–691 (1984).
53. Aggarwal, B. B., Henzel, W. J., Moffat, B., Kohr, W. J., and Harkins, R. N. *J. Biol. Chem.* **260**, 2234–2344 (1985).
54. Gray, P. W., Aggarwal, B. B., Benton, C. V., Bringman, T. W., Henzel, W. J., Jarvett, J. A., Leung, D. W., Moffat, B., Ng, P., Svedersky, L. P., Palladino, M. A., and Nedwin, G. E. *Nature* **312**, 721–724 (1984).
55. Carswell, E. A., Old, L. J., Kassel, L., Green, S., Fiore, N., and Williamson, B. *Proc. Natl. Acad. Sci. USA* **72**, 3666–3670 (1975).
56. Mannel, D. N., Moore, R. N., and Mergenhagen, S. E. *Infect. Immun.* **30**, 523–530 (1980).
57. Nissen-Meyer, J. and Hammerstrom, J. *Infect. Immun.* **38**, 67–73 (1982).
58. Zacharchuk, C. M., Drysdale, B. E., Mater, M. M., and Shein, H. S. *Proc. Natl. Acad. Sci. USA* **80**, 6341–6345 (1983).
59. Matthews, N. *Immunology* **48**, 321–327 (1983).
60. Aggarwal, B. B., Kohr, W. J., Hass, P. E., Moffat, B., Spencer, S. A., Henzel, W. J., Bringman, T. S., Nedwin, G. E., Goddel, D. V., and Harkins, R. N. *J. Biol. Chem.* **260**, 2345–2354 (1985).
61. Pennica, D., Nedwin, G. E., Hayflick, F. S., Seeburg, P. H., Dirynck, R., Palladino, M. A., Kohr, W. J., Aggarwal, B. B., and Goddel, D. V. *Nature* **312**, 724–729 (1984).
62. Shirai, T., Yamaguchi, H., Ito, H., Ito, H., Todd, C. W., and Wallace, R. B. *Nature* **313**, 803–806 (1985).
63. Wang, A. M., Creasey, A. A., Ladner, M. B., Lin, L. S., Stuckler, J., Van Arsdell, J. N., Yamamoto, R., and Mark, D. F. *Science* **228**, 149–154 (1985).

# Human Natural Killer Cytotoxic Factor (NKCF)

## Relevance, Mode of Action, and Relationship to Other Cytotoxic Factors

### JOHN R. ORTALDO

## 1. Introduction

During the past few years, natural killer (NK) cells have attracted considerable attention because of their potential role in antitumor defenses in humans and animals (*1*). Recently, the cells responsible for NK activity in rodents and humans have been shown to be a subset of lymphoid cells termed large granular lymphocytes (LGL) (*2,3*). The mechanism of their lytic activity is still not thoroughly understood, however. Studies of the effects of metabolic inhibitors on NK activity support the stimulation-secretion model originally postulated (*4,5*) to explain the mechanism of killing by cytotoxic T lymphocytes (CTL) (*6*). In addition, Wright and Bonavida (*7*) have recently described a soluble factor that is produced during the interaction of mouse spleen cells and human peripheral blood lymphocytes (*7–10*) and that selectively lyses NK-susceptible target cells. They termed this NK cytotoxic factor (NKCF). Although several lines of correlative evidence suggest a role for NKCF in the mechanism of NK cell-mediated cytolysis, a variety of important issues still remain to be settled. In the present report, NKCF was utilized in an attempt to dissect the various steps that have been postulated to be involved in NK cell-mediated lysis. Studies were performed to examine agents that have been previously demonstrated to inhibit LGL-mediated cytolysis and their effect on NKCF production by LGL and NKCF lysis of tumor target cells. In addition, we initiated biochemical characterization of human NKCF, and because of the recent production of recombinant cytostatic molecules, tumor necrosis factor (TNF), and lymphtoxin (LT), we compared these factors with NKCF.

# 2. Results

## 2.1. Production of NKCF by Human LGL

If NKCF is involved in the mechanism of lysis by human NK cells, one would predict that the factor would be produced from highly purified populations of LGL, the cell responsible for most, if not all, human NK activity. The data indicate that Percoll density gradient fractions containing a high percentage of LGL, upon incubation with K562, produced high levels of NKCF (1–3). In contrast, highly purified T-cell populations (or populations depleted of NK cells) released insignificant levels of NKCF activity. The stimulation of LGL with mitogens, NK-susceptible targets, or membrane fragments of such target cells, resulted in a substantial release of NKCF (7–14). In contrast, an appreciable increase of NKCF production by LGL was not seen when human NK-resistant target cells such as RL(male)1, YAC-1, or Raji were used as stimuli (12). It should be noted that although stimulation of NK cells was usually necessary for obtaining high levels of NKCF, some spontaneous NKCF was produced by the LGL of some donors (data not shown) (12).

Table 1 summarizes some additional general properties of NKCF. In addition to these general properties, some physicochemical properties have also been observed. NKCF produced in serum-free conditions is generally quite stable when maintained at low temperatures (4 °C or lower). In addition, it appears to be protein in nature, since it is inactivated by trypsin treatment and unstable when maintained at high temperatures (56 °C or higher). In addition, data presented by Wright et al. (15) have suggested a disulfide-linked glycoprotein nature of NKCF because of its susceptibility to Na-periodate and reducing agents.

If NKCF plays an important role in NK cell-mediated lysis, then it would be predicted that the factor would bind to the target cells and kill them in a time comparable to that required by intact NK cells (11). In order to test this prediction, target cells were incubated with NKCF for various intervals at 37 °C, and the incubation was either continued in the presence of NKCF or the targets were washed and incubated with culture medium or in the presence of fresh NKCF. At various times thereafter, the level of cytotoxicity was assessed. The results (12) of those experiments indicate that lysis of target cells by NKCF occurred slowly, requiring a period of incubation of approximately 48 h (with [111]In-labeled target cells), although 24 h maximal release has been routinely seen with [51]Cr-labeled targets. These kinetics of lysis were consistent for all of the supernatants tested against [111]In-labeled targets.

In contrast, studies on the kinetics of absorption showed that within 2 h, and at a maximum of between 4 and 6 h after incubation with NK-

Table 1
Characteristics of NKCF

| | | Reference |
|---|---|---|
| *General properties* | | |
| Cellular source | LGL | *10, 13* |
| Stimuli for release | NK-susceptible targets or mitogens | *8, 9* |
| Kinetics of lysis | Slow (> 10 h) required for detectable activity | *8, 10* |
| Pattern of target cell susceptibility | Similar to NK cells | *15* |
| *Biochemical properties* | | |
| Molecular weight | 20–40 $K_d$ | *15* |
| Stability at | | |
| −20 °C | Weeks to months | *8, 10* |
| 4 °C | Days to weeks | *8, 10* |
| 56 °C | Hours | *8, 10* |
| > 56 °C | < 10 Minutes | *8, 10* |
| Inactivation by enzymes | Sensitive to trypsin, | *15* |
| | insensitive to neuraminidase | *15* |

susceptible targets, NKCF activity was removed from supernatants. After incubation of target cells with NKCF, the cells could be washed and lysis proceed with kinetics similar to that observed when the cells were maintained in the presence of NKCF. Addition of fresh NKCF, however, increased the percentage of lysis of target cells, indicating that maximal saturation of the target cells by NKCF was not maintained when the cells were incubated for several hours in the absence of factor. Overall, these results indicated that, in contrast to the rapid killing by NK cells, NKCF requires a longer period of time to produce significant levels of lysis. Optimal binding by NKCF can occur within short periods of incubation (2–4 h of incubation), however, and this exposure is sufficient to cause subsequent lysis of target cells without the continued need for NKCF.

Observations on the inhibition of NKCF might provide an opportunity to dissect, in detail, the proposed step(s) in the lytic process. Therefore, agents known to inhibit NK activity at a postbinding phase have been tested for their ability to block either (1) the production and/or release of NKCF when present during the 24-h period of interaction between the effector cells and target cells, (2) the binding of NKCF to target cells, when present during the 6-h period required for maximal absorption of NKCF (*13*) or (3) during the terminal lytic phase when added to target cells precoated with NKCF. Table 2 summarizes the results obtained with a variety of NK-inhibitory agents (*13–15*). The majority of treatments were found to

Table 2
Effects of Agents (That Inhibit NK Lysis) on NKCF Activity

| | Effect on NKCF[a] | | | |
|---|---|---|---|---|
| Agent | Production and/or release | Binding | Lysis | Reference |
| Sugar-PO₄ | | | | |
| Mannose-PO₄ | — | ↓ | — | 13, 15 |
| Fructose-PO₄ | — | — | — | 13, 15 |
| Antigranule antibody | ? | ↓ | −↑ | 12, 13 |
| Protease inhibitors | — | — | — | 12, 13, 18 |
| Removal of Ca²⁺/Mg²⁺ | ↓ | ? | ? | 13, 18 |
| Strontium chloride | ↓ | — | — | 13 |
| ATP or cAMP | ↓ | — | — | 13 |
| PGE₂ | ↓ | — | — | 13 |
| Ammonium chloride | ↓ | — | — | 13 |
| Monensin | ↓ | — | ↓ | 13 |

[a]The "—" indicates no change, ↑ indicates increase, and ↓ is decrease in NKCF production, binding, or lysis. ? Indicates not evaluable.

be potent inhibitors of production and/or release of NKCF (i.e., the removal of divalent cations or inhibition by the nucleotides ATP or cyclic AMP, prostaglandins, ammonium chloride, strontium chloride, and monensin). Because of their small molecular size, these agents were easily removed from the reaction mixture by dialysis and could therefore be assessed with regard to their effects on factor production or release. Most had no effect on the subsequent binding of NKCF to targets or on the lytic stage itself. The ability of antiserum to isolated cytoplasmic granules from LGL tumors (16) to inhibit production or release of NKCF was not interpretable because of the inability to remove the antibody from the culture medium and because of its ability to inhibit the subsequent binding of NKCF to target cells.

Since the majority of NK-inhibitory agents tested inhibited production and/or release of NKCF, this supports the concept that these NKCF-related processes are key steps in NK activity. These observations also indicate that binding to target cells is not sufficient to activate NK cells, and subsequent postbinding events are necessary for initiation of the lytic process. This hypothesis has been substantiated further by Wright and Bonavida (11), who identified NK-resistant YAC variants that can bind NKCF and are susceptible to lysis by NKCF, but lack the ability to stimulate production and/or release of NKCF.

It is of interest that of all the inhibitory agents tested, only phosphorylated mannose and antibody to LGL granules inhibited the binding of NKCF to target cells. One would predict that antibodies to LGL granules would inhibit the activity of cytotoxic molecules after their release from the effector cells and prior to effective interactions with targets. The inhibition of binding of NKCF by mannose-$PO_4$ also suggests that a carbohydrate-dependent interaction is involved in some way in the binding of NKCF to target cells. This observation is consistent with previous hypotheses regarding the nature of the NKCF receptor on the surface of target cells (7,8,12,13). Further elucidation of the exact chemical nature of the NKCF receptor must await binding studies performed with radiolabeled pure or recombinant NKCF.

## 2.2. Biochemical Characterization of Purified NKCF

In an attempt to determine the molecular weight of NKCF and to begin purification efforts, NKCF was produced in the presence of $^3$H-arginine. Based on size separation, using high-performance liquid chromatography at neutral pH on a molecular sizing column, NKCF activity was observed in the molecular weight range between 18 and 40 $K_d$ (13), with peaks of activity usually seen at approximately 20 and 40 $K_d$. These results suggest the possibility of polymerization of a 20-$K_d$ subunit (13,15). In addition, NKCF activity was consistently found in the void volume (e.g., >300 $K_d$), indicating some high molecular weight aggregates of NKCF.

The above purification methodology provides an approach for the further purification of NKCF and use of radiolabeled factors for subsequent binding studies and/or analysis of the mode of action of NKCF. Preliminary studies with partially purified NKCF indicate that partially purified factor produces an accelerated level of lysis, detected as early as 6 h (12). These results indicate that one reason for the slow rate of lysis of NKCF may be the purity of the factor. Therefore, more highly purified factors may minimize the differences that exist between the kinetics of lysis by intact NK cells versus NKCF.

## 2.3. Relationship of NKCF to Other Cytotoxic or Cytostatic Effectors

In recent years, considerable interest has been centered on a number of cytotoxic and cytostatic proteins (e.g., interferons, TNF, LT) isolated from activated leukocyte populations (17–22). Recently, the availability of an increasing number of genetically engineered homogeneous recombinant molecules with either cytostatic or cytolytic activity, and monoclonal and/or polyclonal antibodies against these defined proteins, has made it possible to analyze the role of these factors in the various forms of cell-mediated cytotoxicity. Our studies (12,13) have focused on the possible relationship of such defined cytotoxic molecules to NKCF and/or granule cytolysin, and on their possible involvement in the cytolytic and/or cytostatic activity of NK cells or other natural effector cells. Particular emphasis has been placed on the possible relationship of lymphotoxin (LT) or tumor necrosis factor (TNF) to NKCF (23).

Lymphotoxin was initially derived from cell supernatants of antigen- or mitogen-stimulated lymphocytes and has been reported to have tumoricidal or cytostatic activity *in situ* (19). TNF has also been shown to have cytostatic or cytolytic activity in vitro against a narrower range of transformed cell lines, whereas most normal cells have been resistant to its effects (20–22).

When comparisons were made between the characteristics of NK activity, ADCC, or cytotoxicity by NKCF, considerable differences were seen. Lymphotoxin and TNF have potent activity against a much narrower range of target cells than NK cells and NKCF, with L-929 being perhaps the most susceptible target available to both recombinant cytokines. We have found that the majority of NK- or NKCF-susceptible human and mouse targets are not susceptible to growth inhibition or cytolysis by either of the recombinant LT or TNF molecules (23). In addition to target susceptibility, the cells producing these various factors and the stimuli needed to induce them vary considerably. Although TNF and LT may be produced by NK cells, these factors are mainly produced by monocyte or B lineage cells, respectively.

In regard to the mechanism of their effects on target cells, LT and TNF also appear to be distinct from NKCF or LGL granule cytolysin. For example, whereas mannose-$PO_4$ inhibits lysis of targets by NK cells and NKCF (12,13), it had no effect on the activity of either LT or TNF (23).

It is possible that NKCF is not one factor, but a functional activity that is the sum of many factors acting synergistically. In order to test this, mixtures of various cytolytic factors were tested. NKCF activity could not be mimicked by various combinations of LT, TNF, and interferon-α or -γ. Therefore, based on the information available, it seems very unlikely that LT, TNF, or interferon, or a combination of these molecules, are involved in the cytotoxic activity mediated by NKCF.

The above results strongly suggested a divergence between NKCF and LT or TNF. In addition the possible role of LT or TNF as a mediator of NK cell activity against the NK-susceptible target cells, K562 or YAC-1 seems unlikely. To more directly examine the possible relationship of the factors and to determine their possible role in NK cell-mediated cytotoxicity, studies have been performed with antibodies produced against recombinant human LT and TNF. A summary of these results is presented in Table 3. The antibodies to LT or TNF strongly inhibited the cytotoxicity by the homologous protein against L-929 cells. In contrast, these antibodies

Table 3
Effects of Antibodies to LT, TNF, or LGL Granules on Cytolysis by
Effector Cells or Cytotoxic Molecules[a]

| Antibody added to assay | Effectors | | | | | |
|---|---|---|---|---|---|---|
| | PBL or LGL | PBL or LGL | NKCF | Granules | LT | TNF |
| | Targets | | | | | |
| | K562[b] | Ab + RLmale1 (ADCC) | K562 | YAC-1 | L-929 | L-929 |
| Rabbit anti-rat LGL granules | ↓ | ↓ | ↓ | ↓ | — | — |
| Monoclonal anti-recombinant human LT | — | — | — | — | ↓ | — |
| Monoclonal or rabbit antirecombinant human TNF | — | — | — | — | — | ↓ |

[a]From refs. (13) and (23).
[b]↓ = significant inhibition of cytolysis; — = no significant effect.

had no detectable effects on the cytotoxicity induced by NKCF or on NK or ADCC activities. For comparison, the effects of antibodies to LGL granules (16) were examined in the same experiments. The anti-granule antibody, as expected, inhibited the cytotoxicity by NKCF and also inhibited NK and ADCC activities, whereas it had no detectable effects on the activity of either LT or TNF. Thus, these results supported the conclusion that NKCF and LGL granule cytolysin are distinct from LT or TNF, and their activity does not depend on the presence of either LT or TNF in the assay. Further, cellular ADCC or NK activity against the prototype target cells does not appear to be mediated by, or dependent on, either LT or TNF since inclusion of antibodies to LT and TNF had no effect on these activities.

It was also of interest to determine the possible relationship of NKCF to leukoregulin, a molecule with cytostatic activity that has been reported to be induced from human PBL by incubation with lectins (24). In contrast, leukoregulin is induced by tumor cells and is highly cytostatic for a number of cells like the mouse lymphoma, MBL2, which has little sensitivity to lysis by human NK cells. As an additional approach to evaluate the possible relationships between NKCF and leukoregulin, the effects of mannose-6-phosphate and antibodies against rat LGL granules were tested.

These reagents, as discussed above, strongly inhibited NKCF, but had no effect on the ability of leukoregulin to mediate growth inhibitory effects on a variety of targets (data not shown) (23).

The availability of antibodies to recombinant LT and TNF allowed for an examination of the possible relationship of these molecules to leukoregulin. No inhibition of cytostasis by leukoregulin was observed, indicating that LT or TNF are not involved in this cytotoxic activity (23).

Therefore, it appears that NKCF is distinct from leukoregulin, LT, or TNF. Further studies are needed to confirm the biochemical identity of NKCF and to determine whether these latter factors are produced by NK cells.

## 3. Discussion

Since the original descriptions of human and mouse NKCF (7–11), several lines of evidence have suggested that this factor might be involved in the mechanism of lysis by NK cells. Studies by Wright et al. (8) and Farram et al. (10) have indicated that NKCF is released during coculture of NK-sensitive target cells with NK cells. Although such evidence is consistent with the hypothesis that NKCF is involved in lysis by human NK cells, little or no information about the actual mechanism of lysis by human NKCF or its relationship to the mechanism of lysis by NK cells has been reported.

First, if human NKCF plays a direct role in a mechanism of cytotoxicity by NK cells, it would be predicted that it would be produced and released by human LGL. Our experiments certainly confirm previous reports that highly purified LGL are responsible for production of NKCF, as well as for NK activity (10).

Second, release of NKCF should be selectively triggered by NK-susceptible targets. Our results (12,13) have shown that production of NKCF was elicited mainly by NK-susceptible target cells, with NK-insusceptible targets inducing little or no NKCF production. Thus, it is possible that the recognition receptors leading to release of NKCF and to binding to susceptible target cells may be very similar or identical.

Studies have indicated that carbohydrate moieties are involved in some postbinding events of cell-mediated lysis (25–27). The present results are consistent with the hypothesis that inhibition of NK activity by phosphorylated sugars occurs by blocking the uptake of NKCF. In addition, the pattern of inhibition of NKCF binding by various sugars was similar to that seen in studies of inhibition of lysis by intact LGL (e.g., mannose-6-phosphate inhibited, whereas nonphosphorylated mannose or phosphorylated fructose did not). These parallel patterns of inhibition by sugars of NK-mediated lysis and of NKCF are consistent with the hypothesis that NKCF is involved in the mechanism of lysis by NK cells. The concept that a sugar-related site is involved in NKCF binding was also supported by the observation that tunicamycin-treated target cells, whose glycosylation of surface lipoproteins or glycoproteins was blocked, demonstrate deficient binding or subsequent lysis of NKCF (*12*). These results indicate that glycosylated materials on the surface of the target are somehow required for lysis by NKCF.

Wright and Bonavida have previously demonstrated removal of the factor by NK-susceptible targets (*7–9*). Our experiments extend these results, however, by indicating that not only is NKCF activity lost upon incubation with NK-susceptible targets, but this interaction leads to subsequent lysis. This rules out the possibility that loss of NKCF activity is caused entirely by inactivation of NKCF by the targets, since factor-independent lysis was seen. Our results also demonstrated that binding occurs gradually, with optimal binding of NKCF occurring by 6 h. After this point, target cells were already programmed for subsequent lysis, with lysis occurring at the same kinetics as those seen in the continued presence of NKCF. In contrast to the rapid killing seen by NK cells, which is detected in short-term Cr-release assays, high levels of NKCF lysis required 48 h with $^{111}$In-labeled targets or 24 h with $^{51}$Cr-labeled targets. These results are consistent with previous results obtained in both the mouse and human (*7–11*). One likely explanation for this slow cytotoxicity is that the rate of lysis of targets is largely controlled by the concentration of available factor.

The events that occur after initial binding of NKCF to targets still remain obscure. The experiments performed here, however, may provide new insights to some of the interactions with NKCF and targets. Inhibition of NKCF by phosphorylated sugars is consistent with the concept that NKCF may recognize sugars on the surface of target cells or, alternatively, may bind to target cells via a receptor in the form of a glycoprotein or glycolipid. Our results with tunicamycin are consistent with the binding of NKCF to glycosylated residues on the target cells.

Although the relationship between the mechanisms of lysis of target cells by NKCF and by NK cells requires further investigation, the production of NKCF under serum-free conditions and further purification of this factor should facilitate its biochemical characterization and help to provide information on mechanisms of lysis by NK cells and NKCF.

# References

1. Herberman, R. B., ed. *NK Cells and Other Natural Effector Cells* Academic, New York (1982).
2. Timonen, T., Ortaldo, J. R., and Herberman, R. B. *J. Exp. Med.* **153**, 569–582 (1981).
3. Reynolds, C. W., Timonen, T., and Herberman, R. B. *J. Immunol.* **127**, 282–287 (1981).
4. Roder, J. C. and Haliotis, T., in *Natural Cell-Mediated Immunity Against Tumors* (Herberman, R. B., ed.) pp. 379–390, Academic, New York (1980).
5. Quan, P. C., Ishizaka, T., and Bloom, B. R. *J. Immunol.* **128**, 1786–1791 (1982).
6. Henney, C. S. *Transplant. Rev.* **17**, 37–52 (1973).
7. Wright, S. C. and Bonavida, B. *J. Immunol.* **126**, 1516–1521 (1981).
8. Wright, S. C. and Bonavida, B. *J. Immunol.* **129**, 433–439 (1982).
9. Wright, S. C., Weitzen, M. L., Kahle, R., Granger, G. A., and Bonavida, B. *J. Immunol.* **130**, 2479–2483 (1983).
10. Farram, E. and Targan, S. R. *J. Immunol.* **130**, 1252–1261 (1983).
11. Wright, S. and Bonavida, B. *Proc. Natl. Acad. Sci. USA* **80**(6), 1688–1692 (1983).
12. Blanca, I., Herberman, R. B., and Ortaldo, J. R. *Natl. Immun. Cell Growth Reg.* **4**, 48–59 (1985).
13. Ortaldo, J. R., Blanca, I., and Herberman, R. B., in *Mechanisms of Cell-Mediated Cytotoxicity* (Henkart, P. and Martz, E., eds.) pp. 203–218, Plenum, New York (1985).
14. Wright, S. C. and Bonavida, B. *J. Immunol.* **130**, 2960–2964 (1983).
15. Wright, S. C., Wilber, S. M., and Bonavida, B., in *Mechanisms of Cell-Mediated Cytotoxicity* vol. II (Henkart, P. and Martz, E., eds.) pp. 179–200, Plenum, New York (1985).
16. Reynolds, C. W., Reichardt, D., Henkart, M., Millard, P., and Henkart, P. *J. Exp. Med.* (submitted).
17. Deem, R. L. and Targan, S. R. *J. Immunol.* **133**, 72–77 (1984).
18. Hiserodt, J. C., Britvan, L. J., and Targan, S. R. *J. Immunol.* **131**, 2710–2713 (1983).
19. Granger, G. A., Shacks, S. J., Williams, T. W., and Kolb, W. P. *Nature* **221**, 1155–1161 (1969).
20. Mathews, N. and Watkins, J. F. *Br. J. Cancer* **38**, 302–309 (1978).
21. Carswell, E. A., Old, L. J., Kassel, R. L., Green, S., Fiore, N., and Williamson, B. *Proc. Natl. Acad. Sci. USA* **72**, 3666–3670 (1975).
22. Aggarwal, B. B., Kohr. Hass, P. E., Moffat, B., Spencer, S. A., Henzel, W. J., Bringman, T. S., Hedwin, G. E., Goeddel, D. V., and Harkins, R. N. *J. Biol. Chem.* **260**, 2345–2354 (1985).
23. Sayers, T. J., Ransom, J. R., Denn, A. C., III, Herberman, R. B., and Ortaldo, J. R. *J. Immunol.* **137**, 385–390 (1986).

24. Ransom, J. H., Evans, C. H., McCabe, R. P., Pomato, N., Heinbaugh, J. A., Chin, M., and Hanna, M. G., Jr. *Cancer Res.* **45**, 851–862 (1985).
25. Forbes, J. T. and Oeltman, T. N., in *NK Cells and Other Natural Effector Cells* (Herberman, R. B., ed.) pp. 977–982, Academic, New York (1982).
26. Ortaldo, J. R., Timonen, T. T., and Herberman, R. B. *Clin. Immunol. Immunopathol.* **31**(3), 439–444 (1984).
27. Stutman, O., Dien, P., Wisum, E., and Lattime, E. C. *Proc. Natl. Acad. Sci. USA* **77**, 2895–2898 (1980).

# Natural Killer Cell Cytotoxic Factor

RICHARD L. DEEM and STEPHAN R. TARGAN

## 1. Introduction

Natural killer cell cytotoxic factor (NKCF) has been biologically defined as a soluble cytotoxic factor produced by natural killer (NK) cells that can lyse NK-sensitive targets. This factor was initially described by Wright and Bonavida (*1*) and has been implicated as the lytic factor responsible for NK cell-mediated cytotoxicity (*1-9*). Although NKCF demonstrates the same target cell specificity of lysis as NK cells (*1-4*), the rate of lysis is extremely slow, requiring 8–12 h, compared to less than 2 h for NK cell-mediated cytotoxicity (*1,4*). NKCF-mediated lysis is also very sensitive to pharmacologic perturbations of target cell functions (*10,11*), whereas NK cell-mediated cytotoxicity is rarely affected by pharmacologic modulation of target cells. Recently, NKCF generation has been associated with the presence of mycoplasma in stimulator cell lines (*12*). The presence of mycoplasma cannot account for all NKCF activity, however, since NKCF can be generated by lectin stimulation of effector cells (*9*).

More recently, cytolysin, a 60 kdalton cytolytic protein isolated from rat large granular lymphocyte (LGL) tumors has been described as the lytic factor responsible for NK cell-mediated cytotoxicity (*13*). The lytic action of cytolysin is $Ca^{2+}$ dependent (*14*), occurs within minutes (*14*), and is relatively target cell nonspecific (*13-15*). In a recent preliminary report, antibody to cytolysin has been reported to inhibit the action of NKCF (*16*). The relationship between cytolysin and NKCF and their role in NK cell-mediated cytotoxicity remains to be determined.

In addition to their ability to produce NKCF, NK cells have been implicated in the secretion of the cytotoxic lymphokines lymphotoxin (LT), tumor necrosis factor (TNF), and leukoregulin (LR) (*17-19*). All of these studies, however, have used at best only partially purified populations of effector cells and have used numerous methods of generation of these factors (using different stimulator lines and/or chemical activators for various periods of time). Until the method of generation of NKCF is standardized, comparison of the properties of these factors is difficult to interpret. It is interesting to note that NKCF, LT, and TNF have similar molecular weights (9,20–22). In addition, both NKCF and TNF are inhibited by monoclonal antibodies to TNF (18). Thus, it appears that these factors may be identical or closely related molecules.

Besides its role in NK cell-mediated cytotoxicity, NKCF has been implicated as a possible immunoregulatory molecule. It has been shown to be able to inhibit bone marrow colony formation (22) and lymphoblastoid antibody production (23) in vitro. Reduced NKCF production has also been correlated with decreased NK and antibody-dependent cellular cytotoxicity (ADCC) function in neonates (24) and in the immune disorder systemic lupus erythematous (25).

## 2. Biology of NKCF

### 2.1. Generation of NKCF

NKCF has been generated in a number of animal systems, mouse (3), rat (3), and human (3,4,20), by incubation with numerous stimulator cells and lectins for various periods of time. The supernatant collected from these cultures has been termed NKCF and is selectively lytic for NK-sensitive cell lines (1–5).

### 2.1.1. Phenotypes of Effector Cells

The generation of NKCF from murine effector cells was shown to be caused by a population of cells that were asialo-$GM_1^+$ and Thy-1.2$^-$, demonstrating that these cells were probably NK cells (5). These observations were extended to human NKCF using Percoll density gradients. Large granular lymphocytes (LGL), the population of human lymphocytes containing the NK population, were shown to be responsible for the generation of NKCF activity (2,4,20). Percoll gradients, however, copurify many other large lymphocytes, such as lymphoblastoid B-cells (M. Brogan, F. Shanahan, and S. Targan, unpublished data). Evidence from this laboratory indicates that non-NK cells also produce factors with lytic potential for NK-sensitive targets. We have used monoclonal antibodies to purify peripheral blood lymphocytes (PBL) subpopulations and have found that NKCF-like activity (using both L-929 and U-937 targets) can be generated from both NKH-1$^+$ and NKH-1$^-$ subpopulations (Deem and Targan, unpublished data).

## 2.1.2. Target Cell Requirements

NK-sensitivity appears to have little or no effect upon the ability of target cell lines to stimulate release of NKCF. Thus, both NK-sensitive lines, U-937, MOLT-4, K562, and HSB-2, and NK-resistant lines, W1-L2 and SGL-1, were able to stimulate release of NKCF from murine effector cells (3). Another study found that NK-sensitive lines, K562 and MOLT-4, but not NK-resistant lines, Raji and YAC-1, were able to stimulate generation of NKCF from human LGL (4). NKCF can also be produced by coculture of effector cells with lectins, such as concanavalin A (Con A) and phytohemagglutinin (PHA) (1,3) or even occasionally without any stimulus (3).

## 2.1.3. Effects of Interferon

Since interferon (IFN) pretreatment of effector cells enhanced NK cell-mediated cytotoxicity, it was expected that IFN pretreatment should also enhance generation of NKCF. Wright and Bonavida found that IFN did increase levels of NKCF generated, and the production of this additional activity required *de novo* protein synthesis (6). It was also noted, however, that IFN by itself enhanced the activity of NKCF, and that supernatants high in IFN activity also possessed high NKCF activity (7). IFN pretreatment of target cells results in reduced susceptibility to NK lysis, and likewise, resulted in a decreased ability of these targets to stimulate release of NKCF (7).

## 2.1.4. Calcium and Magnesium Requirements

Since direct NK cytotoxicity requires $Mg^{2+}$ (for conjugate formation) and $Ca^{2+}$ (for the programming stage), it was hypothesized that NKCF generation would also require the presence of these ions. NKCF generation in HBSS deficient in $Ca^{2+}$ and $Mg^{2+}$ was significantly reduced and only restored by addition of both of these ions to the deficient media (4).

## 2.1.5. Kinetics of NKCF Generation

The kinetics of generation of NKCF appear to coincide approximately with the kinetics of lysis by NK cells. Thus, for human PBLs, maximum levels of NKCF are generated after a period of incubation of 6 h (2,4). In the murine system, generation of NKCF appears to require a longer incubation period (20 h) (5).

## 2.2. NKCF Receptor

The probable existence of an NKCF receptor was first demonstrated by Wright and Bonavida. NK-sensitive target cells were shown to absorb NKCF activity better than NK-resistant targets (5). The absorption of activity occurred at 4, 25, or 37°C and required only a 30-min incubation period (5,26).

### 2.2.1. Target Cell Differences and Susceptibility

Murine NKCF specificity was demonstrated by the ability of NKCF to lyse the NK-sensitive targets YAC-1 and RL(male)1, but not the NK-insensitive targets P815, EL-4, AKSL2, and LA-6 (1). In addition, it was shown that YAC-1 targets were better able to absorb NKCF activity than EL-4 and AKSL2 targets (5). Similar results were seen with NKCF derived from human lymphocytes. Thus, the NK-sensitive target cell lines, K562 and MOLT-4, were lysed by human NKCF, and the NK-resistant lines, Raji, YAC-1, EL-4, and W1-L2, were unaffected by human NKCF (2,4). Both MOLT-4 and K562 targets were able to absorb human NKCF activity, whereas IM-9 and Raji cells were unable to absorb any NKCF activity (4). It appeared from these results that target cell resistance to NKCF and possibly direct NK activity might be caused by reduced or absent NKCF receptors. In addition, YAC-1 clones selected for resistance to NKCF were also resistant to direct NK lysis and unable to absorb NKCF activity, suggesting that they lacked a receptor for NKCF (8).

### 2.2.2. Effects of Monosaccharides and Tunicamycin

The NKCF receptor appears to be a mannose-6-phosphate receptor, since it can be inhibited by mannose-6-phosphate (9,20), fructose-6-phosphate (9), and $\alpha$-methyl-D-mannoside (9). Very high concentrations (25–50 m$M$) of these monosaccharides, however, are required for inhibition of NKCF lysis (9,20) compared to the concentrations (less than 10 m$M$) required for inhibition of lysosomal enzyme uptake (27). In addition, there are conflicting results regarding the ability of one of these monosaccharides (fructose-6-phosphate) to inhibit NKCF binding (9,20).

Experiments using tunicamycin have indicated that the NKCF receptor is probably a glycoprotein. Pretreatment of K562 target cells for 18 h with tunicamycin resulted in decreased susceptibility of these targets to lysis by NKCF and a decreased ability to absorb the factor (20). Since it was not noted whether NKCF absorptions were done at 37 or 4°C, it is possible that the inhibition of NKCF absorption could be caused by inhibition of endocytosis.

### 2.2.3. Effects of Low pH

Since it had been shown that the NKCF receptor might be a mannose-6-phosphate receptor, and lysosomal enzymes can be dissociated from this receptor at low pH (27), it was thought that low pH might also affect binding of NKCF to its receptor. Although pH values between 5 and 6 had no effect upon NKCF directly, when the pH of an NKCF assay was lowered below 6.5, lysis was inhibited (Table 1). Inhibition of lysis occurred, however, only when the pH was lowered soon after addition of NKCF to the target cells. Thus, although lysis was inhibited 65% when the pH was lowered immediately after addition of NKCF, this inhibition was reduced to 32% only 30 min later, and there was no effect after 4 h (Table 1). These results suggested that low pH was affecting an early stage of NKCF-mediated lysis, probably the NKCF-binding stage.

Table 1
Effect of Low pH upon NKCF and NKCF Lysis

| pH | NKCF pretreatment[a] | pH in NKCF assay[b] | pH pulse 7.5 to 6.0[c] | |
|---|---|---|---|---|
| | | | Time, h | Cytotoxicity, % |
| 8.0 | — | $15 \pm 1$ | 0 | $26 \pm 3$ |
| 7.5 | $59 \pm 3$ | $22 \pm 2$ | 0.5 | $50 \pm 16$ |
| 7.0 | — | $14 \pm 1$ | 1 | $54 \pm 13$ |
| 6.5 | — | $10 \pm 1$ | 2 | $61 \pm 2$ |
| 6.0 | $64 \pm 3$ | $2 \pm 1$ | 4 | $70 \pm 14$ |
| 5.5 | — | $0 \pm 0$ | 24 | $74 \pm 6$ |
| 5.0 | $64 \pm 1$ | — | | |

[a]Mean $\pm$ SD, expressed as $LU_{40}$, the reciprocal dilution of NKCF that resulted in lysis of 40% of L-929 target cells. The pH of NKCF dilutions was adjusted with $10N$ HCl or $5N$ NaOH, incubated 8 h at 37°C, and dialyzed for 24 h against PBS, pH 7.4. The NKCF was diluted and added to L-929 target cells for 18 h at 37°C.

[b]Mean $\pm$ SD expressed as $LU_{30}$, the reciprocal dilution of NKCF that resulted in lysis of 30% of L-929 target cells. The pH of NKCF dilutions was adjusted with $10N$ HCl or $5N$ NaOH and added to L-929 target cells for 18 h at 37°C.

[c]Mean $\pm$ SD NKCF (1:20 dilution) was added to L-929 target cells at 37°C and at times indicated, the pH was lowered from 7.5 to 6.0 with $10N$ HCl. All wells were harvested 24 h after addition of NKCF.

To test whether low pH was affecting binding of NKCF to its receptor, pH adjusted NKCF was added to L-929 target cells for various lengths of time at 4°C, washed three times, and incubated for 18 h in the presence of 10 $\mu M$ glutaraldehyde. Less than 10% lysis occurred when NKCF was preincubated with the targets at pH 5.5, compared to over 60% lysis when NKCF was preincubated with targets at pH 7.5 (Table 2). To determine if NKCF could be dissociated from target cells by low pH, NKCF was bound to L-929 target cells for 30–60 min at 4°C, followed by removal of NKCF and addition of RPMI adjusted to either pH 7.5 or 5.5 for 4 h. Following this pH pulse, the target cells were washed and incubated at pH 7.4 for 18 h at 37°C. The low pH pulse resulted in a 60–70% reduction of lytic units, probably because of dissociation of membrane-bound NKCF by low pH (Table 3). Thus, it appears that NKCF–receptor bind-

Table 2
Effect of Low pH upon NKCF Binding

| Time NKCF bound, h | Cytotoxicity[a], % | |
| --- | --- | --- |
| | pH 5.5 | pH 7.5 |
| 1 | 2 ± 4 | 67 ± 4 |
| 2 | 3 ± 3 | 77 ± 4 |
| 3 | −3 ± 1 | 62 ± 2 |
| 4 | 4 ± 3 | 89 ± 1 |
| 5 | 5 ± 3 | 82 ± 4 |
| 6 | 6 ± 3 | 79 ± 2 |
| 7 | 5 ± 4 | 72 ± 1 |

[a]Mean ± SD, the pH of NKCF (diluted 1:20) was adjusted with 10$N$ HCl and added to L-929 target cells at 4°C followed by removal of unbound NKCF, three washings with RPMI, and addition to 10 $\mu M$ glutaraldehyde for 18 h at 37°C.

ing is pH sensitive, since it can be blocked by pH below 6 or, once bound, can be dissociated by low pH. These data, together with the ability of mannose-6-phosphate and tunicamycin to block NKCF binding, suggest that the NKCF receptor may be similar or identical to receptors for lysosomal enzymes.

Table 3
Effect of Low pH upon NKCF Bound to L-929 Target Cells

| Time NKCF bound, min | pH Pulse | NKCF dilution[a] | | | LU$_{30}$[b] |
| --- | --- | --- | --- | --- | --- |
| | | 1:5 | 1:10 | 1:20 | |
| 60 | 7.5 | 71 ± 4 | 61 ± 3 | 39 ± 3 | 32 ± 10 (0) |
| 60 | 5.5 | 46 ± 4 | 33 ± 2 | 22 ± 7 | 12 ± 1 (63) |
| 30 | 7.5 | 58 ± 4 | 44 ± 1 | 25 ± 2 | 17 ± 1 (0) |
| 30 | 5.5 | 29 ± 4 | 19 ± 3 | 9 ± 4 | 5 ± 1 (71) |

[a]Mean % cytotoxicity ± SD, NKCF (diluted 1:20, pH 7.5) was added to L-929 target cells at 4°C followed by removal of unbound NKCF, three washings with RPMI, and addition of RPMI at pH 7.5 or adjusted to pH 5.0 with 10$N$ HCl for 4 h at 4°C. Following this pH pulse, L-929 were washed twice and 10 $\mu M$ glutaraldehyde, pH 7.5 was added for 18 h at 37°C.
[b]Mean ± SD, LU$_{30}$ is the reciprocal dilution of NKCF that results in lysis of 30% of L-929 target cells. Percent inhibition is enclosed in parenthesis.

## 2.3. NKCF as an Immunoregulatory Factor

NK cells and supernatants of mixed cultures of human NK effectors and K562 target cells have been shown to inhibit bone marrow hematopoietic colonies in vitro (28). The supernatants, termed NK cell-derived colony inhibiting activity (NK-CIA), were found to be identical to NKCF with regard to lytic potential for and absorption by NKCF-sensitive targets, inhibition by D-mannose-6-phosphate, and enhancement by IFN (22). In addition, the NKCF and NK-CIA activities coeluted on both gel filtration and ion exchange columns (22).

Not only does NKCF inhibit cell proliferation, but there is evidence that it can effect some immunological functions. Targan et al. found that NKCF could suppress IgG-tetanus production from human lymphoblastoid cells (23). Cold target competition and cold target absorption studies showed that the NKCF-binding target, K562, but not the NKCF-nonbinding target, Raji, was able to reverse this effect, suggesting that NKCF was responsible for this inhibition (23). Thus, it appears that NKCF may act as an immunoregulatory mediator to affect cell function and proliferation.

## 3. Biochemistry of NKCF

Since NKCF has not been purified, its biochemical nature remains largely unknown. Early studies indicated that it was nondialyzable, suggesting a molecular weight greater than 12 kdalton, and inactivated by high temperatures (100°C for 15 min), indicating its proteinaceous nature (1). Recent studies have indicated partial or total homology with the cytotoxic lymphokines TNF and LT (9,18,20–22).

### 3.1. Molecular Weights

HPLC gel filtration chromatography has indicated that NKCF preparations contain lytic molecules in the molecular weight ranges of 20–30 kdalton (9) or 20–40 kdalton (20). In addition, some NKCF activity has been found at higher molecular weights of 50–60 kdalton (29) and greater than 300 kdalton (20), indicating that these molecules may form aggregates. FPLC gel filtration chromatography of NK-CIA supernatants, which were shown to be identical to NKCF, revealed the peak of lytic activity at 17 kdalton. These molecular weights are similar to those observed for LT (21) and TNF (30).

### 3.2. Susceptibility to Chemical Attack and pH

Studies have shown that reducing and alkylating agents irreversibly inhibit NKCF activity, suggesting that disulfide bonds may be required for expression of its lytic potential (9). In addition, oxidation of NKCF supernatants with sodium periodate abrogates its lytic activity, suggesting that NKCF may possess carbohydrate moieties, essential for lysis (9). NKCF is not effected by protease inhibitors, such as $N\alpha$-p-tosyl-L-lysine chloromethyl ketone (TLCK), $N$-tosyl-L-phenylalanine chloromethyl ketone (TPCK), and $N$-acetyl-L-tyrosine ethyl ester (ATEE) (*9,10*), which indicates that it may not have proteolytic activity. NKCF is irreversibly inactivated, however, by glutaraldehyde, a protein crosslinking agent (*5*), and is susceptible to the effects of low pH (*9*).

### 3.3. Temperature Stability

NKCF appears to be relatively temperature stable. At $-20\,°C$ it is stable for weeks (*2*) to months (*4*), and at $37\,°C$ it is stable for at least 24 h (*4*). It is also stable at $56\,°C$ for several hours (*2*), but is inactivated in minutes at $60\,°C$ and above (*4*).

### 3.4. Susceptibility to Enzymatic Attack

NKCF activity is sensitive to the action of the proteolytic enzymes trypsin (*9,26*) and chymotrypsin (*26*). This inhibition could be eliminated by treatment of NKCF with these enzymes in the presence of soy bean trypsin inhibitor (*26*). NKCF is not sensitive to neuraminidase (*9*), suggesting that sialic acid residues are not necessary for activity.

## 4. Mechanism of Action of NKCF

The mechanism of action of NKCF remains the least studied aspect of this cytotoxic lymphokine. Early studies by Wright and Bonavida examined target specificity for generation of NKCF and susceptibility of target cells to lysis. From these studies it was apparent that NKCF first bound to a receptor on a susceptible target cell (*5,8*). Binding of NKCF was rapid (1 h), even at low temperatures (*26*). Following binding was a period (8–12 h) during which little appeared to be happening to the target cell. Target cell lysis began after this and continued for 24–48 h (depending on the target cell) (*1,2,4,5,20*).

### 4.1. Kinetic Model for NKCF-Mediated Lysis

Since NKCF-mediated lysis involved a receptor on susceptible targets, it was hypothesized that membrane active compounds might inhibit the action of NKCF. We chose the protein crosslinking agent glutaraldehyde for further study. Low concentrations of glutaraldehyde (10–100 $\mu M$) did inhibit lysis when added concurrently or prior to the addition of NKCF (*31*). In addition, target cells pretreated with glutaraldehyde and washed were also resistant to the effects of NKCF. This resistance was caused by alteration of the NKCF receptor since glutaraldehyde-treated cold target cells (L-929 or K562) were not as effective cold target competitors. In addition, these pretreated cells were less able than untreated targets to absorb NKCF at 4 °C. Thus, the NKCF receptor could be chemically modified to prevent binding of NKCF (31).

In contrast to these observations, it was found that after NKCF became bound to the target cell, glutaraldehyde did not inhibit lysis, but instead, greatly enhanced the activity of NKCF (31). This enhancement occurred only during a critical period of time; 2–5 h after the addition of NKCF to the target cell. In addition to its ability to enhance the amount of lysis induced by NKCF, glutaraldehyde also enhanced the kinetics of lysis. Thus when glutaraldehyde was added 2 h after addition of NKCF, significant lysis occurred within 3 h, compared to 10 h without addition of glutaraldehyde (31). When added after this critical time, lysis was not affected, even though the actual lytic process did not begin until 10–12 h after addition of NKCF.

Thus, there appear to be at least four substages of NKCF-mediated lysis, as defined by glutaraldehyde modulation of the process. (1) The NKCF binding stage is blocked by alteration of the NKCF receptor; (2) The assembly/activation stage is enhanced by the action of glutaraldehyde; (3) The effector stage is unaffected by glutaraldehyde, although no cell lysis has occurred at this time; and (4) The lysis stage is also unaffected by glutaraldehyde.

## 4.2. Effects of Chemical Crosslinking Agents

In order to further analyze the mechanism by which glutaraldehyde enhanced lysis during the assembly/activation substage of NKCF-mediated lysis, several specific chemical crosslinking agents were chosen for study. Noncrosslinking aldehydes, butryaldehyde and valeraldehyde, had no effect upon NKCF-mediated lysis, demonstrating that enhancement of lysis was not caused merely by the presence of aldehyde functional groups (10). Monofunctional crosslinking aldehydes, formaldehyde and acetaldehyde, however, enhanced NKCF lysis slightly (19–35%), and bifunctional aldehydes, glutaraldehyde and malondialdehyde, enhanced NKCF lysis by greater than 100% (10). The more specific protein crosslinking agents, bis-imidates, dimethyl suberimidate, dimethyl pimelimidate, and dimethyl adipimidate, which react only with primary amino groups, also enhanced NKCF-mediated lysis by greater than 100%. Crosslinking lectins Con A and wheatgerm agglutinin, but not soy bean agglutinin and peanut agglutinin, enhanced NKCF lysis. Pretreatment of L-929 target cells with Con A prior to addition of NKCF also enhanced lysis, but this effect could be eliminated when α-methyl-D-mannoside was also added during the pretreatment period.

These results suggest that chemical crosslinking agents act to enhance NKCF-mediated lysis by crosslinking protein or glycoprotein molecules on the target cell membrane. These agents may enhance lysis by crosslinking the NKCF receptor, or by a generalized crosslinking of membrane proteins, resulting in enhanced uptake of the lytic factors.

### 4.3. Effects of Agents That Break Disulfide Bonds

Reagents that break disulfide bonds, such as 2-mercaptoethanol (2-ME) (5 m$M$) and dithiothrietol (DTT) (0.5 m$M$), inhibited NKCF lysis nearly completely when added concurrently with NKCF (10). Although these agents did not block binding of NKCF to its receptor, their ability to block lysis diminished rapidly after addition of NKCF (10). Thus, within 5 h after addition of NKCF, inhibition of lysis by 2-ME and DTT was reduced to less than half of that which occurred when these agents were added simultaneously with NKCF (10). Thus it appeared that agents that break disulfide bonds act in the early substages of NKCF lysis.

### 4.4. Effects of Inhibitors of Serine Proteases

Inhibitors of serine protease activity did not affect the activity of NKCF directly, but when added to NKCF assays, inhibited subsequent lysis (10). TLCK, an irreversible trypsin alkylating agent, and TPCK, an irreversible chymotrypsin alkylating agent, inhibited NKCF-mediated lysis greater than 50%. These agents also partially inhibited lysis when target cells were pretreated with these agents and washed, however, suggesting that at least part of their inhibitory activities might be caused by alkylation of the NKCF receptor or modification of the cell membrane. In contrast to these results, N$\alpha$-p-tosyl-L-lysine methyl ester (TLME), a reversible trypsin substrate inhibitor, had little or no effect upon NKCF-mediated lysis. Thus it appears likely that NKCF probably does not have trypsin- or chymotrypsin-like activities, although these activities may be required in the target cell for lysis to proceed.

### 4.5. Effects of Membrane Active Agents

Since cross-linking of the target cell membrane after addition of NKCF resulted in enhancement of lysis, it was hypothesized that the opposite effect, increasing membrane fluidity, might inhibit NKCF-mediated lysis. The neutral anesthetic benzyl alcohol was chosen for study, because of its specific fluidizing effect upon the lipid bilayer of biological membranes (32). Benzyl alcohol completely inhibited NKCF lysis, although it had no effect upon NKCF directly and had no effect when target cells were pre-treated with this agent and washed prior to addition of NKCF (*10*). Analysis of the kinetics of inhibition of NKCF lysis by benzyl alcohol indicated that this agent inhibited very late substages of lysis. Thus, even when added 8 h after addiction of NKCF, this agent completely inhibited lysis by NKCF. These results suggest that membrane fluidity plays a major role in the activity of NKCF.

## 4.6. Effects of Inhibitors of Receptor-Mediated Endocytosis

Previous studies (*10,11,31*) have shown that NKCF-mediated cytolysis can be divided into substages that are affected by various pharmacologic agents. In addition, NKCF-mediated lysis is a slow process (8–12 h are required before lysis begins) that is highly temperature dependent (*10*), suggesting that the target cell itself plays an active role during lysis. We examined the possibility that the NKCF lytic process requires active uptake of NKCF by the target cell. Since NKCF has not been purified, receptor-mediated endocytosis of NKCF can not be demonstrated directly. Receptor-mediated endocytosis is known to be influenced by several classes of pharmacologic agents, however, including metabolic inhibitors (*33,34*), microtubule inhibitors (*34,35*), calmodulin inhibitors (*33,35,36*), and lysomotropic agents (*33,34,36–40*). Since it had been shown that crosslinking of the target cell membrane influenced NKCF-mediated lysis (*31,40*), it was thought that other pharmacologic mediators that affect the membrane might affect NKCF lysis.

### 4.6.1. Effects of Metabolic Inhibitors

By reducing cellular ATP levels, metabolic inhibitors reduce the rate of receptor-mediated endocytosis, an energy-requiring process. We examined the effects of inhibitors of glycolysis [2-deoxy-D-glucose (2-DG) and fluoride] and inhibitors of electron transport [dinitrophenol (DNP) and cyanide] on the action of NKCF and a control toxin, *Pseudomonas* toxin A, known to act through receptor-mediated endocytosis. Two inhibitors, 2-DG and cyanide, inhibited both NKCF and *Pseudomonas* toxin activity by greater than 60% at concentrations that effectively reduced ATP levels of the L-929 target cells (ATP levels were reduced by 50% following a 2-h incubation period) (*41*). Both of these metabolic inhibitors have been shown to inhibit toxins that require endocytosis by the target cell for expression of toxicity. Cyanide (1 m*M*) has been shown to provide protection against the plant toxin abrin (*33*). Fluoride had little or no effect upon the activity of *Pseudomonas* toxin or NKCF at concentrations that were not toxic to the target cells. Fluoride (6 m$M$) has been previously shown to be unable to inhibit the action of *Pseudomonas* toxin (*42*), diphtheria toxin (*33*), and the plant toxins abrin, modeccin, and ricin (*33*). DNP provided L-929 target cells partial protection from the action of NKCF, but had no effect upon *Pseudomonas* toxin activity. Since NKCF and *Pseudomonas* toxin have different toxic effects, it is possible that inhibition of NKCF activity by DNP may be caused by inhibition of its specific toxic effect. DNP (0.5 m$N$), however, has been shown to partially inhibit the expression of diphtheria toxin effects against HEp-2 cells (*34*).

Metabolic inhibitors were added to L-929 target cells for various periods of time to determine how rapidly these agents reduced ATP levels. These experiments indicated that reduction of cellular ATP occurred rapidly, with 56–65% of maximal inhibition occurring within 2 h after addition of the agents (*41*). Since metabolic inhibition was rapid, addition of metabolic inhibitors to L-929 target cells at various times after addition of NKCF should indicate the approximate time during which these agents effectively inhibited NKCF activity. These experiments indicated that metabolic inhibitors were most effective during early and middle stages of the NKCF lytic process (*31*). Thus, 8 h after addition of NKCF (before measurable lysis), metabolic inhibition of NKCF-mediated cytolysis was reduced to approximately half of maximal inhibition.

Although metabolic inhibitors reduce endocytosis, the relationship between cellular ATP levels and the rate of endocytosis is complex and not completely predictable (*20*). Thus, although 2-DG inhibits intoxication by abrin, it has no inhibitory effect upon intoxication by modeccin, ricin, and diphtheria toxins (*33*). Likewise, DNP inhibits the action of diphtheria toxin (*34*), but not *Pseudomonas* toxin. Thus the ability of metabolic inhibitors to protect L-929 target cells from the activity of NKCF indicates that an active target cell process is probably required for completion of NKCF-mediated cytolysis, but does not rule out processes other than endocytosis.

### 4.6.2. Effects of Endocytosis Inhibitors

Cytochalasin B, an inhibitor of microtubules, has been shown to inhibit receptor-mediated endocytosis by affecting internalization of coated pits (*35,43*). This agent afforded L-929 cells partial protection from the action of NKCF (50% inhibition) and *Pseudomonas* toxin (24%) (*41*) and had been shown previously to reduce intoxication of HEp-2 cells by diphtheria toxin (*34*). Cytochalasin B can also affect membrane fluidity (*34*), however, which could account for the inhibition of NKCF activity (*10*).

Trifluroperazine (TFP), a calomodulin inhibitor, blocks receptor-mediated endocytosis by preventing clathrin coat formation (*35,36*). The action of both NKCF and *Pseudomonas* toxin was inhibited by greater than 50% by TFP (*41*). It has been shown previously that 25 $\mu M$ TFP inhibited the action of modeccin and diphtheria toxins (*33*).

### 4.6.3. Effects of Lysomotropic Agents

Lysomotropic amines are regarded as the most specific pharmacologic modulators of receptor-mediated endocytosis. These agents inhibit receptor-mediated endocytosis by blocking the action of the protein crosslinking enzyme transglutaminase (*37*) and by preventing recycling of receptors (*27,38*). In this study, three lysomotropic agents were chosen for examination; chloroquine, ammonium chloride, and dansylcadavarine. In addition, cadavarine was chosen as a control reagent, since it is similar in structure to dansylcadavarine, but has a slow rate of lysosomal uptake and reduced lysosomal inhibitory activity (*39*). All three lysomotropic agents tested inhibited both NKCF activity (by greater than 90% based upon lytic units or greater than 50% based upon percent cytotoxicity, $p < 0.001$) and the effects of *Pseudomonas* toxin (by greater than 50%), whereas the control reagent, cadavarine, had no effect upon NKCF lysis or *Pseudomonas* toxin activity (*41*). In previous studies, it has been shown that chloroquine (10–100 $\mu M$) inhibits the action of both *Pseudomonas* toxin (*42*) and diphtheria toxin (*33,35*). Dansylcadavarine (100 $\mu M$) has been shown to inhibit receptor–ligand clustering and internalization of $\alpha_2$-macroglobulin (*37*). In addition to its lysomotropic effects, chloroquine has been shown to inhibit protease activity and to increase membrane fluidity (*39*), both side effects of which have been shown to inhibit NKCF activity (*10*). Ammonium chloride has none of these side effects (*39*), however, and thus it is likely that the inhibitor effects of this agent are caused by inhibition of some stage of receptor-mediated endocytosis (i.e., receptor clustering and internalization or receptor recycling from the lysosome). Lysomotropic agents also increase the pH of endosomes and lysosomes by as much as 1.5 pH units, which reduces the activity of several lysosomal enzymes (*44*). The pH elevating properties of lysomotropic agents have been shown to inhibit the activity of diphtheria toxin by inactivating proteases that are required to cleave the toxin to produce the active fragment A (*45*). Thus, it is possible that lysomotropic agents might inhibit "activation" of NKCF once it enters the lysosome.

Since NKCF-mediated lysis is blocked by agents that inhibit the action of many protein synthesis inhibitory toxins, it was decided to examine the effects of NKCF on target cell protein synthesis. Target cell protein synthesis, cellular ATP levels, and the rate of DNA and RNA synthesis remained at control levels up until the time of cell death. Thus, the mechanism of action of NKCF remains to be determined, but does not involve inhibition of protein synthesis.

These results suggest that some stage of NKCF-mediated cytolysis requires active target cell participation for lysis to be completed. This target cell participation probably requires energy, since inhibitors of energy metabolism block NKCF lysis. In addition, an intact microtubule system seems to be necessary, since cytochalasin B also inhibits lysis. Inhibitors of receptor-mediated endocytosis, trifluoperazine and lysomotropic agents, block the action of NKCF, as has been shown for other protein toxins that must be endocytosed for their activities to be expressed. Thus, although not directly demonstrated, it seems likely that receptor-mediated endocytosis of NKCF is required for expression of toxicity.

## 5. Future Studies

The primary questions that need to be addressed concerning NKCF are whether it is the lytic factor responsible for direct NK cell-mediated lysis, or whether it is merely one of several lymphokines released by NK cells in response to a variety of stimuli. The answers to these questions will ultimately require biochemical purification, development of monoclonal antibodies, and tracking of this factor during the stages of the NK lytic process. Generally, the action of NKCF mirrors that seen in NK cell-mediated cytotoxicity. NK-sensitive targets are also more able to absorb NKCF activity and are better lysed by NKCF. Both NKCF-mediated cyto-toxicity and NK cell-mediated cytotoxicity are inhibited by phosphorylated monosaccharides, reducing agents, membrane active compounds, metabolic inhibitors, and inhibitors of receptor-mediated endocytosis. When com-paring the action of pharmacologic probes in NKCF-mediated lysis with NK cell-mediated cytotoxicity, it must be shown that the agent affects only the terminal stage of lysis, killer cell-independent lysis. For many of these studies, this has not been done. In addition, many of these agents have broad effects on NK cells and inhibit secretory and other processes unrelated to lysis. We have used the monoclonal antibody 13.3, which specifically inhibits the NK cell trigger mechanism of cell-mediated cytotoxicity (45), to further examine the role of NKCF in NK cell-mediated cytotoxicity. This antibody completely inhibited NK lysis by NKH-1[+] effector cells in an 18-h assay, but failed to inhibit generation of NKCF by these same cells during this same period of time (Deem and Targan, unpublished data). NKCF-mediated lysis is also unlike NK cell-mediated cytotoxicity in the kinetics of lysis and the requirement for active participation (probably in-volving endocytosis) of the target cell in its own death. In view of these data, we seriously question the role NKCF plays in NK cell-mediated cytotoxicity.

NKCF may exhibit regulatory functions involving cell proliferation and immune function, however. These activities have been demonstrated in vitro by its ability to inhibit bone marrow colony formation and antibody production by lymphoblastoid B-cells.

NKCF appears to be closely related to both LT and TNF. All three of these cytotoxic lymphokines have similar molecular weights and are produced by the same populations of lymphocytes. In addition, the cytotoxic activities of these factors are enhanced by the action of γIFN (*7,47,48*). Initial reports have suggested that NKCF activity is inhibited by antibody to TNF (*18,22*) or is not inhibited by antibody to TNF (*16,49*). NKCF may also be related to cytolysin, since its activity can be inhibited by anti-granule antisera (*16,20,49*). The relationship among these factors is complex and will require further biochemical characterization and studies utilizing more highly purified subpopulations of effector cells to clarify the nature and in vivo significance of NKCF.

## References

*1.* Wright, S. C. and Bonavida, B. *J. Immunol.* **126**, 1516–1521 (1981).

*2.* Wright, S. C., Weitzen, M. L., Kahle, R., Granger, G. A., and Bonavida, B. *J. Immunol.* **130**, 2479–2483 (1983).

*3.* Wright, S. C. and Bonavida, B. *J. Immunol.* **133**, 3415–3423 (1984).

*4.* Farram, E. and Targan, S. R. *J. Immunol.* **130**, 1252–1256 (1983).

*5.* Wright, S. C. and Bonavida, B. *J. Immunol.* **129**, 433–439 (1982).

*6.* Wright, S. C. and Bonavida, B. *J. Immunol.* **130**, 2960–2964 (1983).

*7.* Wright, S. C. and Bonavida, B. *J. Immunol.* **130**, 2965–2968 (1983).

*8.* Wright, S. C. and Bonavida, B. *Proc. Natl. Acad. Sci. USA* **80**, 1688–1692 (1983).

*9.* Wright, S. C. and Bonavida, B., in *Mechanisms of Cell-Mediated Cytotoxicity* vol. II (Henkart, P. and Martz, E., eds.) Plenum, New York (1985).

*10.* Deem, R. L. and Targan, S. R., in *Mechanisms of Cell-Mediated Cytotoxicity* II (Henkart, P. and Martz, E., eds.) Plenum, New York (1985).

*11.* Targan, S. R. and Deem, R. L., in *Natural Cell-Mediated Immunity* (Herberman, R., ed.) Academic, New York (1985).

*12.* Wayner, E. A. and Brooks, C. G. *J. Immunol.* **132**, 2135–2142 (1984).

*13.* Millard, P. J., Henkart, M. P., Reynolds, C. W., and Henkart, P. A. *J. Immunol.* **132**, 3197–3204 (1984).

*14.* Henkart, P. A., Millard, P. J., Reynolds, C. W., and Henkart, M. P. *J. Exp. Med.* **160**, 75–93 (1984).

*15.* Blumenthal, R., Millard, P. J., Henkart, M. P., Reynolds, C. W., and Henkart, P. A. *Proc. Natl. Acad. Sci. USA* **81**, 5551–5555 (1984).

*16.* Ortaldo, J. R., Palladino, M., Sayers, T., Denn, A. C., Shepard, M., and Herberman, R. B. *J. Leuk. Biol.* **38**, 161 (1985).

17. Weitzen, M. L., Yamamoto, R. S., and Granger, G. A. Cell. Immunol. 77, 30–41 (1983).
18. Svedersky, L. P., Nedwin, G. E., Bringman, T. S., Shalaby,, M. R., Lamott, J. A., Goeddel, D. V., and Palladino, M. A. Fed. Proc. 44, 589 (1985).
19. Evans, C. H., Ransom, J. H., and Heinbaugh, J. A. P. Am. Assoc. Ca. 25, 268 (1984).
20. Ortaldo, J. R., Blanka, I., and Herberman, R. B., in Mechanisms of Cell-Mediated Cytotoxicity vol. II (Henkart, P. and Martz, E., eds.) Plenum, New York (1985).
21. Stone-Wolff, D., Yip, Y. K., Kelker, H. C., Le, J., Henriksen-Destafano, D., Rubin, B. Y., Rinderknecht, E., Aggarwal, B. B., and Vilcek, J. J. Exp. Med. 159, 828–843 (1984).
22. Degliantoni, G., Murphy, M., Kobayashi, M., Francis, M. K., Perussia, B., and Trinchieri, G. J. Exp. Med. 162, 1512–1530 (1985).
23. Targan, S., Brieva, J., Newman, W., and Stevens, R. J. Immunol. 134, 666–669 (1985).
24. Nair, M. P. N., Schwartz, S. A., and Menon, M. Cell. Immunol. 94, 159–171 (1985).
25. Sibbitt, W. L., Mathews, P. M., and Bankhurst, A. D. Arthritis Rheum. 27, 1095–1100 (1984).
26. Hiserodt, J. C., Britvan, L., and Targan, S. R. J. Immunol. 131, 2705–2709 (1983).
27. Gonzalez-Noriega, A., Grubb, J. H., Talkad, V., and Sly, W. S. J. Cell Biol. 85, 839–852 (1980).
28. Degliantoni, G., Perussia, B., Mangoni, L., and Trinchieri, G. J. Exp. Med. 161, 1152–1168 (1985).
29. Thomas, K. R., Scribner, C. L., Kay, H. D., and Klassen, L. W. Clin. Res. 32, 759A (1984).
30. Wang, A. M., Creasy, A. A., Ladner, M. B., Lin, L. S., Strickler, J., Van Arsdell, J. N., Yamamoto, R., and Mark, D. F. Science 228, 149–154 (1985).
31. Deem, R. L. and Targan, S. R. J. Immunol. 133, 1836–1840 (1984).
32. Shibata, T., Sugiura, Y., and Iwayanagi, S. Chem. Phys. Lipids 31, 105–116 (1982).
33. Sandvig, K. and Olsnes, S. J. Biol. Chem. 257, 7504–7513 (1982).
34. Ivins, B., Saelinger, C. B., Bonventre, P. F., and Woscinski, C. Infect. Immun. 11, 665–674 (1975).
35. Salisbury, J. L., Condeelis, J. S., and Satir, P. J. Cell. Biol. 87, 132–141 (1980).
36. Van Berkel, J. C., Nagelkerke, J. F., and Kruijt, J. K. FEBS Lett. 132, 61–66 (1981).
37. Davies, P. J. A., Davies, D. R., Levitzki, A., Maxfield, F. R., Milhaud, P., Willingham, M. C., and Pastan, I. H. Nature 283, 162–167 (1980).
38. King, A. C., Hernaez-Davis, L., and Cuatrecasas, P. Proc. Natl. Acad. Sci. USA 77, 3283–3287 (1980).
39. Seglen, P. O., Meth. Enzymol. 96, 737–764 (1983).

40. Deem, R. L. and Targan, S. R. *J. Immunol.* **133**, 72-77 (1984).
41. Deem, R. L., Niederlehner, A., and Targan, S. R. *Cell. Immunol.* **102**, 187-197 (1986).
42. Michael, M. and Saelinger, C. B. *Curr. Microbiol.* **2**, 103-108 (1979).
43. Silverstein, S. C., Steinman, R. M., and Cohn, Z. A. *Ann. Rev. Biochem.* **46**, 669-722 (1977).
44. Ohkuma, S. and Poole, B. *Proc. Natl. Acad. Sci. USA* **75**, 3327-3331 (1978).
45. Collier, R. J. *Bacteriol. Rev.* **39**, 54-85 (1975).
46. Targan, S. R. and Newman, W. *J. Immunol.* **131**, 1149-1153 (1983).
47. Soehnlen, B., Liu, R., and Salmon, S. E. *P. Am. Assoc. Ca.* **26**, 303 (1985).
48. Svedersky, L. P., Nedwin, G. E., Goeddel, D. V., and Palladino, M. A. *J. Immunol.* **134**, 1604-1608 (1985).
49. Sayers, T., Ransom, J. H., Denn, A. C., Shepard, M., Herberman, R. B., and Ortaldo, J. R. *J. Leuk. Biol.* **38**, 88 (1985).

# Leukoregulin

# Leukoregulin

## Biology, Biochemistry, and Mode of Action

JANET H. RANSOM and RANDALL E. MERCHANT

## 1. Introduction

The first evidence demonstrating that leukoregulin is a unique lympho-kine was found during the study of the biologic effects of Syrian hamster lymphotoxin (*1*). Hamster lymphotoxin preparations, in addition to the ability to lyse the murine L-929 cell line, also inhibited the growth of hamster tumor cells and could inhibit the chemical or radiation-induced carcinogenic transformation of normal hamster fetal fibroblasts (*2–5*). This activity was initially attributed to lymphotoxin, but after extensive bio-chemical characterization, an anti-hamster tumor cell and anticarcinogenic activity could be physically separated from lymphotoxin as well as inter-feron, interleukins, and macrophage activity factor (*1*). Subsequent studies of human lymphokine preparations also demonstrated that a unique molecular species was responsible for the cytotoxicity of numerous human tumor cell lines (*6*). This lymphokine was termed leukoregulin. This chapter discusses the evidence supporting the unique identity of human leukoregulin and its effects on human tumor cells.

## 2. Biology of Leukoregulin

### 2.1. Cell Source of Leukoregulin

Leukoregulin is a secreted product of lymphoblastoid cell lines or mitogen- or lectin-stimulated lymphocytes (Table 1). Leukoregulin has not been detected in supernatants of lectin-stimulated mononuclear or poly-morphonuclear leukocytes. Phytohemagglutin (PHA) is the most potent stimulator of leukoregulin secretion by normal lymphocytes. The total

Table 1
Human Cell Source of Leukoregulin

| Cell type | Stimulating agent | Leukoregulin, units/mL |
|---|---|---|
| *Experiment 1*[a] | | |
| Unfractionated PBL | 5 μg PHA/mL | 13 |
| Adherent cells | 5 μg PHA/mL | 0 |
| Nonadherent cells | 5 μg PHA/mL | 50 |
| T-cells | 5 μg PHA/mL | 5 |
| Null cells | 5 μg PHA/mL | 34 |
| Polymorphonuclear leukocytes | 5 μg PHA/mL | 0 |
| *Experiment 2* | | |
| PBL | 5 μg PHA/mL | 74 |
| PBL | 1000 units IL-2/mL | 44 |
| PBL | 5 μg PHA/mL + 1000 units IL-2/mL | 119 |
| *Experiment 3*[b] | | |
| PBL | Media | 0 |
| PBL | K562 cells | 5 |
| PBL | HT-29 cells | 0 |
| PBL | WiDr cells | 0 |
| *Experiment 4*[c] | | |
| PBL | 5 μg PHA/mL | 25 |
| PBL | 100 ng PMA/mL | 1 |
| PBL | 5 μg PHA + 10 ng PMA/mL | 20 |
| PBL | 0.1–10 μg LPS (serotype 0111:B4)/mL | 0 |
| PBL | 0.1–10 μg LPS (serotype 055:B5)/mL | 0 |
| PBL | 0.1–10 μg SEB/mL | 0 |

[a]Cellular fractionation was described in ref. (*4*). Adherent cells were 85% monocytes, nonadherent cells were 98% lymphocytes, T-cells were 99% E-rosette positive, null cells were 100% E-rosette negative and displayed NK activity. Cell media was RPMI 1640 with 5% fetal bovine serum (FBS).

[b]Media was serum-free RPMI 1640.

[c]PBL was added to stimulator cells at a ratio of 50:1 in RPMI 1640 containing insulin, transferrin, selenium (Collaborative Research, Lexington, MA), and 0.25% bovine serum albumin and incubated 24 h.

amount and time course of leukoregulin secretion upon PHA stimulation vary among individuals; generally, however, maximal secretion is found after 2 d (Fig. 1). Recombinant interleukin-2 also stimulates leukoregulin

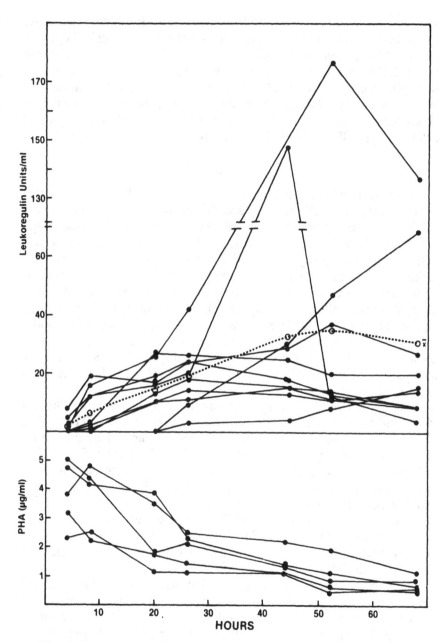

Fig. 1. Time course of leukoregulin production and PHA depletion from human peripheral blood leukocytes from individual donors. The dashed line indicates the mean production.

secretion and in combination with PHA gives additive, but not synergistic, production. A leukoregulin-like activity has also been found in the supernatants of human peripheral blood lymphocytes stimulated with the human erythroleukemia cell line K562 (7). We have not detected leukoregulin when lymphocytes were stimulated with natural killer cell (NK)-insensitive targets such as HT-29 and WiDr cells. Other agents that fail to induce leukoregulin secretion include lipopolysaccharide (LPS), staphylococcal enterotoxin B (SEB), and phorbol 12-myristate 13-acetate (PMA).

## 2.2. Bioassays

Leukoregulin has three distinct modes of action on human tumor target cells: (1) cytostasis, (2) cytolysis, and (3) enhancement of target cell sensitivity to NK-mediated cytotoxicity. Specific details of assay methodology are covered in ref (6) and in the next chapter by Evans. We routinely use both inhibition of dye uptake and $^3$H-thymidine incorporation to measure leukoregulin's growth inhibitory activity. Inhibition of $^3$H-thymidine incorporation is two- to five-fold more sensitive than the dye-uptake assay for some target cell lines; the dye-uptake assay can be performed more rapidly, however, and is more amenable to assessment of the large number of samples that are generated during biochemical purification. These assays do not discriminate between cell cytostasis and cytolysis. A specific assay to measure cytolysis only is measurement of $^3$H-thymidine release in prelabeled target cells.

The most sensitive and specific target cell used to measure human leukoregulin's effect is the human nasopharyngeal carcinoma cell line RPMI 2650 (6). The effects of leukoregulin on this cell line include growth inhibition, lysis, and increased sensitivity to NK cell cytolysis. RPMI 2650 cells are not sensitive to interferon-γ or -α, lymphotoxin, or tumor necrosis factor, either alone or in combination. Another cell line used extensively to study leukoregulin is the human colon adenocarcinoma cell line HT-29. There is a disadvantage to using HT-29 cells, however, in that these cells, although sensitive to leukoregulin, are also sensitive to interferon-γ when combined with lymphotoxin, but to neither cytokine alone (see the next section for details).

Leukoregulin enhancement of tumor cell susceptibility to NK-mediated cytotoxicity is a unique activity because it occurs in the absence of a direct leukoregulin-induced target cell cytolysis and is opposite the inhibitory effect that the interferons have on NK-sensitive targets. Leukoregulin may function two ways to enhance NK killing: (1) by increasing NK cell–target cell conjugation (8) and (2) by increasing target cell membrane permeability (6). Leukoregulin-induced target cell enhancement to NK-mediated killing occurs rapidly (within 0.5 h of expoure to leukoregulin) and, during concomitant treatment of target cells with leukoregulin and interferon, leukoregulin's enhancing effect overrides interferon's inhibitory effect. Lymphotoxin neither enhances nor inhibits the tumor cells' sensitivity to NK cells.

We also sought to determine whether the NK-enhancing activity plays a role in vivo using a guinea pig model system (9). A guinea pig NK-sensitive tumor cell line, 104C1, either untreated or incubated with a guinea pig lymphokine preparation containing a leukoregulin-type activity, was mixed with guinea pig NK cells and injeted subcutaneously. Tumor growth was assessed, and that of cells treated with leukoregulin and mixed with NK cells was inhibited significantly compared to that of tumor cells not treated with leukoregulin, but mixed with NK cells. This inhibition occurred only with NK cells and not with activated macrophages. This result suggests that under appropriate circumstances leukoregulin may aid NK killing in vivo.

## 2.3. Target Cell Sensitivities

Leukoregulin inhibits the growth of a large number of different types of malignant cells, including gastrointestinal, lung, and bladder carcinomas, glioblastoma, and leukemia (Table 2). Tumor cell lines vary in their susceptibility to leukoregulin's growth-inhibitory effect. Some cell lines such as RPMI 2650 are readily lysed (measured by $^3$H-thymidine release over 3 d, whereas others such as K562 are growth-inhibited, but not lysed. The differences in target cell sensitivities are not a function of the different growth rates of the cells, because HT-29 and LoVo cells have a 31–32 h doubling time, yet HT-29 cells require 1.7 units, and LoVo cells require 200 units, of leukoregulin to cause a 50% growth inhibition. Normal skin fibroblasts, colonic mucosal cells, and lectin-stimulated normal lymphocytes are not inhibited by up to 1000 units of leukoregulin.

## 2.4. Relationship of Leukoregulin to Other Cytotoxic Lymphokines

Supernatants of PHA-stimulated human peripheral b' od leukocytes inhibit the growth of L-929 cells and numerous human tumor cells and contain interferon-$\gamma$ and -$\alpha$. The L-929 inhibitory activity is related to lymphotoxin and/or tumor necrosis factor (TNF). The anti-human tumor cell inhibitory activity was shown to be biochemically separable from L-929 inhibitory activity and was attributed to leukoregulin. Lymphotoxin, TNF, and interferon-$\gamma$ have been shown to act synergistically to inhibit the growth of some human tumor cells (10); therefore, experiments were performed to determine whether leukoregulin activity could be the result of the synergy

Table 2
Relative Susceptibilities of Human Tumor Cells to Leukoregulin

| Cell line | Type | Units causing 50% cytostasis | Units causing 50% cytolysis | Population doubling time, h |
|---|---|---|---|---|
| *Gastrointestinal carcinomas* | | | | |
| HT-29 | Colon | 1.7 | 53 | 31 |
| Sw-480 | Colon | 2.7 | | 23 |
| SW-948 | Colon | 4.8 | | |
| HUTU-80 | Duodenum | | | 3.7 |
| LS-174 | Colon | 22 | | 26 |
| SW-1463 | Rectum | 140 | | |
| LoVo | Colon | 200 | | 32 |
| CaCo | Colon | 1200 | | 45 |
| *Head and Neck* | | | | |
| RPMI 2650 | Nasal carcinoma | 1.0 | 5 | |
| KB | Mouth epidermoid carcinoma | 13 | | |
| Hep-2 | Larynx epidermoid carcinoma | 83 | | |
| *Bladder Carcinomas* | | | | |
| HT-1376 | | 5.7 | | 35 |
| RT-4 | Transitional cell | 3 | | |
| J-82 | Transitional cell | 650 | | 40 |
| T24 | Transitional cell | 517 | | |
| SCABER | Squamous | No effect | | 33 |
| *Lung Carcinomas* | | | | |
| CaLu-3 | Adenocarcinoma | 3.7 | | |
| A-427 | Adenocarcinoma | 18 | | |
| SK-Lu-1 | Adenocarcinoma | 120 | | |
| CaLu-1 | Epidermoid carcinoma | 130 | | |
| *Brain* | | | | |
| LN-71 | Glioblastoma | 8 | | |
| LN-18 | Glioblastoma | 8 | | |
| LN-235 | Glioblastoma | 80 | | |
| U-251 | Glioblastoma | 800 | | |
| *Leukemia* | | | | |
| K562 | Erythroleukemia | 17 | | |
| MOLT-4 | T-Cell leukemia | 20 | | |
| CEM | T-Cell leukemia | 60 | | |

(*continued*)

Table 2 (*continued*)
Relative Susceptibilities of Human Tumor Cells to Leukoregulin

| Cell line | Type | Units causing 50% cytostasis | Units causing 50% cytolysis | Population doubling time, h |
|---|---|---|---|---|
| *Others* | | | | |
| MCF-7 | Breast carcinoma | 1.7 | | |
| A375 | Melanoma | 1.8 | | |
| PC-3 | Prostatic carcinoma | 7.7 | | |
| 769 | Renal carcinoma | 20 | | |
| DX-3 | Melanoma | 35 | | |
| Du145 | Prostatic carcinoma | 48 | | |
| OST | Osteosarcoma | 590 | | |

of these other cytokines. Sayres et al. (*7*) and Ortaldo et al. (*11*) found that leukoregulin was not inhibited by neutralizing antibodies to lymphotoxin, tumor necrosis factor, interferon-γ, or anti-NK granule antibodies that neutralize natural killer cell cytotoxic factor. We also sought to determine whether lymphotoxin and interferon-γ could mimic leukoregulin's growth-inhibitory activity of nine human tumor cell lines (Fig. 2). Lymphotoxin alone did not inhibit any of the tumor cells tested. Only the WiDr cells were inhibited by interferon-γ with 240 units causing a 50% growth reduction. Interferon-γ and lymphotoxin in combination, however, inhibited WiDr, HT-29, HT-1376, SW-948, and LN-71 cell lines. At the highest units tested, the combined lymphokines had no effect on the leukoregulin-sensitive cell lines RPMI 2650, K562, CEM, and MOLT-4. Therefore, these four cell lines can be used to distinguish leukoregulin from interferon-γ and lymphotoxin.

We also sought to determine whether the PHA used to induce leukoregulin secretion interfered with measurement of leukoregulin's biological effects. Using a capture ELISA assay for PHA sensitive to 20 ng/mL, we found that about 80% of the PHA added to lymphocyte cultures was depleted from the medium during cell stimulation. The remainder could be removed during biochemical fractionation of leukoregulin using either gel filtration, DEAE anion exchange, or thyroglobulin-Sepharose affinity chromatography. Therefore, partially purified leukoregulin preparations did not contain detectable PHA. We also determined whether low amounts of PHA had any synergistic effect with leukoregulin (Fig. 3). PHA alone at 10 μg/mL or greater significantly inhibited the growth of HT-29 cells. When PHA (at 0.01–1.0 μg/mL) was added to leukoregulin, no effect on

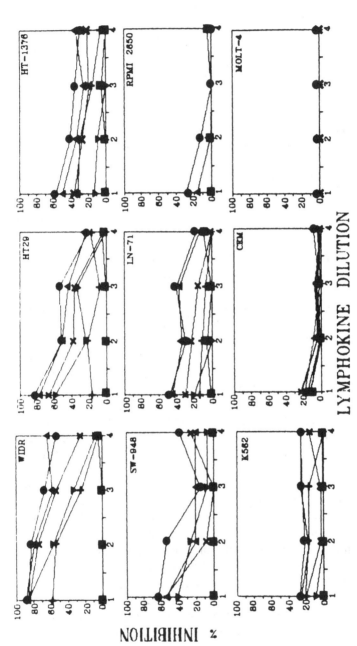

Fig. 2. Growth inhibitory effects of gamma interferon (IFNγ) and lymphotoxin (LT) alone or in combination on human tumor cell targets in a 3-d MTT dye hydrolysis assay. Lymphokine dilution: (1) 300 units LT or 3600 units IFNγ; (2) 30 units LT or 360 units IFNγ; (3) 3 units LT or 36 units IFNγ; (4) 0.3 units LT or 3.6 units IFNγ; ■, LT alone, dilutions 1–4; +, IFNγ alone, dilutions 1–4; ○, 300 units LT, dilutions 1–4 IFNγ; △, 30 units LT, dilutions 1–4 IFNγ; X, 3 units LT, dilutions 1–4 IFNγ; ▼, 0.3 units LT, dilutions 1–4 IFNγ.

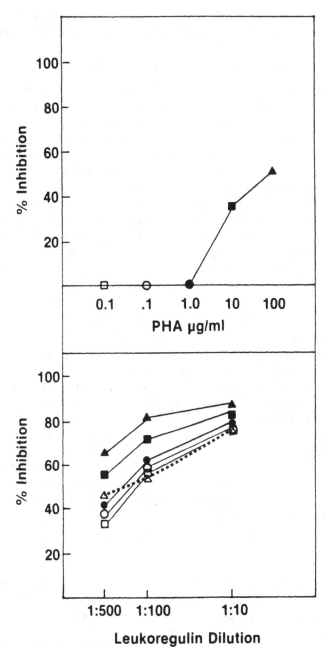

**Leukoregulin Dilution**

Fig. 3. Effect of PHA on the growth inhibition of HT-29 cells alone or in combination with leukoregulin. PHA alone (top) and PHA at 100 µg/mL (△), 10 µg/mL (■), 1 µg/mL (●), 0.1 µg/mL (□) added to different dilutions of leukoregulin (△) and assayed on HT-29 cells in a 3-d MTT dye hydrolysis assay.

the biological activity was observed. Therefore, PHA did not synergistically enhance or decrease leukoregulin's inhibition of HT-29 cell growth.

## 2.5. Leukoregulin Species Specificity

Supernatants of PHA-stimulated leukocytes from human, hamster, guinea pig, or rat inhibit the growth of tumor cells, but not normal cell counterparts within the same species. Lymphokines from the hamster, guinea pig, and rat have similar effects when tested on tumor cells among these three species; when human leukoregulin is added to tumor cells from the three animal species, however, no growth inhibition occurs (12). Similarly, lymphokine preparations from the hamster, guinea pig, and rat do not inhibit the growth of human tumor cell targets sensitive to human leukoregulin (12). Human leukoregulin also does not inhibit several mouse tumor cell lines, including L-929, EL-4, P815, and YAC. This observation is in contrast to a number of other mouse and human lymphokines, such as lymphotoxin, TNF, and interferons, IL-1, IL-2, and the B-cell growth factors, whose activities cross species.

## 2.6. Mechanism of Action

We have examined the morphology of HT-29 cells and four human glioblastoma cell lines (13) following exposure in vitro to various concentrations of partially purified leukoregulin. Direct examination of these cultures by phase contrast microscopy provided evidence of cell lysis in all leukoregulin-treated cultures, the degree of which was dependent on the units of leukoregulin used and the time of exposure. Cultured HT-29 cells are adherent and form small, cobblestoned islands before reaching confluency (Fig. 4). Ultrastructurally, HT-29 cells form a homogeneous population of rounded cells with variable numbers of short microvilli on their surface (Fig. 5). Underlying the highest point of each cell is a large, euchromatic nucleus with frequent indentations. Their cytoplasm is composed of an extensive concentration of polyribosomes and other organelles, including large-diameter mitochondria, inclusions of variable electron density, microfilaments, and microtubules. Mitotic figures are also occasionally observed.

Following an exposure to 100 units leukoregulin/mL culture medium, HT-29 cells appear to draw in their cytoplasmic processes, round up, and become detached from their substrate (Fig. 6). Both direct examination and colorimetric assay reveal that this concentration of leukoregulin causes a pronounced decrease in the number of cultured HT-29 cells. Inspection of HT-29 tumor cell targets by transmission electron microscopy at various time points following exposure to 100 units of leukoregulin revealed a

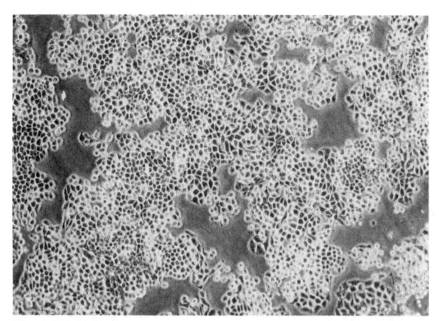

Fig. 4. HT-29 control culture (×86).

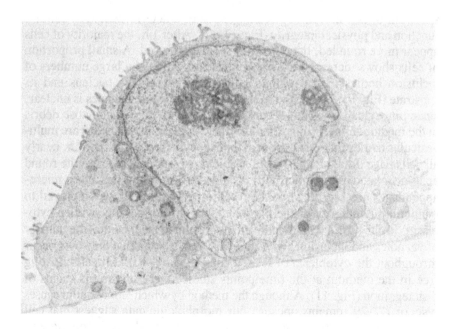

Fig. 5. Normal HT-29 cell (×4600).

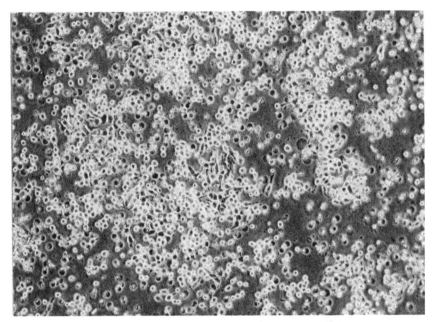

Fig. 6. HT-29 cells exposed to 100 U leukoregulin/mL for 24 h (×86).

spectrum of cell morphologies suggestive of a deteriorization in cellular function and physical integrity (Figs. 7–11). After 1 h, the majority of cells appear more rounded, but otherwise seem unaffected. A small proportion of cells shows increased cytoplasmic vacuolization and large numbers of inclusion bodies in the region of the cell between the nucleus and its substrate (Fig. 7). The origin of the membrane-bound vacuoles is unclear, since pinocytosis does not occur. HT-29 cells do not phagocytose debris in the medium either, suggesting that the cytoplasmic inclusions are multi-vesicular bodies that result from autophagocytic processes. By 4 h, nearly all cells have drawn in their cytoplasmic processes and appear quite round and vacuolated. Most microvilli disappear, suggesting that these micro-appendages are sacrificed so their cell membranes may be employed to maintain the integrity of the plasmalemma enveloping the swollen cyto-plasm. From 4 to 24 h after adding leukoregulin to the medium, the number of vacuoles and inclusion bodies increases to the point that they now occur throughout the cytoplasm of HT-29 cells (Figs. 8–10). All cells floating free in the medium at the time points studied were in various stages of disintegration (Fig. 11). Although the method by which leukoregulin causes lysis of HT-29 remains unclear, our morphologic data suggest that cell death results from increased absorption of fluid by the cells, possibly as a result of a defect in the plasmalemmal structure or function. Irreversi-

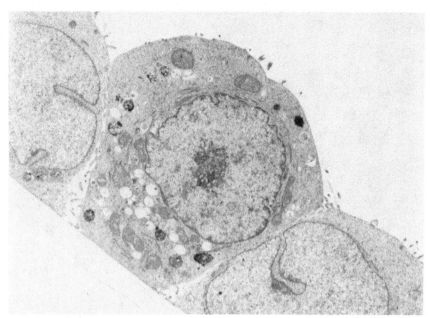

Fig. 7. HT-29 cell 1 h after addition of leukoregulin to culture medum; vacuoles appear in an infranuclear position (×5760).

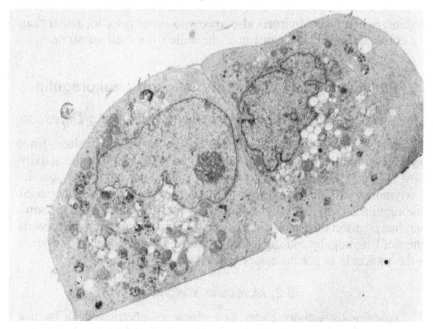

Fig. 8. Pair of HT-29 cells exposed to leukoregulin for 4 h (×4030).

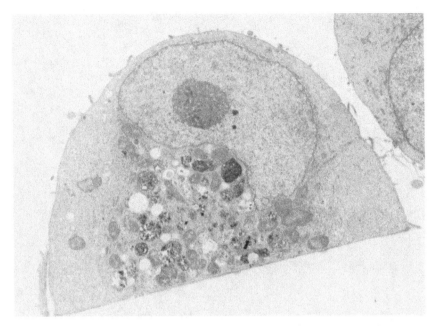

Fig. 9. HT-29 cell after 6 h in the presence of leukoregulin possesses numerous clear and autophagic vacuoles (×6048).

ble damage and lysis of targets also appear to occur prior to, rather than as a consequence of, detachment of the cells from their substrate.

# 3. Physicochemical Characteristics of Leukoregulin

## 3.1. Leukoregulin Sensitivity to pH and Enzymatic Digestion

Leukoregulin activity is stable over a wide range of pH values, from 2 to 8; when maintained at pH 10 for 1 h, however, 77% of the activity is lost (Table 3). Digestion of leukoregulin with 32 units of trypsin, 6 units of chymotrypsin, or 6 units of pronase for 1 h at 37°C decreased leukoregulin activity from 32 to 48% (6). Neuraminidase digestion, however, had no effect on leukoregulin activity. This confirms the proteinaceous nature of leukoregulin and suggests that the presence of sialic acid residues on the molecule is not necessary for activity.

## 3.2. Molecular Weight

Leukoregulin activity elutes as a single symmetrical peak from a Sephacryl S-200 column (Fig. 12) or a TSK G-3000 HPLC gel filtration

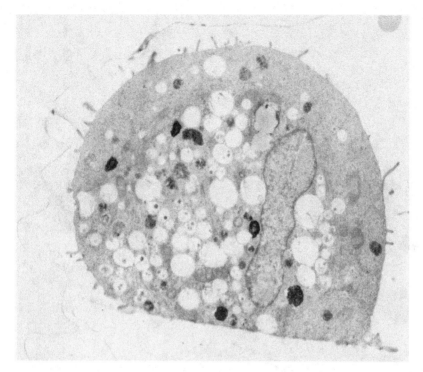

Fig. 10. Vacuoles and multivesicular bodies increase in number with time of leukoregulin exposure, 12 h (×6300).

column (6) with an apparent molecular weight of 50,000. When this type of chromatographic separation is performed in the presence of 0.1% polyethylene glycol, leukoregulin can be separated from lymphotoxin and interferon (6).

A much larger apparent molecular weight is observed for leukoregulin, 140,000 $K_d$, when separation is performed by linear gradient polyacrylamide gel electrophoresis (a nondenaturing system), probably because of aggregation.

### 3.3. Isoelectric pH

Leukoregulin activity can be separated by isoelectric focusing into species with IpH values of about 5.3 and 7.5 (6). Each of the two isoelectric species displays similar bioactivities, tumor cell cytostasis, cytolysis, and target cell enhancement for NK-mediated cytoxicity. The major difference between the two isoelectric species seems to be that some donors produce more of one type than the other.

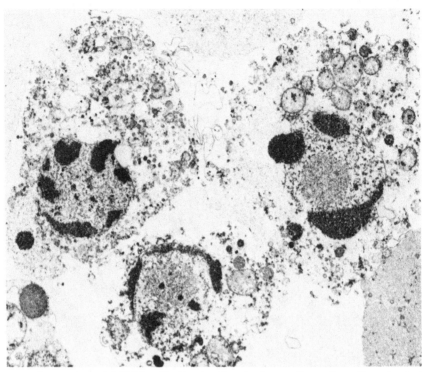

Fig. 11. Lysed HT-29 cells floating free in the medium of a culture treated with leukoregulin for 24 h ($\times 4200$).

Table 3
pH Stability of Leukoregulin[a]

| Sample treatment | LR units/mL | % of pH 7.2 |
|---|---|---|
| pH 2.0 | 25.2 | 62% |
| pH 3.0 | 23.5 | 58% |
| pH 4.0 | 23.0 | 57% |
| pH 5.0 | 24.9 | 61% |
| pH 6.0 | 32.0 | 79% |
| pH 7.2 | 40.5 | |
| pH 8.0 | 31.0 | 77% |
| pH 10.0 | 9.4 | 23% |

[a]A partially purified sample of leukoregulin was adjusted to the appropriate pH by addition of HCl or NaOH, held for 1 h at room temperature, then neutralized. The pH 7.2 sample was held as a reference and was diluted with 20 m$M$ Tris, pH 7.2, to equal treated sample volumes before assay.

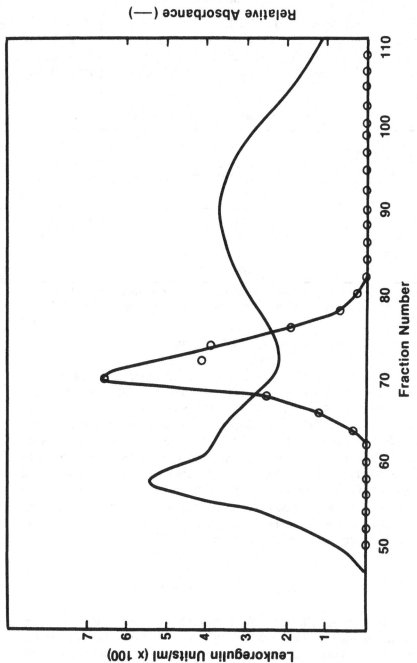

Fig. 12. Sepharcyl S-200 gel filtration chromatography of leukoregulin. Human serum albumin and ovalbumin elute at fractions 68 and 74, respectively.

## 3.4. Stability

Leukoregulin was stored at 37, 4, $-20$, and $-70\,°C$ to determine the stability at various temperatures (Table 4). The activity had a half-life of 3 d at 37 °C, 2 wk at 4 °C, and greater than 6 mo at $-20\,°C$ or below when stored at a protein concentration of 1 mg/mL 20 m$M$ tris-HCl pH 7.4.

Table 4
Temperature Stability of Leukoregulin[a]

| Storage temperature, °C | | | | |
|---|---|---|---|---|
| 37 | $t_{½}$ relative to 4 °C = 4 d | | | |
| | Units/mL | | | |
| | 1 wk | 2 wk | 3 wk | 4 wk |
| 4 | 100 | 49 | 38 | 31 |
| $-20$ | 73 | 63 | 41 | 80 |
| $-80$ | 98 | 65 | 42 | 79 |

[a]A partially purified leukoregulin preparation at a protein concentration of 1 mg/mL was aliquoted, stored at the indicated temperature, and assayed daily (37 and 4 °C) and weekly.

# 4. Conclusions

Leukoregulin was identified as a unique cytotoxic immunologic hormone because it is biochemically separable from lymphotoxin and interferon, is not neutralized by antisera to lymphotoxin, tumor necrosis factor, interferon, or NKCF, and possesses biological activities distinct from these other cytokines. Leukoregulin inhibits the growth and lyses a wide variety of tumor cell lines and can enhance tumor cells' susceptibility to lysis mediated by NK cells. Leukoregulin cellular toxicity is accompanied by changes in cell membrane permeability, increase in cell volume, and intracellular vacuole formation. We have also tested leukoregulin's potential as a cancer therapeutic agent in a variety of preclinical screens. These results are discussed in a later chapter.

# Acknowledgments

We thank Linda Cleveland for her excellent technical assistance and Dr. Nicholas Pomato for the thoughtful discussions provided during this research. This work was supported in part by a grant from the Jeffress Memorial Trust.

# References

*1.* Ransom, J. H. and Evans, C. H. *Cancer Res.* **43**, 5222–5227 (1983).
2. Ransom, J. H., Evans, C. H., and DiPaolo, J. A. *J. Natl. Cancer Inst.* **69**, 741–744 (1982).
*3.* Ransom, J. H., Evans, C. H., Jones, A. E., Zoon, R. A., and DiPaolo, J. A. *Cancer Immunol. Immunother.* **15**, 126–130 (1983).
*4.* Evans, C. H. and DiPaolo, J. A. *Int. J. Cancer* **27**, 45–49 (1981).
*5.* Evans, C. H., Heinbaugh, J. A., and DiPaolo, J. A. *Cell Immunol.* **76**, 295–303 (1983).
*6.* Ransom, J. H., Evans, C. H., McCabe, R. P., Pomato, N., Heinbaugh, J. A., Chin, M., and Hanna, M. G., Jr. *Cancer Res.* **45**, 851–862 (1985).
*7.* Sayres, T. J., Ransom, J. H., Denn II, A., Herberman, R. B., and Ortaldo, J. R. *J. Immunol.* **137**, 1–6 (1986).
*8.* Ransom, J. H., Evans, C. H., McCabe, R. P., and Hanna, M. G., Jr., in *Mechanisms of Cell Mediated Cytotoxicity II* pp. 281–287 (Henkart P. and Martz, E., eds.) Plenum, New York (1985).
*9.* Ransom, J. H., Pintus, C., and Evans, C. H. *Int. J. Cancer* **32**, 93–97 (1983).
*10.* Williams, T. W. and Bellanti, J. A. *J. Immunol.* **130**, 518–520 (1983).
*11.* Ortaldo, J. R., Ransom, J. H., Herberman, R. B., and Sayres, T. J. *J. Immunol.* **137**, 2857–2863 (1986).
*12.* Rundell, J. O. and Evans, C. H. *Immunopharmacology* **3**, 9–18 (1981).
*13.* Merchant, R. E., Ransom, J. H., and Young, H. F. *J. Neuroimmunol.* **13**, 31–45 (1986).

# Leukoregulin Mechanisms of Anticancer Action

## CHARLES H. EVANS

## 1. Discovery of Leukoregulin

Leukoregulin is an immunologic hormone possessing distinct and unique regulatory activities for cells undergoing transformation to the neoplastic state as well as for fully neoplastic cells. The anticancer activities (Fig. 1) include (1) prevention of chemical carcinogen- as well as radiation-induced transformation, (2) inhibition of neoplastic cell proliferation, (3) augmentation of target cell sensitivity to natural killer cell cytotoxicity, and (4) lysis of neoplastic cells (*1*). Unlike many lymphokines, which function primarily to activate, stimulate, or otherwise regulate cells within the immune system, leukoregulin has no identified immunoregulatory role for cells in the normal immune system. Instead, leukoregulin directly induces an anticarcinogenic state in normal cells and directly regulates the integrity and proliferative ability of abnormal target cells.

Leukoregulin was first identified (*2*) and named (*3,4*) in 1984 as a unique target cell-directed immunologic hormone able to both prevent the development of a cancer cell as well as control the proliferation of fully developed tumor cells (*1*). The identification of leukoregulin as a new direct-acting anticancer lymphokine brought into focus a number of observations made during the previous decade that the native or natural immune system possesses the ability to interact with and directly modulate the development of neoplasia (reviewed in ref. *5*). Early in the 1970s, normal macrophages (*6*) and lymphocytes (*7*) were recognized as possessing the inherent capacity to inhibit the growth of tumor cells. The ability of lymphocytes to inhibit proliferation and integrity of tumor cells was shortly, thereafter, demonstrated to be effected, at least in part, by secretory products of the lymphocytes, i.e., lymphokines (reviewed in ref. *5*). With the develop-

189

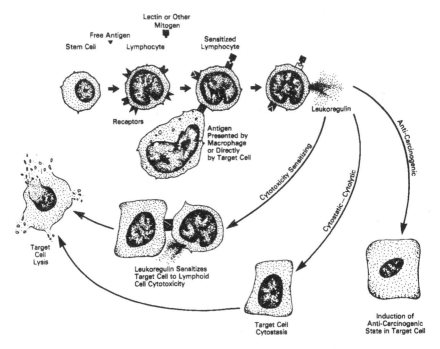

Fig. 1. The direct antitumor cell activities of leukoregulin.

ment of cell culture model systems to study the transition of target cells to the neoplastic state, i.e., carcinogenesis, the lymphokine-directed inhibition of tumor cell proliferation was shown to develop in close association with acquisition during the carcinogenic process of the ability of cells to grow progressively to form a tumor (8). The lymphokine inhibition was also demonstrated to be independent of the presence of tumor-specific transplantation antigens (9) and type of chemical carcinogen or form of radiation (10–11) that had induced the transformation. Subsequent findings that susceptibility to the anticancer lymphokine(s) can develop during preneoplastic stages of carcinogenesis (12–13) and that the lymphokine or lymphokines were able to prevent radiation as well as chemical carcinogenesis in vivo (14) indicated a truly unique target cell-directed activity for this immunologic hormone.

In the guinea pig and Syrian hamster, the anticarcinogeneic and antitumor lymphokine activities parallel and copurify with lymphotoxin activity during conventional molecular sizing and molecular charge fractionation procedures (15–16). The anticancer lymphokine activities up to 1983, therefore, were attributed to lymphotoxin until the combined use of isoelectric focusing and molecular sizing chromatography separated the hamster and human anticancer lymphokine activities from lymphotoxin (1,17). Additional evidence supporting the presence of a distinct new lymphokine was the more than 1000-fold variation in leukoregulin and lymphotoxin activity in lymphokine preparations prepared from normal human lymphocytes of different individuals (Table 1) and the differential sensitivity of lymphotoxin and leukoregulin activities to proteases and neuraminidase

Table 1
Relative Lymphotoxin Cytolytic and Human Target Cell Cytostatic Activities
in Individual Human Lymphokine Preparations

| Leukoregulin preparation | Alpha-L-929 cytolytic units[a] | K562 cytostatic units[a] | Ratio L-929/K562 units |
|---|---|---|---|
| PBL Hu-838C | 25,000 | 20 | 1,250 |
| PBL Hu-8311C | 2,428 | 105 | 23 |
| PBL Hu-8312C | 12,500 | 10 | 1,250 |
| PBL Hu-8313C | 3,750 | 232 | 16 |
| PBL Hu-8317C | 13,538 | 50 | 271 |
| RPMI 1788 | 1,000 | 10 | 100 |

[a]Total activity secreted by $10^8$ Ficoll-Hypaque prepared fresh human mononuclear leukocytes or by RPMI 1788 lymphoblast-like cells following 48 h of culture in serum-free RPMI 1640 medium at 37°C with 10 $\mu$g phytohemagglutinin-L/$10^6$ cells/mL.

(1,17). The combined evidence from the hamster and human lymphokine studies demonstrated that the activities were separable from lymphotoxin as well as interferons, interleukins-1 and -2, and from macrophage migration inhibitory factor. The new lymphokine was named leukoregulin (3,4) to signify that it is a leukocyte hormone with growth regulatory actions for a wide variety of preneoplastic and neoplastic cells. The major importance of this finding in addition to the discovery of a new lymphokine is the identification of a remarkable new class of molecules intrinsic to the normal immune system that possess the ability to directly affect the growth and function of tumor cells and that offer the potential for new insights into differentiation, cell physiology and biochemistry, and homeostasis (18).

The purpose of this article is to describe the assays being used to characterize the biological actions of leukoregulin, and methodology known at present capable of producing biologically active leukoregulin, and the current information regarding pathways of leukoregulin action. The assays, actions, and molecular pathways of leukoregulin activity are presented not as definitive information, but as our current state of knowledge to facilitate the more rapid exploration of the identity of the physiologic role and potential usefulness of this unique and powerful immunologic hormone.

# 2. Assays Defining Leukoregulin Activity

The cell proliferation inhibitory (cytostatic), destructive (cytolytic), augmentation of sensitivity to natural killer lymphocyte cytotoxicity and anticarcinogenic activities of leukoregulin (Fig. 1) can be measured using a variety of diverse biological assays. Each is a well-established target cell assay in which either inhibition or enhancement of a specific parameter is quantitated in the presence of serially diluted leukoregulin. Some of the analytical/quantitative advantages and disadvantages of each assay are described in the following section.

## 2.1. Cytostasis—Inhibition of Cell Proliferation

Three general methods are available to measure target cell proliferation: enumeration of cell number, cell colony growth, and radionuclide incorporation.

### 2.1.1. Enumeration of Cell Number

*2.1.1.1. Direct Cell Counting.* Assays that directly or colorimetrically measure cell number can be employed to quantitate the number of target cells for calculation of the proliferation inhibitory action of leukoregulin (*1*). Direct cell counts obtained with a hemocytometer or by an electronic (Coulter) cell counter are the simplest and the most widely used methods. They are the most important assays of leukoregulin cytostatic activity since they directly measure actual target cell number and, in turn, leukoregulin activity with a high degree of reproducibility, i.e., with a standard error of less than 5% (*19*). Human leukoregulin cytostatic activity was defined using these assays with one leukoregulin unit being the amount of leukoregulin producing a 50% inhibition in the proliferation of $10^4$ human K562 leukemia cells in 1 mL of cell culture during 3 d of cell growth (*1*). Direct target cell enumeration remains the reference to which all other assays must be compared or calibrated with when assessing leukoregulin activity.

Visual examination of individual cells in the presence of trypan blue during the target cell enumeration process also allows for simultaneous evaluation of alterations in target cell membrane integrity. Direct cell counting is unable, however, to measure detachment of target cells from the substratum in monolayer culture or the presence of cytolysis, either of which if present at levels above that in cultures of cells not exposed to leukoregulin erroneously increases the apparent level of leukoregulin cytostatic activity. Measurement of radionuclide release into the culture medium from radiolabeled target cells in conjunction with target cell enumeration, however, permits measurements of both cytostasis and cytolysis in the same assay of lymphokine or other effector functions (*1,19*).

***2.1.1.2. Colorimetric Assays.*** Colorimetric quantitation of target cell proliferation by spectrophotometric evaluation of cellular dye uptake provides a sensitive alternative to direct cell counting (*1*). Colorimetric assays, moreover, can be performed in 96-well microcytotoxicity plates, resulting from the reduction in culture volume in a fivefold increase in sensitivity of lymphokine measurement and in the rapid sampling of many assays on the same and related culture plates by obtaining spectrophotometric measurements with a micro ELISA recording spectrophotometer. The attributes of increased sensitivity, rapidity, and automation make colorimetric microcytotoxicity assays particularly useful for following leukoregulin activity in the numerous samples generated during fractionation/purification procedures (*1*). The same considerations present in direct cell counting with regard to detection of combinations of cytostasis, cytolysis, and monolayer target cell detachment present in direct cell counting assays apply as well to colorimetric assays of target cell proliferation.

In direct colorimetric cytotoxicity assays, the degree of target cell proliferation is readily obtained by measuring the absorbance of dyes such as methylene blue or crystal violet following their addition to and uptake by methanol-fixed target cells in monolayer culture (*20*). This method stains all cells, live and dead, and the target cells must be washed free of extracellular dye before spectrophotometic measurement of the precipitated dye within the cells or, more preferably, the released solubilized dye following addition of ethanol, methanol, or another solvent to the stained cells. Direct colorimetric cytotoxicity assays are fast, inexpensive, and sensitive. The disadvantages are that the cells must first be washed to remove unbound dye and care must be taken to keep to a minimum the number of stained cells dislodged and lost during the washing process.

Indirect colorimetric methods measure the absorbance of a dye that is metabolically converted by the target cells to a derivative with a maximum absorbance at a wavelength different from that of the precursor dye. MTT (3-[4,5-Dimethylthiazol-2-y1],5-diphenyltetrazolium bromide), which possesses a yellowish color, is reduced intracellularly to a blue terazolium derivative that can be spectrophotometrically quantitated after solubilization of the blue terazolium derivative in isopropyl alcohol (*21*). Assay of leukoregulin using MTT (*1*) has a sensitivity comparable to that obtained by crystal violet staining of whole cells. The MTT assay also has the advantage that washing of the cells is not required because it is the reduced intracellular derivative possessing a divergent wavelength of maximum absorbance from the original dye that is measured. Any substance or condition that interferes with either MTT uptake or metabolism, however, may alter the dye derivative absorbance/target cell relationship necessary for reproducible quantitation of cell proliferation. For this reason this type of indirect colorimetric cytotoxicity assay requires periodic calibration with a direct cell-counting assay to ensure that the measured absorbance of the dye derivative accurately reflects the number of cells in the assay.

### 2.1.2. Measurement of Cell Colony Growth

Evaluation of the number and size of target cell colonies after a period of 7–14 d growth is a particularly good way to quantitate the rate and percent growth of target cells either in adherent cell culture or as colonies in semisolid medium suspension culture (*19*). This method is useful in measuring the extent of cell detachment from monolayer culture (*see* section 2.1.1.1) and is the best means of assessing the homogeneity of growth inhibitory response within the target cell population. It is also a very useful technique for determining the reversibility of growth inhibition (*19*). The major disadvantage of quantitating cell growth in colony growth culture is that it requires a large cell culture surface area or volume to permit development of sufficient colonies for examination and therefore requires considerably more lymphokine and cell culture materials than does the other assays, e.g., up to 30-fold or more lymphokine.

### 2.1.3. Radionuclide Incorporation

Measurement of radiolabeled amino acids and nucleotides is particularly useful in evaluation of protein synthesis and nucleic acid synthesis in relation to cell proliferation (*19*). Radionuclide incorporation, however, is expensive compared to direct enumeration or dye assays and is a specialized cytotoxicity assay that often is best reserved for metabolic rather than routine lymphokine bioassay. Radionuclide incorporation may also be useful in conjunction with indirect cell enumeration measurement, e.g., the MTT dye reduction assay, to monitor the metabolic state of the cells.

### 2.1.4. Spectrum of Cell Response to Leukoregulin

Each tumor cell line possesses a unique sensitivity to leukoregulin. The range of sensitivity from the least to the most sensitive tumor cell, moreover, is greater than a 1000-fold in terms of the amount of the lymphokine necessary to effect a 50% reduction in the proliferation of target cells over a 72-h period in cell culture (*1*). Carcinoma, leukemia, and sarcoma cells can possess similar (*1*) as well as widely divergent sensitivities (Table 2) that are distinct not only for leukoregulin, but also from each cell line's response to other potentially direct inhibitory lymphokines, including interferon and tumor necrosis factor (Table 3). Normal cells are at least 10,000-fold more resistant to leukoregulin cytostatic activity (*1*) demonstrating the extraordinarily high specificity of leukoregulin for preneoplastic and neoplastic cells.

Table 2
Comparative Sensitivity of Human K562 Myelocytic Leukemia, HT-29 Colon
Carcinoma, RPMI 2650 Nasal Septum Squamous Carcinoma, and U937
Histiocytic Lymphoma Cells to Leukoregulin Cell Proliferation Inhibitory Activity

| Target cell[a] | Approximate relative sensitivity to leukoregulin growth inhibition[b] |
|---|---|
| K562 Chronic myelocytic leukemia (CCL243) | 1 |
| HT-29 Colon adenocarcinoma (HTB38) | 10 |
| RPMI 2650 Nasal septum squamous cell carcinoma (CCL30) | 20 |
| U937 Histiocytic lymphoma (CRL1593) | 40-fold more sensitive |

[a]Target cells from the American Type and Culture Collection, Rockville, Maryland.
[b]Calculated from the ability of DEAE-ion exchange purified, p*I* 5.3, 50,000 HPLC mol. wt.$_{avg}$ leukoregulin to inhibit the growth of $10^4$ target cells by 50% in a 72-h Coulter counter cell enumeration assay.

Table 3
Comparative Growth Inhibitory Activity of Human Leukoregulin,
Interferon, and Tumor Necrosis Factor for U937 Lymphoma Cells

| Dilution | Inhibition of U937 cell growth at 3 d[f], % | | | | | | Tumor necrosis factor[e] |
|---|---|---|---|---|---|---|---|
| | Leukoregulin | | | Interferon | | | |
| | 85D | 85G | 85H | $\gamma$[b] | LB[c] | LK[d] | |
| 1:10,000 | 0 | 0 | 0 | 0 | 0 | 0 | 0 |
| 5,000 | 1 | 0 | 0 | 0 | 0 | 1 | 0 |
| 2,000 | 2 | 6 | 37 | 0 | 0 | 3 | 0 |
| 1,000 | 7 | 7 | 54 | 0 | 0 | 3 | 0 |
| 500 | 9 | 14 | 69 | 0 | 0 | 11 | 0 |
| 200 | 30 | 41 | 81 | 0 | 0 | 10 | 0 |
| 100 | 51 | 55 | 91 | 0 | 0 | 22 | 0 |
| 50 | 68 | 73 | 94 | 0 | 1 | 16 | 0 |
| 20 | 84 | 90 | 93 | 0 | 4 | 22 | 0 |
| 10 | 90 | 93 | 93 | 2 | 9 | 25 | 0 |
| 5 | 92 | 94 | 93 | 2 | 11 | 30 | 0 |

[a]Leukoregulin was isolated by DEAE-ion exchange chromatography (*1*).
[b]$\gamma$ interferon at $10^6$ units/mL was obtained from Sigma Chemical Co., St. Louis, MO.
[c]Lymphoblastoid interferon at $10^6$ units/mL from Sigma Chemical Co.
[d]Leukocyte interferon at $0.25 \times 10^6$ units/mL from Sigma Chemical Co.
[e]Recombinant human tumor necrosis factor (lot 3056-63) at 1.0 mg/mL generously provided by Genentech, Inc., So. San Francisco, CA.
[f]Growth inhibition of $2 \times 10^4$ lymphokine treated U937 cells was measured using a Coulter counter (*1*).

## 2.2. Cytolysis—Target Cell Dissolution

A number of membrane, cytoplasmic, or nuclear radionuclide release assays can be used to measure the degree of leukoregulin or other lymphokine-induced target cell lysis (*19*). It must be remembered, however, that loss of radionuclides such as $^{51}$Cr and those incorporated within radiolabeled amino acids from lymphokine-treated target cells, although indicative of cell damage, does not necessarily signify cell lysis and death. Release of target cell radiolabeled DNA containing a covalently incorporated nucleotide such as $^3$H-TdR or $^{131}$I-UdR is, therefore, preferred as a measure of true target cell cytolysis. When this form of target cell radiolabel release is measured in combination with a target cell enumeration assay (section 2.1.1.1), both cytostasis and cytolysis can be quantitated within the same cell population. Using this technique, leukoregulin has been observed to be more cytostatic than cytolytic for most tumor cells (*1*).

Treatment of tumor target cells with x-irradiation or with metabolic inhibitors fails to induce cytolysis or to increase the degree of proliferation inhibition induced by leukoregulin (Table 4) to the extent that treatment of murine L-929 cells with the same metabolic inhibitors greatly increases the cytotoxic response of L-929 cells to lymphotoxin (*19,22*) or to tumor necrosis factor (*23*). Some enhancement of leukoregulin-treated human K562 leukemia cells is observed, however, following exposure of the cells to x-irradiation, whereas treatment with metabolic inhibitors may decrease the response to leukoregulin (Table 4). These contrasting responses indicate that target cell metabolic activity is required for leukoregulin to function, a finding consistent with the generally nonlytic activities of leukoregulin (*1*) and series of transmembrane signals, increased intracellular calcium ion flux, and alterations in target cell plasma membrane permeability (*18*) that occur after leukoregulin interaction with the target cell and prior to increase in target cell sensitivity to natural killer lymphocyte cytotoxicity and cessation of target cell proliferation.

## 2.3. Inhibition of Target Cell Transformation and Tumor Cell Outgrowth

Quantitative short-term cell culture model systems of carcinogenesis or cancer development in which radiation or chemical carcinogen insult induces morphologic and other phenotypic markers of neoplastic transformation can be used to evaluate the ability of lymphokines such as leukoregulin to prevent, suppress, or otherwise inhibit target cell transition to the neoplastic state (*10,11,14,16,17*). Investigations using these models of neoplasia induction reveal that leukoregulin is able to inhibit X-, gamma-,

Table 4
Susceptibility of x-Irradiated and Antimetabolite-Treated Target Cells
to Leukoregulin Proliferation Inhibitory Activity[a]

| | Percent inhibition in the number of | |
|---|---|---|
| Treatment | K562 cells | U937 cells |
| Leukoregulin alone | 16 | 22 |
| Leukoregulin + 125 rads | 17 (7) | 31 (5) |
| Leukoregulin + 250 rads | 20 (43) | 38 (40) |
| Leukoregulin + 500 rads | 7 (76) | 38 (74) |
| Leukoregulin + 0.25 $\mu$g mitomycin C/mL | 2 (91) | 16 (93) |
| Leukoregulin + 0.50 $\mu$g mitomycin C/mL | 0 (95) | 13 (94) |
| Leukoregulin + 1.0 $\mu$g mitomycin C/mL | 0 (95) | 0 (96) |
| Leukoregulin + 0.5 $\mu$g actinomycin D/mL | 17 (95) | 21 (97) |
| Leukoregulin + 1.0 $\mu$g actinomycin D/mL | 11 (95) | 22 (98) |
| Leukoregulin + 2.0 $\mu$g actinomycin D/mL | 0 (95) | 21 (98) |

[a]Irradiated (16) or nonirradiated target cells were plated at $2 \times 10^4$ cells/1 mL well in 24-well cluster plates in RPMI 1640-10% fetal bovine serum medium containing the indicated concentrations of mitomycin C (19) or actinomycin D (13) and a 1:20 dilution of leukoregulin for K562 and 1:500 dilution of leukoregulin for U937 cells. Three days later the cells in each well were enumerated using a Coulter counter and the percent inhibition in relation to nontreated cells calculated. Values in parentheses are the percent inhibition for cells treated with irradiation or metabolic inhibitor alone.

and UV-irradiation or chemical carcinogen-induced morphologic transformation of mammalian cells. Leukoregulin possesses the ability, moreover, to inhibit transformation at several points or stages in the transition from the growth controlled target cell to a neoplastic cell (14,16). Exposure of the cells of leukoregulin shortly before, at the time of, or shortly after carcinogen treatment, furthermore, completely prevents transformation (10,11,14,16,24).

The antitransformation studies in Syrian hamster cells reveal that there is a critical temporal relationship between the leukoregulin-induced target cell anticarcinogenic state and the carcinogen transformation-inducing insult (16,24). The anticarcinogenic state induced by leukoregulin, moreover, is transient, but the inhibition of the initiation of transformation is irreversible if the anticarcinogenic state is present at an appropriate time in relation to carcinogen insult either in vitro (10,11,16) or in vivo (14,24). The anticarcinogenic action of leukoregulin in cell culture and in vivo, furthermore, occurs without affecting the proliferation of or exerting any detectable toxicity on the normal target cells. The anticarcinogenic action of hamster leukoregulin is, therefore, both irreversible and noncytolytic. Comparable studies with human leukoregulin and human cells remain to be performed once quantitative cell culture models of human carcinogenesis are developed.

The ability of leukoregulin to affect tumor proliferation in vivo can be examined by following the outgrowth of transplanted tumor cells in local and/or distant sites in syngeneic or other appropriate hosts. In the thymic deficient nu/nu mouse, which readily accepts xenotransplants, leukoregulin is able to diminish the outgrowth of intravenously injected xenogeneic human colon adenocarcinoma cells in the lungs and liver (1). Assays of this type complement those evaluating the ability of leukoregulin to prevent carcinogenesis and modulate the growth of carcinogen-initiated cells during the transition to the neoplastic state in syngeneic if not autologous hosts or using in vitro or combined in vivo–in vitro models of cancer development. By using a combination of such assays it is possible to extend evaluation of leukoregulin anticancer actions to all stages of carcinogenesis and tumor growth, including metastasis.

## 2.4. Augmentation of Target Cell Sensitivity to Natural Killer Lymphocyte Cytotoxicity

In addition to leukoregulin prevention of carcinogenesis and modulation of preneoplastic and neoplastic target cell proliferation, the exposure of preneoplastic and neoplastic cells to leukoregulin increases the sensitivity of the target cells to natural killer lymphocyte cytotoxicity (1,13). The increase in target cell sensitivity to natural killer cell cytotoxicity is approximately twofold (Fig. 2). Leukoregulin increases target cell sensitivity; it does not make nonresponsive target cells sensitive to natural killer lymphocyte cytotoxicity. The increase in sensitivity to leukoregulin, furthermore, occurs within approximately 30 min of leukoregulin treatment and is reversible. It is, moreover, opposite to the target cell desensitizing or protective action of interferon (2). Leukoregulin, unlike interferon, also does not directly stimulate natural killer lymphocyte activity and at the target cell level negates the desensitization to natural killer cytotoxicity induced by interferon, i.e., even in the presence of interferon leukoregulin enhances the sensitivity of the target cell to natural killer lymphocyte cytotoxicity (C. H. Evans, unpublished).

## 2.5. Destabilization of the Target Cell Membrane

The ability of leukoregulin to directly induce lysis of some target cells (1) and increase the sensitivity of cells to natural killer lymphocyte cytolysis (Fig. 2) suggests that leukoregulin directly or indirectly perturbs the target cell plasma membrane. Flow cytometric measurements confirm this

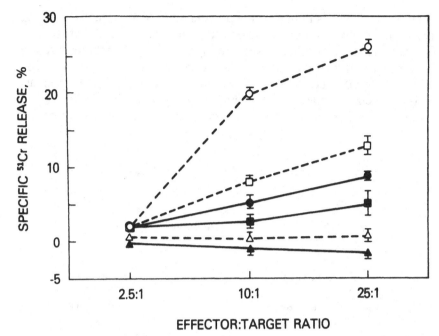

EFFECTOR:TARGET RATIO

Fig. 2. Leukoregulin increases the sensitivity of target cells to natural killer lymphocyte cytotoxicity. $^{51}$Cr-Labeled K562 cells were treated with RPMI 1640-10% FBS medium (solid symbols) or with medium containing 1 unit of leukoregulin/mL (open symbols) for 30 min and mixed with Ficol-Hypaque nylon wool nonadherent unsorted lymphocytes (square symbols), Leu-7$^+$ (natural killer) FACS-sorted (*see* Table 5) lymphocytes (round symbols), or Leu-3a$^+$ (helper) FACS-sorted lymphocytes (triangle symbols) for a 4-h $^{51}$Cr release assay (*1*).

hypothesis by revealing that leukoregulin induces a series of alterations in target cell membrane physiology. Changes in cell surface conformation as indicated by the fluorescence depolarization of fluorochrome-labeled lectins bound to the cell surface and in membrane fluidity as indicated by fluorescence depolarization of 1,6-diphenylhexatriene (*2*), and increases in membrane permeability measureable by the influx of propidium iodide or efflux of intracellular fluorescein (*1*), occur within 30 min and reach a maximum by several hours after leukoregulin treatment of K562 cells. The membrane changes, in addition, correlate well in their time of appearance and in their reversibility with leukoregulin-induced target cell increased sensitivity to natural killer lymphocyte cytotoxicity.

    Flow cytometric measurement of the efflux of intracellular fluorescein has proven to be a valuable method to examine the molecular pathway(s) of leukoregulin action. Target cells rapidly assimilate nonfluorescent fluorescein diacetate and hydrolyze the esterified fluorochrome to fluorescein, which is fluorescent, a process referred to as fluorochromasia (Fig. 3). Fluorescein remains localized within the cell unless there is an increase in plasma membrane permeability. Leukoregulin treatment results in coordinate decreases in intracellular fluorescein and in cell volume (18), which are easily detectable in a flow cytometer (Fig. 4). The decrease in fluorescein diacetate fluorochromasia also parallels the influx of propidium iodide (18), indicating that the decrease in fluorescein fluorescence

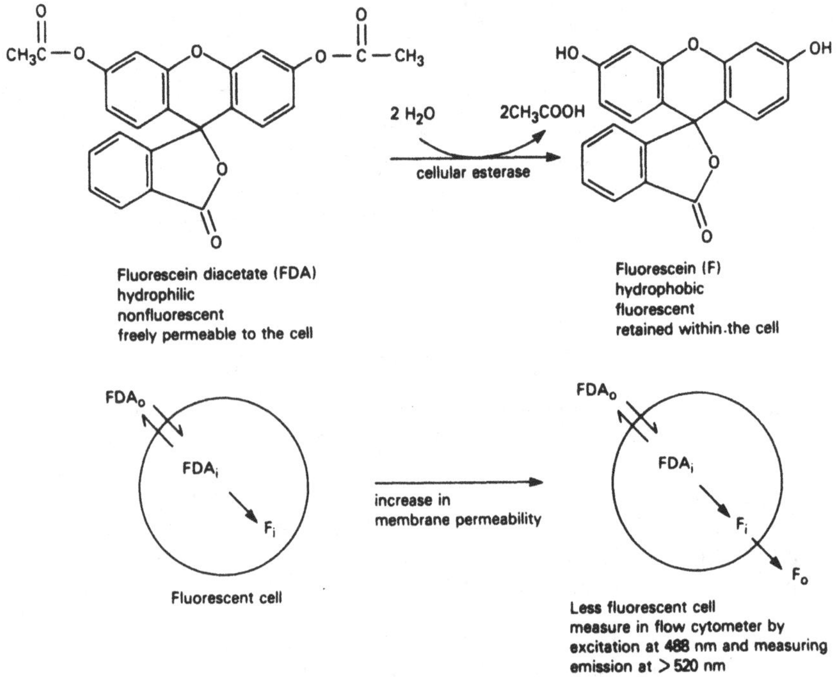

Fig. 3. Use of fluorescein diacetate for measurement of increased target cell plasma membrane permeability as indicated by loss of intracellular fluorescein.

is proportional to the increase in target cell membrane permeability. The changes in membrane permeability and cell volume or forward light scatter are proportional to leukoregulin concentration and are highly reproducible (Figs. 5 and 6). The increase in membrane permeability also correlates closely with the ability of leukoregulin to inhibit the proliferation of K562 leukemia cells (Fig. 7).

The coordinate changes in membrane permeability and in cell volume detectable by reduced fluorescein diacetate fluorochromasia and forward light scatter in leukoregulin-treated target cells also occur in target cells

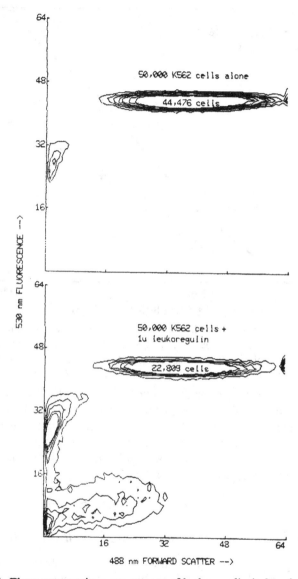

Fig. 4. Flow cytometric measurement of leukoregulin-induced plasma membrane perturbations of K562 leukemia cells. Following a 2-h incubation with medium or medium containing leukoregulin, K562 cells were treated with 6.25 μg fluorescein diacetate per mL for 5 min. Fluorescence and forward light scatter were immediately measured in a FACS IV flow cytometer using 488 nm Argon laser excitation (1).

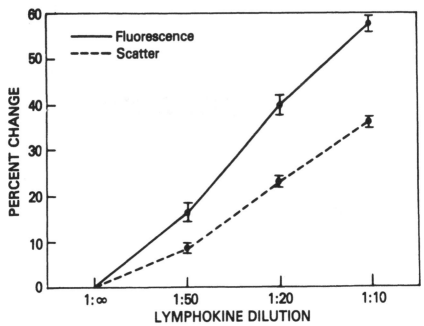

Fig. 5. Reproducibility of flow cytometric measurement of leukoregulin-induced K562 target cell plasma membrane perturbations. Values are the mean $\pm 2$ standard errors of 10 replicate assays (*see* Fig. 4) during a 1-mo period of aliquots from the same leukoregulin preparation stored at $-35\,°C$.

during a natural killer cytotoxicity reaction (Fig. 8) in the absence of added exogenous leukoregulin. The similarity of the changes in leukoregulin-treated and natural killer cell-treated target cells demonstrates the usefulness of flow cytometry in resolving the components present within a cytotoxicity reaction and suggests that leukoregulin is one of the mediators in natural killer lymphocyte cytotoxicity.

# 3. Preparation of Leukoregulin

## 3.1. Cell Sources and Stimuli for Induction

Leukoregulin is readily produced following phytohemagglutinin stimulation of fresh human peripheral blood lymphocytes (Fig. 9). Ficoll-Hypaque-isolated lymphocytes from buffy coats or from apheresis preparations produce similar quantities of leukoregulin. Cells may be stimulated immediately after separation with Ficoll-Hypaque or anytime during the next 24 h if kept refrigerated in the interim (*25*). Less leukoregulin is secreted by lymphocytes isolated from buffy coats that have not been refrigerated for 6 h or more. Antigen stimulation, e.g., tetanus toxoid or

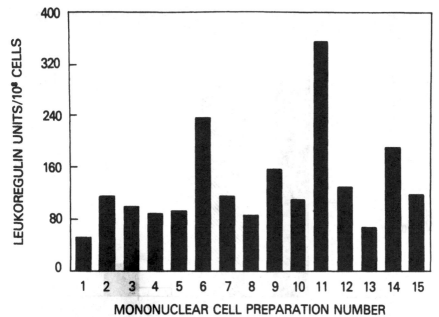

Fig. 6. Range of target cell plasma membrane perturbing activities in 15 leukoregulin preparations from different human peripheral blood lymphocyte samples. Leukoregulin was prepared as in Table 1 and assayed for the ability to increase K562 leukemia plasma membrane permeability as measured by the loss of intracellular fluorescein (Fig. 4). One unit in this assay is defined as the amount of leukoregulin producing a 50% decrease in the fluorescence at 530 $\pm$ 10 nm after incubation of $10^6$ cells with leukoregulin in 1 mL RPMI 1640-10% FBS medium for 2 h at 37°C (18).

tumor target cells, also induces leukoregulin secretion. The amount of leukoregulin produced, however, is greater with phytohemagglutinin stimulation, presumably because more cells are stimulated by the mitogen.

Leukoregulin is produced primarily, if not solely, by lymphocytes (1) and is secreted by Leu-7[+] (natural killer type) (Table 5) and by other still-to-be-defined T- and null lymphocyte subsets. Leukoregulin may be produced in Petri dish and in roller bottle culture using serum-free RPMI 1640 medium. Inclusion of 5–10% fetal bovine serum results in a slightly higher level of leukoregulin production, but also increases the concentration of other proteins that must be removed during purification steps. Phorbol-12-myristate-13-acetate (TPA) may also be substituted for phytohemagglutinin to generate leukoregulin secretion (Table 6). Concanavalin A (Con A), however, is a poor inducer compared to phytohemagglutinin, possibly because Con A and leukoregulin bind to one another. Insufficient data are currently available to determine if combinations of lectin(s) and TPA and/or

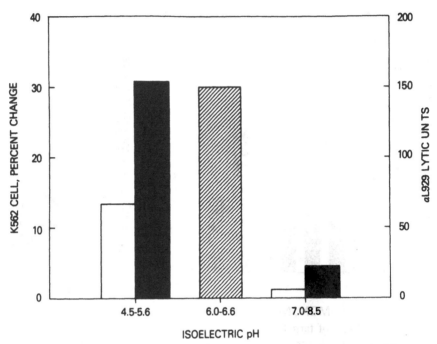

Fig. 7. Copurification of K562 target cell plasma membrane perturbing activity (open bars) and proliferation inhibitory activity (solid bars) from lymphotoxin cytolytic activity for murine alpha-L-929 cells (hatched bars) from the 40,000–60,000 HPLC mol wt $_{avg}$ lymphokines obtained from phytohemagglutinin-L-stimulated peripheral blood lymphocytes. The 40,000–60,000 HPLC mol wt $_{avg}$ lymphokines were obtained as described in Table 7, focused on a pH 3–10 1% ampholine gradient containing 0.1% mol wt 3000 polyethylene glycol, and assayed for leukoregulin activity against human K562 leukemia and for lymphotoxin activity against murine alpha-L-929 cells.

other inducers such as INF$\gamma$ or interleukin-2 induce higher levels of leukoregulin secretion.

Few cell lines have been found that secrete leukoregulin (1). The RPMI 1788 lymphoblast-like cell line originally derived from normal human peripheral blood lymphocytes (26) when stimulated with either phytohemagglutinin or TPA produces about one-tenth the amount of leukoregulin secreted by freshly isolated peripheral blood lymphocytes (Table 6). Unfortunately, in terms of a uniform and continuous source for producing large quantities of leukoregulin, no other cell line has yet proven to be more reliable than RPMI 1788 in producing leukoregulin.

Table 5
Leukoregulin Secretion by Leu-7[+] Natural Killer Lymphocytes[a]

| | Percent decrease induced by a 1:5 dilution of lymphokine produced by natural killer cells |
|---|---|
| Proliferation of RPMI 2650 cells | 47 |
| Membrane integrity of RPMI 2650 cells | 71 |

[a]Fresh Ficoll-Hypaque separated mononuclear human leukocytes were labeled at 4 °C for 30 min with 5 $\mu$g FITC-conjugated anti-Leu[7] monoclonal antibody (Becton Dickinson Immunocytometry Systems, Mountain View, CA) per 10[6] cells. Natural killer lyphocytes were then purified by fluorescence-activated cell sorting at 4 °C using a FACS IV sorting flow cytometer. Sorted cells were washed with RPMI 1640 medium and 2.5 × 10[5] cells/mL incubated with 10 $\mu$g phytohemagglutinin-L per mL for 48 h in serum-free RPMI 1640 medium at 37 °C. The cell culture medium was then concentrated 10-fold and assayed for proliferation inhibitory activity and by flow cytometry for membrane destabilizing activity (1).

Table 6
Leukoregulin Production by Mitogen versus TPA-Stimulated Lymphocytes

| Cells and inducing stimulus | K562 cell cytostatic units/mL of stimulated lymphocyte culture medium[a] |
|---|---|
| Fresh human Ficoll-Hypaque isolated Mononuclear leukocytes | |
| + Phytohemagglutinin-L 10 $\mu$g/mL | 0.1–1 |
| + Phytohemagglutinin-L and TPA 10 ng/mL | Approximately twofold higher |
| + TPA 10ng/mL alone | Approximately 10-fold lower |
| RPMI 1788 lymphoblast-like cells | |
| + Phytohemagglutinin-L 10 $\mu$g/mL | Approximately 0.2 |
| + TPA 10 ng/mL alone | Approximately 0.2 |

[a]10[6] Fresh leukocytes or 5 × 10[5] RPMI 1788 lymphoblast-like cells/mL serum-free RPMI 1640 medium were incubated with the indicated mitogen and/or TPA concentration in roller bottle culture at 37 °C. After 48 h the cell culture medium was concentrated 50-fold and assayed (1) for its ability to inhibit the proliferation of K562 cells by enumerating the number of K562 cells 72 h after incubation with the concentrated lymphokine using a Coulter counter.

CONTROLS                           NK CYTOTOXIC REACTION

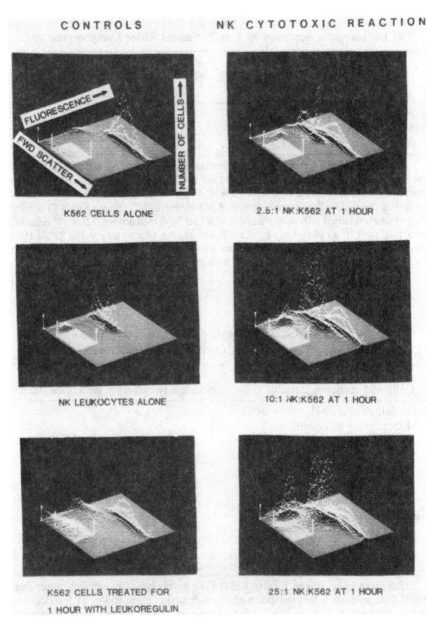

Fig. 8. Three-dimensional flow cytometric analysis of leukoregulin versus nylon wool nonadherent natural killer cell lymphocyte cytotoxicity. K562 cells ($10^6$ per mL) were treated for 1 h with 1 unit leukoregulin/mL or with nylon wool nonadherent lymphocytes at the indicated concentrations. Target, effector, and target-effector cell mixtures were then analyzed by dual parameter forward light scatter and fluorescein diacetate fluorochromasia flow cytometry (18). Each

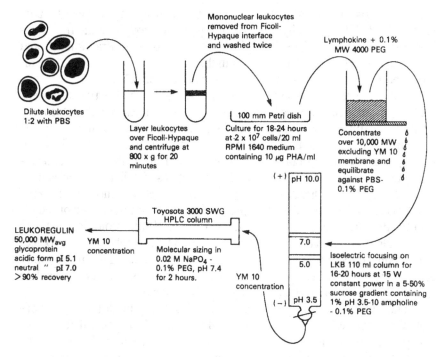

Fig. 9. Sequential ultrafiltration (diafiltration), column isoelectric focusing, and HPLC molecular sizing chromatographic steps in the isolation of leukoregulin (1).

## 3.2. Isolation Procedures and Retention of Biological Activity

Many lymphokines in addition to leukoregulin are present in the culture medium of stimulated peripheral blood lymphocytes. Fractionation of lymphokine mixtures to obtain a specific lymphokine generally requires a multistep procedure resulting in loss of most of the biological activity of the desired lymphokine. A major advance in the isolation and study of leukoregulin has been the finding that the addition of mol wt 3000 polyethylene glycol results in retention of lymphotoxin and leukoregulin activity during processing of the lymphokines (5,15). As much as 95% of the leukoregulin activity is recovered after ultrafiltration, molecular siz-

---

← Fig. 8. (continued)

histogram represents 50,000 K562 target cells (50,000 lymphocytes in the NK leukocytes alone histogram). The highlighted region was selected as one location within which leukoregulin-exposed K562 cells, but not natural killer lymphocytes, are found. Treatment of K562 cells with leukoregulin alone or with increasing numbers of K562 cells results in K562 cells appearing in the highlighted region.

ing chromatographic, and column isoelectric focusing steps when 0.1 percent mol.wt. 3000 polyethylene glycol is present throughout the fractionation procedure (*1,17*). The biological activity of both nonfractionated and purified leukoregulin, however, even in the presence of polyethylene glycol, has a half-life of about 4 mo when stored at −35°C (Fig. 10).

The character of labware and matrix materials in the fractionation steps is also important in retaining high leukoregulin biological activity. Recovery of leukoregulin activity is maximized when plasticware and low retention ultrafiltration membranes such as the Amicon YM10 are used. Good recovery has also been obtained using tangential ultrafiltration to concentrate culture medium from stimulated lymphocytes. Similar recoveries have been obtained from silica versus agarose matrix HPLC molecular sizing columns (Table 7), although comparative studies with a number of leukoregulin preparations have yet to be performed. Little biological activity has to date been recovered from polyacrylamide electrophoresis or isoelectrofocusing polyacrylamide gels. This problem needs much more study since these preparative methods offer some of the best means to isolate and characterize biologically active macromolecules.

The biochemical properties of leukoregulin pertinent to its purification are described elsewhere in this volume (*27*). The general fractionation procedure in this author's laboratory consists initially of batch DEAE-ion exchange chromatography followed by column isoelectric focusing and HPLC molecular sizing chromatography with concentration by ultrafiltration between each step (*1,18*). The main points from our experience are that the majority of guinea pig, hamster, and human leukoregulin activity has a molecular sizing chromatographic elution molecular size of approximately 50,000, which, at least for human leukoregulin, is the same on silica or agarose matrix HPLC molecular sizing columns (Table 7). Several molecular forms of leukoregulin with mildly acidic to neutral isoelectric points in the range of pH 5–7 are present in each species. The ratio of molecules, however, with isoelectric points near 5, to those with isoelectric points near 7, varies widely from one human leukoregulin sample to another, as does the amount of leukoregulin activity that is step-eluted from a DEAE-ion exchange column using 0.1$M$ NaCl–20 m$M$ TrisCl–0.1% polyethylene glycol, pH 7.4 versus 0.2$M$ NaCl–20 m$M$ TrisCl–0.1% polyethylene glycol. These differing physicochemical forms of leukoregulin may result from variations in posttranslational glycosylation, and the specific activity of the different isoelectric leukoregulin forms remains to be defined.

## 4. Pathways of Leukoregulin Action

Leukoregulin inhibits radiation as well as chemical carcinogen-induced morphologic transformation of Syrian hamster fetal cells in vitro (*10,11,*

Table 7
Recovery of Leukoregulin Activity from Silica-Based Versus Agarose-Based
Matrix HPLC columns[a]

| HPLC | Recovery of leukoregulin activity, % |
|---|---|
| Spherogel-TSK 3000 SWG 2.15 × 60 cm (rigid, hydrophilic, spherical silica packing of 13 ± 2 $\mu$m silica particles coated with hydrophilic hydroxyl groups) | 90 |
| Superose 12 HR 10/30 1 × 30 cm (beaded crosslinked agarose-based matrix 10 ± 2 $\mu$m diameter) | 88 |

[a]Leukoregulin was purified by DEAE-ion exchange, isoelectric focusing, and HPLC molecular sizing chromatography (18), and 100 K562 cytostatic leukoregulin units in 100 $\mu$L were applied to the Spherogel-TSK 3000 SWG column in 0.02$M$ sodium phosphate, pH 7.4–0.1% mol. wt. 3000 polyethylene glycol and eluted at 4 mL/min. 50 Leukoregulin units were applied to the Superose 12 column and eluted at 0.5 mL/h using the same buffer and HPLC system. Fractions containing molecules with molecular weights between 40,000 and 60,000 based upon calibration of the HPLC columns with protein standards were pooled, concentrated, and analyzed for their ability to inhibit the proliferation of K562 cells in a 3-d cell growth assay (1).

16,17) and in vivo (14,24). Leukoregulin is able to inhibit transformation at several points or stages in the transition from a growth-controlled to a neoplastic cell (11,16). Exposure of the cells to leukoregulin shortly before, at the time of, or shortly after carcinogen treatment, moreover, completely prevents transformation. The anticarcinogenic activity of leukoregulin, furthermore, is blocked by D-galactose and phytohemagglutinin, but not by Con A (16), suggesting that leukoregulin binds to the cell membrane through a D-galactose-containing receptor or other related glycosyl-containing cell surface structural moiety. The prevention or inhibition of the transformation process occurs, moreover, without the increase in target cell plasma membrane permeability or inhibition of cell division seen in leukoregulin-susceptible preneoplastic and neoplastic cells.

Little is known as yet concerning the molecular events in transmembrane signaling and intracellular biochemical pathways following leukoregulin interaction with the target cell plasma membrane. This is caused largely by the small quantities of homogeneous leukoregulin that so far are available to pursue in depth the molecular aspects of leukoregulin's biological activities. The results ascribed to leukoregulin, although distinct from other direct-acting lymphokines, may, therefore, reflect in part contributions from contaminating sensitizing, synergistic, or antagonistic lymphokines or other still-to-be-recognized cofactors. Nevertheless the current data demonstrate that leukoregulin exerts a dramatic and transient ef-

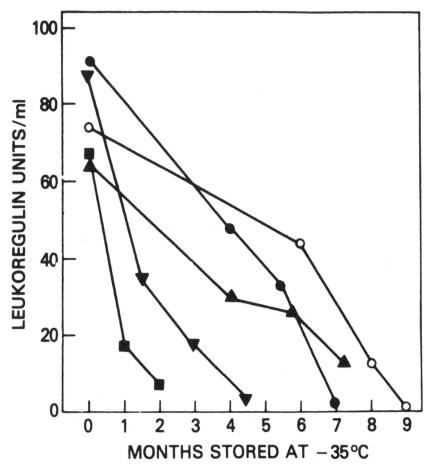

Fig. 10. Storage stability of leukoregulin. Five preparations of Ficoll-Hypaque prepared peripheral blood lymphocytes were stimulated with phytohemagglutinin-L for 48 h (Table 1), concentrated 50-fold by diafiltration over a YM10 membrane, frozen at −35 °C, and aliquots assayed at the indicated times for the ability to induce membrane permeability changes (Fig. 4) in K562 leukemia cells. Proliferation inhibitory activity for K562 cells also declined during leukoregulin storage with a mean half-life of approximately 4 mo.

fect upon target cell membrane integrity that is temporally closely associated with the biological actions of the hormone. Changes in ion membrane permeability, measured by influx of propidium iodide or efflux of fluorescein (1,18), and in membrane fluidity, identified by depolarization of fluorescence from membrane-localized diphenylhexatriene, occur within minutes of tumor target cell exposure to leukoregulin, reaching a maximum and returning to constitutive levels within hours. Similar changes in permeability induced by calcium ionophores and other stimulators of increased intracellular ionic calcium (18) suggest that leukoregulin exerts its action through rapid changes in calcium ion flux.

Increases in intracellular ionic calcium are detectable using the fluorescent calcium chelator indo-1 within seconds after tumor target cell exposure to leukoregulin (28). The rise in intracellular ionic calcium following leukoregulin binding and transmembrane signaling is largely independent of extracellular calcium concentration and may be caused primarily by calcium release from intracellular endoplasmic reticulum calcium stores. The increase in target cell intracellular ionic calcium, moreover, precedes leukoregulin-induced alterations in membrane fluidity, permeability, and surface conformation. The latter in turn antedate release of $^{51}$Cr from the target cells in a natural killer cell cytotoxicity reaction and leukoregulin-induced cessation of target cell proliferation. The sequence in the molecular pathway of leukoregulin action in preneoplastic and tumor cells thus may be: (1) leukoregulin interaction with the target cell plasma membrane, (2) transmembrane signaling resulting in increased intracellular ionic calcium, (3) increased plasma membrane fluidity, permeability, and cell surface conformational change, and (4) inhibition of cell division. Leukoregulin induction of an anticarcinogenic target cell state in target cells for transformation may traverse the same molecular pathway from (1) through (2), but diverges in a still-to-be-defined direction before reaching (3) and (4).

How may an increase in intracellular $Ca^{2+}$ flux and membrane permeability specifically relate to the anticarcinogenic and the cytostatic actions of leukoregulin? A reduction in extracellular ionic calcium concentration inhibits transformation of Syrian hamster cells (29) and is accompanied by an increase in intracellular ionic calcium in human K562 leukemia cells (28). A rise in intracellular calcium has been shown to be a common end-point for toxic cell death (30), although the question of whether the rise in intracellular $Ca^{2+}$ is the causative or a secondary event in the mechanism leading to target cell lysis remains to be defined. An increase in intracellular calcium by itself, however, is insufficient to cause cell destruction since increased intracellular calcium is important in the activation of cell responses without cell death and in the maintenance of cell proliferation (31–33). Increased $Ca^{2+}$ influx also leads to formation of a calcium-dependent regulator protein–$Ca^{2+}$ complex that stimulates $Ca^{2+}$-ATPase, cyclic $3',5'$-nucleotide phosphoesterases, and protein kinases, which in combination with extracellular $Ca^{2+}$ are important, although as yet incompletely understood, in regulating cell proliferation and growth (33). In contrast, the antiproliferative action of partially purified lymphotoxin has been shown to involve creation of an ionic imbalance within the target cell, including an increase in intracellular $Ca^{2+}$ associated with lysis of the cell (34,35). Lysis may, however, be a secondary event of lymphokine target cell interaction resulting from the inability of the target cell to repair the cell membrane destabilization because of lymphokine–target cell interaction. Ionic calcium can thus dramatically affect carcinogenesis and cell proliferation, although the pathways of calcium metabolism are incompletely understood and the points of leukoregulin modulation of calcium metabolism remain to be fully defined.

## 5. Role of Leukoregulin in Homeostasis and Pathophysiology

Leukoregulin destabilization of the cell membrane, along with its associated change in membrane permeability and membrane fluidity (2,18), are major alterations in cell physiology capable by themselves of leading to inhibition of cell proliferation and to conditioning of the cell to cytolytic destruction by direct-acting lytic molecules, including lymphotoxin and tumor necrosis factor or cellular effectors such as natural killer lymphocytes and their lytic molecular mediators. Cells resistant to the direct cytolytic action of leukoregulin (1) may either be able to repair leukoregulin-induced membrane damage or, by as-yet-undefined means, counteract the leukoregulin-directed events associated with increased intracellular calcium and cell destruction. Further definition of the intricacies in the pathways of $Ca^{2+}$ metabolism and their interrelationship with membrane integrity will permit more specific molecular assignment of the role of $Ca^{2+}$ in the anticancer action of leukoregulin. These are important avenues to pursue in the definition of cellular homeostasis in order to understand the molecular pathways by which lymphokines and cellular effector and target cell mechanisms operate to maintain and alter plasma membrane stability.

Leukoregulin may be the critical early mediator in natural killer-type lymphocyte cytotoxicity, serving by its induction of plasma membrane perturbations to "soften up" the target cell membrane to the action of subsequent components in the cytotoxic reaction that lead to lysis of the target cell. A sequence of such events with leukoregulin controlling the specificity of the reaction would be a very important homeostatic mechanism for controlling the proliferation and continued function of a variety of abnormal cells. Impairment or loss of this type of homeostatic surveillance, such as may occur in certain primary immunodeficiency states and in secondary immunodeficiency conditions induced by immunodepressive drugs or by disease as in the acquired immunodeficiency syndrome (AIDS), would allow even cells with normally nonlethal intracellular infectious micro-organisms to survive and, as a result of unchecked microbial proliferation and cellular dysfunction, lead to multifocal pathology, including death.

## 6. Therapeutic Implications and Research Directions

Leukoregulin is the only recognized lymphokine that acts directly at the target cell to specifically prevent the development of chemical- as well as radiation-induced carcinogenesis at several stages in the transition to neoplasia and to specifically inhibit proliferation of preneoplastic and neoplastic cells. The specificity of action, although incomplete, is of such magnitude (greater than four logs difference in the response of the least-sensitive tumor cell lines compared to nontumor cells) that it makes leukoregulin an extremely potent new probe for investigating the process of carcinogenesis and the formation of tumors. This is particularly important in view of the hormone's synergistic and antagonistic potential, as evidenced by its ability to increase the sensitivity of target cells to natural killer-type cytotoxicity, and at the same time counteracting interferon's desensitization of the target cell. Leukoregulin, moreover, is effective in inhibiting the continued proliferation of tumor cells during each phase of the cell cycle and rapidly facilitates the influx of pharmacologically active molecules, such as doxorubicin, into the target cell (C. H. Evans unpublished).

Thus, in addition to being a valuable new probe to study development of neoplasia, leukoregulin provides an additional means to evaluate the process of cytotoxicity and the mechanisms of immunoregulation. Leukoregulin's specificity, moreover, provides a possible new agent for use in the prevention, control, and cure of cancer. Leukoregulin has the potential to prevent carcinogenesis in individuals at high risk because of environmental/occupational, therapeutic, and other forms of carcinogen exposure and to increase the sensitivity of tumor cells to therapeutic attack. The clinical usefulness of leukoregulin is, however, dependent upon the availability of large quantities of biologically active molecules. Gene cloning and DNA recombinant technology will lead to the production of sufficient quantities of recombinant leukoregulin for in vivo preclinical evaluation. For recombinant leukoregulin to be clinically successful, however, it is necessary to determine if each of its anticancer actions is present in the different molecular forms of natural (native) leukoregulin. This is particularly important, since most recombinant molecules are not glycosylated and the degree of glycosylation may be an important factor in determining the solubility and bioactivity of the molecule. It is equally important to know which lymphocyte subsets can produce leukoregulin and which forms of the hormone are produced by a given subset, to be able to determine the functional ability of the lymphocytes in any preparation to produce the hormone as part of evaluating the risk of an individual to develop cancer and his/her potential for a therapeutic response. These are some of the avenues that need to be pursued in establishing the biological role and therapeutic usefulness of leukoregulin. The biochemical basis for leukoregulin activity is just beginning to be revealed. As the biochemical pathways of leukoregulin anticancer action are understood, so in turn will the biological role of this unique lymphokine.

# References

1. Ransom, J. H., Evans, C. H., McCabe, R. P., Pomato, N., Heinbaugh, J. A., Chin, M., and Hanna, M. G., Jr. *Cancer Res.* **45**, 851–862 (1985).
2. Evans, C. H. and Ransom, J. H., in *Thymic Hormones and Lymphokines* (Goldstein, A. L., ed.) Plenum, New York (1984).
3. Cleveland, L., Ransom, J. H., and Evans, C. H. *Fed. Proc.* **43**, 1931 (1984).
4. Evans, C. H. *Fed. Proc.* **43**, 1970 (1984).
5. Evans, C. H. *Cancer Immunol. Immunother.* **12**, 181–190 (1982).
6. Hibbs, J. B., Lambert, L. H., and Remington, J. S. *Proc. Soc. Exp. Biol. Med.* **139**, 1049–1052 (1971).
7. Svedmyr, E. A., Deinhardt, F., and Klein, G. *Int. J. Cancer* **13**, 891–903 (1974).
8. Evans, C. H., Cooney, A. C., and DiPaolo, J. A. *Cancer Res.* **35**, 1045–1052 (1975).
9. Ohanian, S. O., McCabe, R. P., and Evans, C. H. *J. Natl. Cancer Inst.* **67**, 1363–1368 (1981).
10. Evans, C. H. and DiPaolo, J. A. *Int. J. Cancer* **27**, 45–49 (1981).
11. DiPaolo, J. A., Evans, C. H., DeMarinis, A. J., and Doniger, J. A. *Int. J. Cancer* **30**, 781–786 (1982).
12. Evans, C. H., Rabin, E. S., and DiPaolo, J. A. *Cancer Res.* **37**, 898–903 (1977).
13. Ransom, J. H. and Evans, C. H. *Int. J. Cancer* **29**, 451–458 (1982).
14. Ransom, J. H., Evans, C. H., Jones, A. E., Zoon, R. A., and DiPaolo, J. A. *Cancer Immunol. Immunother.* **15**, 126–130 (1983).
15. Ransom, J. H., Rundell, J. O., Heinbaugh, J. A., and Evans, C. H. *Cell. Immunol.* **67**, 1–13 (1982).
16. DiPaolo, J. A., Evans, C. H., DeMarinis, A. J., and Doniger, J. *Cancer Res.* **44**, 1465–1471 (1984).
17. Ransom, J. H. and Evans, C. H. *Cancer Res.* **43**, 5222–5227 (1983).
18. Barnett, S. C. and Evans, C. H. *Cancer Res.* **46**, 2686–2692 (1986).
19. Evans, C. H. and Heinbaugh, J. A. *Immunopharmacology* **3**, 347–359 (1981).

20. Khan, A., Weldon, D., DuvVall, J., Pichangkul, S., Hill, N. O., Mutx, D., Lanius, R., and Ground, M., in *Human Lymphokines: The Biological Immune Response Modifiers* (Kahn, A. and Hill, N. O., eds.) Academic, New York (1982).

21. Green, L. M., Reade, J. L., and Ware, C. F. *J. Immunol. Meth.* **70**, 257-268 (1984).

22. Spofford, B. T., Daynes, R. A., and Granger, G. A. *J. Immunol.* **112**, 2111-2116 (1974).

23. Aggarwal, B. B. and Kohr, W. J. *Meth. Enzymol.* **116**, 448-456 (1985).

24. Ransom, J. H., Evans, C. H., and DiPaolo, J. A. *J. Natl. Cancer Inst.* **69**, 741-744 (1982).

25. Evans, C. H. *J. Immunol. Meth.* **67**, 13-20 (1984).

26. Huang, C. C. and Moore, G. E. *J. Natl. Cancer Inst.* **43**, 1119-1128 (1969).

27. Ransom, J. H. (this volume).

28. Barnett, S. C. and Evans, C. H. *Fed. Proc.* **45**, 488 (1986).

29. Evans, C. H. and Boynton, A. L. *Cancer Lett.* **15**, 271-279 (1982).

30. Schanne, F. A. X., Kane, A. B., Young, E. E., and Farber, J. L. *Science* **206**, 700-703 (1979).

31. Campbell, A. K. and Luzio, J. P. *Experientia* **37**, 1110-1112 (1981).

32. Hallett, M. B., Luzio, J. P., and Campbell, A. K. *Immunology* **44**, 569-576 (1981).

33. Whitfield, J. F., Boynton, A. L., Macmanus, J. P., Rixon, R. H., Sikorska, M., Tsang, B., Walker, P. R., and Swierenga, S. H. H. *Ann. NY Acad. Sci.* **339**, 216-240 (1980).

34. Okamoto, M. and Mayer, M. M. *J. Immunol.* **120**, 272-278 (1978).

35. Okamoto, M. and Mayer, M. M. *J. Immunol.* **120**, 279-285 (1978).

# Lymphotoxins

## Mediators of Cellular Activation, Inflammation, and Cell Lysis That Are Immunologically Related to Macrophage Toxins and Tumor Necrosis Factors

ROBERT S. YAMAMOTO, BRUCE J. AVERBOOK,
MARY T. FITZGERALD, IRENE K. MASUNAKA,
SALLY L. ORR, and GALE A. GRANGER

## 1. Introduction

In the late 1960s it was reported that lymphoid cells from humans and experimental animals could be stimulated in vitro with immunogens and mitogens to release materials that caused cytotoxic and cytostatic effects on continuous nucleated mammalian cells in vitro (1–4). The molecules released by lymphocytes and macrophages were termed lymphotoxins (LT) and macrophage cytotoxins (MCT) respectively (1,2,5). In the mid 1970s, it was reported that the serum of mice infected with bacillus Calmatte-Guerin and then stimulated with endotoxin induced the hemorrhagic necrosis of the murine tumors in vivo; the active component(s) were termed tumor necrosis factors (TNF) (6). It is now clear that LT, MCT, and TNF form an interrelated system of effector molecules.

Subsequent studies of LT found in supernatants from stimulated human lymphocytes revealed that they are heterogeneous and can be grouped into different molecular weight (mol.wt.) classes and charged subclasses (7). Immunological studies indicated that certain different mol.wt. classes were a subunit system of interrelated forms and others were discrete (8,9). In addition, two groups reported on the immunological relationship between lymphocyte- and macrophage-derived cytotoxic forms from both mice and guinea pigs (5,10). These studies all lead to the obvious conclusion that investigators should focus on pure populations of effector cells to determine if different LT forms are from a single cell. Studies were initiated to examine molecules released by separated populations of human lymphocytes (11-13). These studies demonstrated that different kinds of effector cells release common and distinct LT forms that change depending on the kind of stimulus applied. It soon became obvious, however, that primary cells could not provide the quantity of supernatant necessary for biochemical characterization of the LT form (11,12). We turned our attention to the use of continuous lymphoid cell lines as a primary source of these molecules. The two major problems with using continuous cell lines as the source of these molecules were the very low levels of LT spontaneously produced and the failure of these cells to respond to stimulation with lectins. These problems were resolved when it was reported that phorbol myristate acetate (PMA) would induce high levels of LT release by continuous cell lines in vitro (14). These studies revealed that PMA enhanced the production of LT molecules by 10- to 20-fold. In addition, the use of PMA allowed for the release of LT under serum-free culture conditions and at a low cell density (14). The studies presented in this chapter deal with the biochemical purification and the in vitro and in vivo lytic capabilities of LT forms isolated from either PMA-stimulated continuous human B- or T-cell lines.

## 2. Studies of Lymphotoxin from Normal Lymphocytes

Characterization and purification of LT has been difficult because of major impediments such as: minute quantities of these mediators found in lymphocyte supernatants, the polymorphism of the LT system, and the instability of some of the LT classes toward biochemical manipulation (13). Lymphotoxins represent a heterogenous family of glycoproteins with regard to both size and charge (7). Walker and Lucas (15) were the first investigators to show that there were different mol.wt. LT forms from lectin-stimulated human lymphocytes; a 70,000-90,000 mol wt form and a 30,000-50,000 mol wt LT form, termed alpha- and beta-LT, respectively (15). Shortly after this report, Granger et al. and Harris et al. identified additional mol wt LT classes; complex (200,000 mol wt ), alpha heavy (140,000-160,000 mol wt ), and gamma (12,000-20,000 mol wt ) (7,11). The alpha molecule secreted by normal human lymphocytes is a major component in the human LT system (7-9). We subsequently found the alpha-LT can assemble with lytic and nonlytic peptides to form the larger complexes; albeit, the study of these complexes has been difficult because they dissociate into smaller subunits upon routine biochemical manipulation (11,16). Therefore, we proposed to term members of this family of molecules LT-1, because of the immunological cross-reactivity of antibody to different purified LT molecules that express an alpha antigen (8,9). These studies characterized a heterogenous family of LT forms from a heterogenous lymphocyte population; however, recent breakthroughs in biological and biochemical procedures have made it possible to examine the different components of LT forms from the continuous human lymphoid cell lines.

## 2.1. Human B-Cell Lymphotoxin

Our early studies demonstrated that many different continuous human B-lymphoblastoid cell lines release the alpha-LT form (17–19). We developed a subclone of the continuous human B-cell line GM3104A termed IR 3.4 that can be induced to release high levels of alpha-LT when cocultured with PMA in vitro (14). A low mol wt serum substitute, lactalbumin hydrolysate, was used in these studies because it maintained cell viability, protected the LT molecule from proteolytic degradation, and was easily removed during the biochemical separation procedures. The LT-1 in these supernatants was purified to homogeneity by a combination of the following procedures: (1) controlled pore glass beads, (2) DEAE ion exchange chromatography, (3) lentil lectin affinity chromatography, and (4) native preparative polyacrylamide gel electrophoresis (PAGE) (20). Biochemical homogeneity of the LT-1 preparation in the preparative PAGE fractions was verified by comigration of radioactivity and bioactivity on native 5 and 7% PAGE gels as a single peak (20). There is an apparent yield of 1–1.5% of the starting material with a specific activity of $10^6$–$10^7$ units/mg. The LT-1 molecule from the IR 3.4 cell line has an isoelectric point of 5.8–6.3 and exists in two forms: (1) a 90,000–100,000 mol wt molecule composed of a 27,000 mol wt peptide (21) and (2) a 27,000 mol wt peptide in association with the Fc region of IgM. Scientists at Genentech have purified to homogeneity, amino acid sequenced, and cloned the LT-1 molecule from the continuous human B-cell line RPMI 1788 (22). The LT-1 from the RPMI 1788 cell line is composed of a nonglycosylated 25,000 mol wt noncovalent subunit that has an isoelectric point of 5.8 (22). The LT-1s from each of these cell lines are immunologically related because antibodies made against each cell line LT-1 form will neutralize the lytic activity of both cell line LT-1 forms in vitro.

## 2.2. Human T-Cell Lymphotoxin

Primary human T-cells, when stimulated in an allogeneic non-T mixed lymphocyte reaction (AMLR) or against class I or II antigens expressed on certain continuous B-cell lines, evolve into an effector cell population of T killers termed the anomolous T killer and specific cytotoxic T killer (CTL) (23–25). In extensive studies we have found that these T killers spontaneously release LT-1 in vitro when proliferating in the presence of IL-2. These cytotoxic T killers, when stimulated with lectins or in contact with target cells, release LT forms that are immunologically and functionally distinct from the LT-1 family of cell toxins (12). Further studies of the LT forms in supernatants from these effector T-cells presented several serious problems. Although AMLR cultures are a source of enough supernatant for preliminary biochemical studies, these cultures are not satisfactory, for they represent a mixture of effector cells. In contrast, the CTLs are a homogeneous cell population, but there are not enough cells to produce the necessary quantities of supernatant for biochemical analysis.

Our identification of a subline of the continuous human T-cell line, HUT-102, made it possible to examine these T-cell-derived LT forms (26). A subclone of the parental HUT-102 cell line, termed YM 1.2, releases molecules with biochemical similarity to LT forms released by primary cytotoxic T-killers. In a fashion similar to primary T-cells, the YM 1.2 cell line, when cultured spontaneously, produces LT-1; however, when stimulated with PMA in vitro this cell line releases molecules that are similar to LT forms released by lectin or antigen-stimulated T killers (26). The biochemical regimen for the purification of these molecules to homogeneity included; (1) DEAE ion exchange chromatography, (2) column isoelectric focusing, and (3) polyacrylamide gel electrophoresis. Molecules responsible for lytic activity have been purified to homogeneity and were resolved into two proteins upon isoelectric focusing, one at pH 5.6–5.8 and a second at pH 5.0–5.3. The pH 5.6–5.8 and pH 5.0–5.3 molecules were subjected to electrophoresis on native PAGE slab gels, and comparison of silver-stained gels and position of bioactivity showed a single protein band that coincided with bioactivity (26). The materials with an isoelectric point of 5.6–5.8 and 5.0–5.3 were termed LT-2 and LT-3, respectively. There is an apparent yield of 1–5% of the starting material with a specific activity of about $10^7$ units/mg. The LT-2 and LT-3 were subjected to reducing SDS PAGE gels, and the results of these procedures demonstrated that the LT-2 is a multimeric protein composed of covalent 20,000 mol wt subunits, and the LT-3 is composed of a single peptide of 69,000 mol wt. Neither of these two forms reacts with serum that neutralizes LT-1 molecules, yet it is apparent the LT-1, -2, and -3 forms are composed of peptides of similar molecular weight.

## 3. Immunological Relationships of LT-1, LT-2, LT-3, MCT, and TNF

Studies were conducted to establish if anti-LT-1 and anti-TNF could neutralize the lytic activity of the various LT forms in vitro. Monospecific rabbit antibody made against either recombinant TNF (rTNF) or purified LT-1 demonstrated that these antibodies recognized antigens distinct to each molecule and specifically inhibited 100% of the lytic activity of the inducing antigen (12). The in vitro lytic activity in the supernatants from stimulated T-cell lines was not neutralized by either anti-LT-1 or anti-TNF antibody alone; however, the activity was totally neutralized by a mixture of the two antisera, as shown in Table 1. In addition, lytic activity of supernatants from lectin or antigen-stimulated human NK cells containing NK-LT forms (27–30) was also neutralized by a mixture of these antisera (12). These data support the recent reports that anti-TNF or anti-LT-1 antibody neutralized NK-CF and NK cell-mediated cytotoxicity (CMC) of NK-sensitive target cells in vitro (31,32). Collectively, these data suggest that the lytic forms in supernatants released by stimulated NK and T effector cells are related to LT and MCT. Lymphotoxin-2, and -3 were subjected to neutralization of lytic activity by the antisera made against the rTNF or LT-1. The anti-LT-1 and anti-TNF partially neutralized the lytic activity expressed by the LT-2 and LT-3, but when each of the antibodies was added together to these LT forms, 100% of the lytic activity was neutralized. Since the lytic activity of the LT-2 and LT-3 were neutralized by the combination of the two antisera together, these LT forms were subjected to immunoprecipitation. If these LT forms are a mixture, then immunoprecipitation with a single antibody should remove only one form; although if both determinants are expressed on one molecule, then the immunoprecipitation will remove all the lytic activity. The results of these studies, shown in Table 2A, indicate that immunoprecipitation of LT-2 with anti-LT-1 did not remove a significant amount of activity; however, when the nonprecipitated lytic activity was tested with anti-TNF, a significant amount of lytic activity was neutralized, as shown in Table 2B. The opposite results were observed when the two antisera were tested in reverse order with LT-2, as shown in Table 2. Thus, this particular LT-2 fraction contains an "alpha-like" and a "TNF-like" molecule because the removal of one of the LT-2 forms by one antibody was followed by almost complete neutralization by the opposite antibody. The same immunoprecipitation procedures were performed on LT-3, and the results of these studies indicate that a majority of the lytic activity was removed with the anti-TNF and second antibody, but not affected by anti-LT-1 and second antibody. The LT-3 appears to be an "LT-TNF-like" form that expresses TNF,

Table 1
Effect of Anti-LT-1 and Anti-TNF Sera on the Cell Lytic Activity of
Supernatants Derived from Stimulated Normal and Continuous Human Lymphoid
Cells In Vitro[a]

| | Antiserum employed | | |
|---|---|---|---|
| Supernatant source | Anti-LT-1, % | Anti-TNF, % | Anti-LT-1 + Anti-TNF, % |
| *Spontaneous release* | | | |
| Continuous B-cells | 100 | NE[b] | ND[c] |
| Continuous T-cells | 100 | NE | ND |
| *Lectin stimulated* | | | |
| Anomalous T killer | NE | NE | 100 |
| Specific T killer | NE | NE | 100 |
| Natural killer | NE | NE | 100 |
| *Antigen stimulated* | | | |
| Anomalous T killer | NE | NE | 100 |
| Specific T killer | NE | NE | 100 |
| Natural killer | NE | NE | 100 |
| *PMA stimulated* | | | |
| Continuous B-cell | 100 | NE | ND |
| Continuous T-cell | NE | NE | 100 |

[a]Five units of supernatant activity from the different cell cultures were added to: (1)
5 μL of anti-LT-1 or anti-TNF serum or (2) 5 μL composed of 2.5 μL of anti-LT-1 and
2.5 μL of anti-TNF. The mixture was tested for lytic activity on the L-929 cells in the
microplate assay (*34*). After 16 h at 37°C the percent neutralization was calculated by
the following formula:

$$\frac{(L\text{-}929 + LT + \text{antibody}) - (L\text{-}929 + LT + \text{control serum})}{(L\text{-}929 + \text{control serum}) - (L\text{-}929 + LT + \text{control serum})} \times 100$$

[b]NE, no effect.
[c]ND, not done.

but not LT, antigens. Immunologically the LT-2 and -3 and NK-CF are
each related to the TNF-like molecules, but the LT-1 is antigenically
distinct. Yet recent biochemical evidence indicates that human LT-1 derived
from the continuous B-cell line RPMI 1788 and human TNF derived from
the monocytic-like cell line HL-60 are related since they share a 36% amino
acid sequence identity and 51% homology (*33*).

## 4. Effects of Lymphotoxins on Cells In Vitro

Continuous mammalian cells exhibit a spectrum of sensitivities to each
of the human LT molecules in vitro (*27*). Sensitive cells can be lysed in

Table 2
Removal of LT-2 In Vitro Lytic Activity by Immunoprecipitation with
Rabbit Anti-LT-1 or Anti-TNF Followed by Sheep Anti-Rabbit Serum

*Table 2A*

| | Neutralization of LT-2 activity after treatment with the indicated reagent followed by sheep anti-rabbit serum, % | | | |
|---|---|---|---|---|
| | PBS | NRS | Anti-LT-1 | Anti-TNF |
| | 2[a] | 4 | 28 | 12 |

*Table 2B*

| | Neutralization of nonprecipitated LT-2 activity, % | | | |
|---|---|---|---|---|
| Antibody | PBS | NRS | Anti-LT-1 | Anti-TNF |
| 1. Anti-LT | 23[b] | 22 | 10 | 95 |
| 2. Anti-TNF | 8 | 14 | 92 | 12 |
| 3. Anti-LT + anti-TNF | 88 | 93 | 96 | 97 |

[a]Sample of 50 units of LT-2 was incubated with 25 $\mu$L of either phosphate-buffered saline (PBS), normal rabbit serum (NRS), anti-LT-1, or anti-TNF for 30 min at 37 °C, then 25 $\mu$L of sheep anti-rabbit serum was added and incubated for an additional 30 min at 37 °C. The precipitate was removed by centrifugation at 12,500$g$ for 5 min and percent neutralization calculated as described in Table 1.

[b]Sample 5 units of the nonprecipitated LT-2 activity was mixed with either (1) 5 $\mu$L of anti-LT-1 and 5 $\mu$L of NRS, (2) 5 $\mu$L of anti-TNF and 5 $\mu$L of NRS, or (3) mixture of 5.0 $\mu$L of each anti-LT-1 and anti-TNF. The supernatants were then tested in the microplate assay on L-929 cells for LT activity and the percent neutralization calculated as described in Table 1.

2–24 h, moderately sensitive cells are permanently growth inhibited and cellular death occurs in 3–4 d, and resistant cells are reversibly growth inhibited or unaffected. Strains of the murine L-929 fibroblasts were initially identified as target cells that are sensitive to all the different LT forms and have consequently been used as target cells by most investigators studying these cell toxins. A highly sensitive microassay has been developed to allow for the detection and quantitation of minute amounts of these molecules in vitro (*34*). The amount of LT activity in a sample is usually expressed as units of cell lytic activity per milliliter. A unit of activity is defined as the amount of material necessary to destroy 50% of L-929 cells in a 16–24 h period (*34*). These lymphotoxin assays require internal standards because the sensitivity of the L-cells can vary with time.

Recent studies in our laboratory have compared the cell lytic ability of LT-1 from the IR 3.4 cells and the LT-2 and LT-3 from the YM 1.2 cells on a variety of transformed and primary target cells in vitro (*26*). The specific activities of these three forms are quite similar when tested on L-929 cells ($10^6$–$10^7$ units/mg protein). The results of these studies are shown in Table 3 and indicate that the LT-1 form is the least effective

Table 3
The Effect of LT-1, LT-2, and LT-3 on Various Target Cells In Vitro[a]

| Target cell | Units of LT causing 50% lysis | | |
|---|---|---|---|
| Continuous human | LT-1 | LT-2 | LT-3 |
| HeLa | 550 | 25 | 10 |
| Melanoma | 850 | 35 | 25 |
| Breast carcinoma | NE[b] | 725 | 25 |
| Colon carcinoma | 1050 | 825 | 75 |
| K562 | NE | 180 | 100 |
| Raji | NE | 925 | 85 |
| MOLT-4 | NE | 85 | 15 |
| *Nontransformed human* | | | |
| WI-38 Fibroblasts | NE | NT[c] | NT |
| GM3468 Fibroblasts | NE | NT | NT |
| *Continuous murine* | | | |
| Meth A fibrosarcoma | NE | 425 | 125 |
| B-16 melanoma | NE | 115 | 30 |
| Rift fibrosarcoma | NE | 140 | 40 |
| *Nontransformed murine* | | | |
| 3T3 Fibroblasts | NE | NT | NT |
| Primary fetal cells | NE | NT | NT |

[a]Cells (10,000/well) were established in microplates, then exposed to various dilutions of sample containing 0–2000 units of LT activity. After incubation for 72 h, the number of viable cells remaining was determined as described by Yamamoto et al. (*34*). The number of LT units causing a 50% reduction in cell numbers is expressed. These are the average of two separate studies and four individual microplate wells.
[b]NE, no effect with 2000 units.
[c]NT, not tested.

molecule, the LT-2 form was the next most effective, requiring from 20 to 900 units to lyse the target cells tested, and the LT-3 form was effective on all the continuous target cells tested at levels of 10–100 units. These data give the first quantitative results that indicate that each LT form is effective on only a selected family of target cells and appears to be more effective on transformed than primary cells in vitro. The LT-1, 2, and 3 forms caused lysis of L-929 and HeLa cells within the first 24 h; however, the other target cells required an additional 24–48 h before they were affected.

## 5. Antitumor Effects of Lymphotoxins In Vivo

Lymphotoxin forms have a combination of cytolytic and growth inhibitory effects on transformed cells in vitro; and yet under the same conditions exhibit no adverse affect on primary cells. There is evidence that these molecules have antitumor effects in vivo. Papermaster et al. reported that injection of unseparated supernatants or partially purified LT preparations from continuous B-cell lines into human patients with melanomas and carcinomas caused regression of the tumors (35). Kahn et al. reported the regression of a canine malignant melanoma after the intratumor injection of partially purified human LT from lectin stimulated human lymphocytes (36). Williamson et al. reported supernatants from several continuous human B lymphoid cell lines caused hemorrhagic necrosis of subcutaneous methylcholanthrene (meth A)-induced tumors in Balb/C mice when injected intravenously (37). These studies were important preliminary work and demonstrated tumor necrosis factors could be obtained from activated lymphoid cells, but it was still necessary to obtain purified molecules.

Two groups have examined the activity of human LT-1 from the RPMI 1788 and IR 3.4 cells in the murine assay for TNF activity. Gray et al. found the LT-1 from the RPMI 1788 cell line caused necrosis of meth A-induced tumor cells growing subcutaneously in the Balb/C mice when 10,000–100,000 units were injected directly into the tumor (38). Orr et al. found that as few as 200–300 units of LT-1 from the IR 3.4 cells injected intravenously caused partial regression and growth inhibition of 8 d subcutaneous meth A-induced tumors in the Balb/C mice (21). Our experiments indicate that the LT-1 has a 2–3 h functional half life in the blood stream of Balb/C mice (39). Animals can receive up to 200,000 units of LT-1 in a single injection or 50,000 units given every other day for five injections without showing any overt signs of discomfort. The LT-1 from the IR 3.4 cell line causes a dose-dependent growth inhibition or necrosis of 8–10-d-old subcutaneous meth A tumors growing in Balb/C mice. Low levels of LT-1 administered via intraperitoneal, intravenous, or intratumor routes caused growth inhibition of tumor, and high levels of LT-1 induced necrosis and tumor destruction. As shown in Fig. 1, total tumor necrosis was induced by injection with 30,000–50,000 units intraperitoneally, 6,000–10,000 units intravenously, and 800–1000 units given by intratumor route. The most effective route is repeated injection into or around the base of the tumor. Necrosis became evident at 8–12 h and increased over a 48-h period. Over the next 5–7 d, host tissue grew under the necrotic tumor and the lesion healed. Animals were tumor-free up to 1 yr and appeared to develop a significant resistance to the meth A cells when compared to control animals that had the tumor surgically removed. In the control, the inhibition of tumor growth with low doses of LT-1 only lasted from 7 to 14 d after a single injection of LT, but these tumors eventually regrew and resulted in death of the animal.

Lymphotoxin 3 was examined in the meth A TNF assay system as described previously. The effectiveness of LT-3 was determined by the

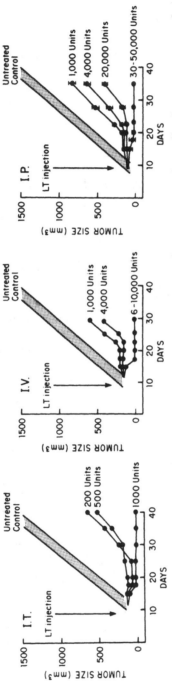

Fig. 1. The effects of LT-1 administered intratumor (it), intravenously (iv), or intraperitoneally (ip) on cutaneous 8-d Meth-A tumors in Balb/C mice. Five mice bearing single cutaneous Meth-A tumors of 0.8-1.0 cm in diameter received a single it, iv, or ip injection of LT-1 at various dose levels. Tumor size was measured every 3 d and volume calculated by the following formula:

$$(\text{length} \times \text{width} \times \text{height} \times \text{pi})/6 = \text{volume}$$

dosage and route of injection, as was demonstrated with LT-1. Quantitative comparison of LT-3 and LT-1 revealed that LT-3 is from 3 to 10 times more effective on a unit basis in causing necrosis and total regression of these meth A tumors. Moreover, the LT-3 induces necrosis more rapidly than LT-1. Necrosis begins within 2–4 h after injection, and the tumor is totally destroyed by 24–36 h. The material is effective regardless of route of injection, though much less material is required when administered directly into the tumor. Shown in Fig. 2 is the necrosis of a meth A tumor on a Balb/C mouse after 4 h.

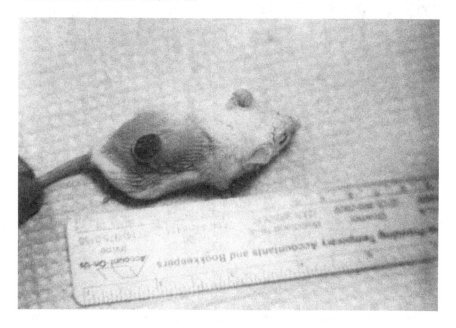

Fig. 2. The effects of 100 units of LT-3 4 h after it injection on a cutaneous 8-d Meth-A tumor on a Balb/C mouse.

## 6. Lymphotoxins as Inducers of Inflammation

In the previous section LT-1 was shown to be active in the TNF assay. Figure 3 shows the histologic examination of 8–10-d-old meth A tumors injected with either 3000 units of LT-1 or control buffer. It reveals the infiltration of polymorphonuclear neutrophils (PMN) into the base and border of the tumor that was concurrent with necrosis in the first 24–48 h. There was evidence of PMN death and the loss of their cytoplasmic constituent with associated tumor cell death by 24 h. In 48–72 h there is a diminishing number of PMNs, along with a few mononuclear cells.

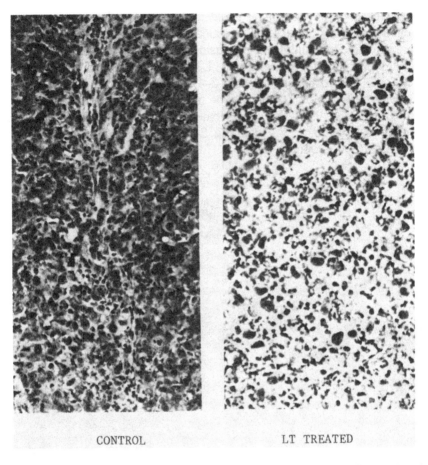

CONTROL                                          LT TREATED

Fig. 3. Microscopic hematoxylin- and eosin-stained section of control and lymphotoxin-treated 10-d old Meth-A tumor 48 h after direct it injection (magnified 25×. Control tumors were injected with 10 μL of 1% BSA in PBS. Lymphotoxin-treated tumors were injected with 3000 units (10 μL) of LT-1. The LT-treated tumor showed an increased number of dead and dying tumors cells intermixed with an inflammatory cell infiltrate.

Microscopic examination of all these LT-1-treated tumors indicated that inflammation and necrosis can coexist.

The identification of host inflammatory cells in the tumor site leads to the question of whether the influx of inflammatory cells was not caused by LT, but was caused by the necrosis. In order to examine this question, LT-1 was injected into normal tissue. In both mouse and rabbit skin, LT-1 appears to induce an inflammatory process characterized by rapid polymorphonuclear cellular infiltrate seen as early as 3 h after inoculation. Visible evidence of inflammation was not present in the mouse, but rabbits responded with erythema and local warmth or hyperthermia 20 h after the LT-1 inoculation, as shown in Fig. 4. Histologic correlation at 20 h in the rabbit demonstrated increased leukocyte infiltration and tissue changes compatible with acute inflammation. The skin reaction in rabbits peaked between 24 and 48 h. At the site of repeated LT-1 inoculation over a 3-d period the rabbit visibly demonstrated all the characteristics of a delayed type hypersensitivity (DTH) response, including palpable induration up to 1 cm. Histology of these specimens showed a combination of acute and chronic inflammation along with focal areas of tissue destruction. It has been thought that LT would only cause destruction of malignant cells in vitro; however, it appears that this may not be the case in vivo. Mobilization of a host inflammatory response and release of leukocyte cytoplasmic granules may be responsible, in part, for tissue necrosis.

## 7. Conclusion

Human lymphotoxins represent a family of cell toxins that are released when lymphocytes are stimulated in vitro (7). Subsequent studies of supernatants from unseparated cell populations revealed that these supernatants contained distinct, individual LT forms and an interrelated subunit system of LT forms of different MW (8,9). Cell separations led to the concept that different lymphocyte subpopulations could release different LT forms (11–13). The studies presented in this chapter examines the LT forms released by purified lymphocyte cell populations when a particular stimulus is applied. Normal and continuous T- and B-cell lines spontaneously release in vitro a common LT form, LT-1. Normal B-cells, when stimulated with mitogens, or continuous B-cell lines, cultured in the presence of PMA, continue to release the LT-1 form in vitro. The anomalous and specific T killer or the continuous T-cell line, YM 1.2, when stimulated with the proper inducing signal, releases new LT forms that are immunologically and functionally distinct from the LT-1 family of cell toxins. These T-cell LT forms, termed LT-2 and LT-3, have a shared immunological identity with cytotoxins that were thought to be released only by macrophages. In addition, these preparations of T-cells release cytolytic forms that express different cell lytic abilities in vitro and in vivo when compared to LT-1 and TNF (40). Although each of the LT forms affects different cells in vitro, they appear to be more effective on transformed cells in comparison to primary fibroblasts. The order of lytic effectiveness of these forms, going from the least to most effective, appears to be LT-1, LT-2, and LT-3. We find that the LT-3 form is the most effective in vitro and

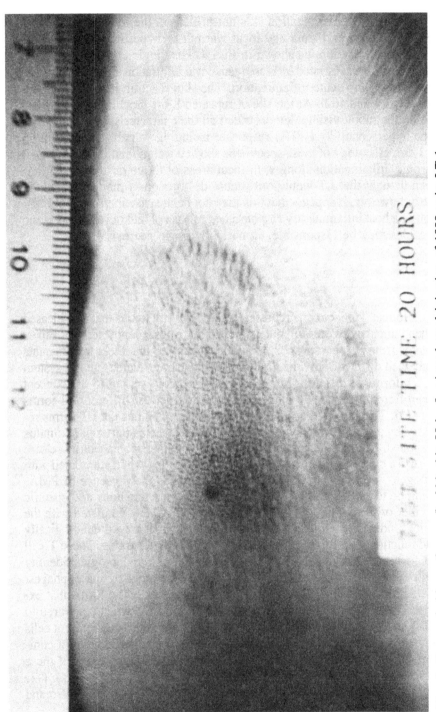

Fig. 4. Gross, visable erythema of rabbit skin 20 h after intradermal injection of 1000 units LT-1.

that it lyses all transformed target cells that have been tested to date. These studies are still in the early stages and must be expanded to include tests on both transformed and primary cells from many different tissue sources to clearly define the effectiveness of these toxins and their "selectivity" for transformed cells in vitro.

Immunological and biochemical evidence indicates that LT-1 from the IR 3.4 human B-cell line is distinct from the LT-2 an LT-3 form from the YM 1.2 human T-cell line. The LT-2 is similar, but not identical, to TNF released by macrophages and macrophage-like cell lines. The LT-2 molecule expresses antigens in common with TNF and is composed of small mol.wt. subunits, but the LT-2 is slightly larger and has an increased lytic capacity for continuous human cells over TNF. The LT-3 molecule appears to be an "LT-TNF-like" form, since it expresses TNF antigens and not LT antigens in aqueous solutions; LT antigens are present, however, but are apparently masked, for they are expressed under other conditions. The LT antigens are expressed during the cell lytic reaction, since anti-LT serum is required to neutralize all the LT-3 lytic activity. Several observations support the concept that TNF and LT antigens coexist on the same protein: (1) most of the LT-3 was immunoprecipitated with anti-TNF and second antibody, (2) the LT-3 preparations contain a single 69,000 mol wt peptide that does not dissociate into smaller subunits, and (3) LT-3 has a different isoelectric point than either TNF or LT. Thus, LT-3 is either a composite of TNF and LT peptides or a single peptide that shares immunologic determinants with both these molecules. A comparison of peptide maps and amino acid sequence will be required to resolve these questions.

The LT-1 and LT-3 has antitumor effects on murine tumor cells in vivo. Either local or systemic injections of LT-1 or LT-3 affected the growth and viability of subcutaneous meth A-induced tumors in the Balb/C mouse. The destruction of a tumor by injection of toxin into the tumor mass is understandable; yet this material was also found to be active when injected intravenously. This latter observation is especially interesting, for it implies that the LT molecule was able to exit the blood vascular system and selectively alter tumor growth and viability without detectable effects on the host. In this situation the LT could only have a direct effect on the tumor for a short interval, since it is cleared from the blood stream of normal animals after 8 h. The LT treatment may also have induced participation of host resistance mechanisms, in that a small amount of LT was able to induce dramatic effects on a relatively large mass of tumor cells. Moreover, studies indicate that the meth A-induced tumor is not highly sensitive to the LT-1 molecule in vitro. These observations indicate that the LT-1 molecule may be more active in vivo than in vitro. Clearly, these studies are in the preliminary stage and must be extended to other tumors, dosages, and routes.

Both native and recombinant LT-1 induces a host-inflammatory response in normal and malignant tissue. This is the first evidence demonstrating LT to be an inflammatory agent and possibly a mediator in other tissue-destructive processes involved with autoimmunity. Recombinant TNF does not give rise to skin reactions in rabbits. This suggests a different mechanism of action of in vivo tumor cell destruction when comparing TNF to LT-1. The LT-1 effects on tissue may involve and interact with other mediators, such as interferons, kinins, chemotactic factors, interleukins, prostaglandins, and macrophage activation factors. Further studies will need to be done to adequately understand the mechanisms and cellular components involved.

Human lymphotoxins represent an inducible family of cell lytic effector molecules, and it is now apparent that individual lymphocytes can release different LT forms in response to stimulation with different agents. In addition, each of these toxins is effective on different types of continuous cell lines in vitro. The finding that lymphotoxins have selectivity for transformed cells in vitro makes it plausible to propose that these effector cells are the source of these molecules in vivo. Moreover, they may employ these proteins as a mechanism for control and destruction of transformed cells in vivo. Thus, the inducing signal (i.e., antigens, mitogens, phorbal esters) has a role in selecting which toxins are secreted by the stimulated lymphocyte. This is an important concept, for it implies that effector lymphocytes may have a role in host resistance to neoplasms. The finding that each LT form affects different families of target cells also lends support to the concept that effector cells may employ different toxins to deal with the heterogeneous cell populations present in a tumor mass.

# References

1. Ruddle, N. H. and Waksman, B. H. *J. Exp. Med.* **128**, 1267–1279 (1968).
2. Granger, G. A. and Kolb, W. P. *J. Immunol.* **101**, 111–120 (1968).
3. Jeffes, E. W. B. and Granger, G. A. *J. Immunol.* **114**, 64–69 (1975).
4. Kramer, S. and Granger, G. A. *Cell. Immunol.* **15**, 57–68 (1975).
5. Kramer, J. J. and Granger, G. A. *Cell. Immunol.* **3**, 88–100 (1972).
6. Carswell, E. A., Old, L. J., Kassel, R. I., Green, S., Fiore, N., and Williamson, B. *Proc. Natl. Acad. Sci. USA* **72**, 3666–3670 (1975).
7. Granger, G. A., Yamamoto, R. S., Fair, D. S., and Hiserodt, J. C. *Cell. Immunol.* **38**, 388–402 (1978).
8. Lewis, J. E., Carmack, C. E., Yamamoto, R. S., and Granger, G. A. *J. Immunol. Meth.* **14**, 163–176 (1977).
9. Yamamoto, R. S., Hiserodt, J. C., Lewis, J. E., Carmack, C. E., and Granger, G. A. *Cell. Immunol.* **38**, 403–416 (1978).

10. Zacharchuk, C. M., Drysdale, B. E., Mayer, M. M., and Shin, H. S. *Proc. Natl. Acad. Sci. USA* **80**, 6341-6345 (1983).
11. Harris, P. C., Yamamoto, R. S., Crane, J., and Granger, G. A. *J. Immunol.* **126**, 2165-2170 (1981).
12. Yamamoto, R. S., Ware, C. F., and Granger, G. A. *J. Immunol.* **137**, 1878-1884 (1986).
13. Devlin, J. J., Klostergaard, J., Orr, S. L., Yamamoto, R. S., and Granger, G. A., in *Lymphokines* (Pick, E., ed.) Academic, San Diego (1984).
14. Yamamoto, R. S., Johnson, D., Masunaka, I., and Granger, G. A. *J. Biol. Resp. Modif.* **3**, 76-87 (1984).
15. Walker, S. M. and Lucas, Z. J. *J. Immunol.* **109**, 1233-1243 (1972).
16. Hiserodt, J. C., Yamamoto, R. S., and Granger, G. A. *Cell. Immunol.* **38**, 417-433 (1978).
17. Granger, G. A., Moore, G. E., White, J. G., Matzinger, P., Sundsmo, J. S., Shupe, S., Kolb, W. P., Kramer, J., and Glade, P. R. *J. Immunol.* **104**, 1476-1485 (1970).
18. Papermaster, B. W., Holterman, O. A., Klein, E., Djerassi, J., Rosner, D., Dao, T., and Costanzi, J. *Clin. Immunol. Immunopathol.* **5**, 31-47 (1976).
19. Fair, D. S., Jeffes, E. W. B., and Granger, G. A. *Mol. Immunol.* **16**, 185-192 (1979).
20. Johnson, D. L., Yamamoto, R. S., Masunaka, I. K., Plunkett, J. M., and Granger, G. A. *Mol. Immunol.* **20**, 1241-1244 (1983).
21. Orr, S. L., Plunkett, M., Masunaka, I., and Granger, G. A., in *Cellular and Molecular Biology of Lymphokines.* (Sorg, C. and Schimpl, A., eds.) Academic, Orlando (1985).
22. Aggarwal, B. B., Moffat, B., and Harkins, R. N. *J. Biol. Chem.* **259**, 686-691 (1984).
23. Muul, L. M. and Gately, M. K. *J. Immunol.* **132**, 1202-1207 (1984).
24. Meur, S. C., Schlossman, S. F., and Reinherz, E. L. *Proc. Natl. Acad. Sci. USA* **79**, 4395-4399 (1982).
25. Krensky, A. M., Clayberger, C., Reiss, C. S., Strominger, J. L., and Burakoff, S. J. *J. Immunol.* **129**, 2001-2003 (1982).
26. Granger, G. A., Kobayashi, M., Plunkett, J. M., Masunaka, I. K., and Yamamoto, R. S. *J. Immunol.* **137**, 1885-1892 (1986).
27. Yamamoto, R. S., Hiserodt, J. C., and Granger, G. A. *Cell. Immunol.* **45**, 261-275 (1979).
28. Yamamoto, R. S., Weitzen, M. L., Miner, K. M., Devlin, J. J., and Granger, G. A., in *NK Cells and Other Natural Effector Cells* (Herberman, R. B., ed.) Academic, New York (1982).
29. Wright, S. C., Weitzen, M. L., Kahle, R., Granger, G. A., and Bonavida, B. *J. Immunol.* **130**, 2479-2483 (1983).
30. Weitzen, M. L., Yamamoto, R. S., and Granger, G. A. *Cell. Immunol.* **77**, 30-41 (1983).
31. Svedersky, L. P., Nedwin, G. E., Bringman, T. S., Shalaby, M. R., Lamott, J. A., Goeddel, D. V., and Pallidino, M. A. *Fed. Proc. Abs.* **44**, 589 (1985).
32. Weitzen, M. L., Innins, E., Yamamoto, R. S., and Granger, G. A. *Cell. Immunol.* **77**, 42-51 (1983).

*33.* Aggarwal, B. B., Kohr, W. S., Hass, P. E., Moffat, B., Spencer, S. A., Henzel, W. J., Bringman, T. S., Nedwin, G. S., Goeddel, D. V., and Harkins, R. N. *J. Biol. Chem.* **260**, 2345-2354 (1985).

*34.* Yamamoto, R. S., Kobayashi, M., Plunkett, J. M., Masunaka, I. K., Orr, S. L., and Granger, G. A., in *Practical Methods in Clinical Immunology* (Yoshida, T., ed.) Churchill Livingstone, London (1985).

*35.* Papermaster, B. W., Holterman, O. A., Klein, E., Parnett, S., Dobkins, D., Laudio, R., and Djerassi, J. *Clinical Immunol. Immunopathol.* **5**, 48-59 (1976).

*36.* Kahn, A., Martin, E., Webb, K., Weldon, D., Hill, N., Duvall, J., and Hill, J. *Proc. Soc. Exp. Biol. Med.* **169**, 291-294 (1982).

*37.* Williamson, B., Carswell, A., Rubin, B., Prendergast, J., and Old, L. *Proc. Natl. Acad. Sci. USA* **80**, 5397-5401 (1983).

*38.* Gray, P. W., Aggarwal, B. B., Benton, C. V., Bringman, T. S., Henzel, W. J., Jarrett, J. A., Leung, D. W., Moffat, B., Ng, B., Pallidino, M. A., and Nedwin, G. E. *Nature* **312**, 721-724 (1984).

*39.* Granger, G. A., Averbook, B., Orr, S., Yamamoto, R. S., and Masunaka, I., in *Second International Research Symposium on Cellular Oncology.* (in press).

*40.* Wang, A. M., Creasey, A. A., Ladner, M. B., Lin, L. S., Strickler, J., Van Arsdell, J. N., Yamamoto, R., and Mark, D. F. *Science* **228**, 149-154 (1985).

# Tumor Necrosis Factors Alpha and Beta

## A Family of Biochemically Related Cytokines

MICHAEL A. PALLADINO, JR. and ARTHUR J. AMMANN

## 1. History of Tumor Necrosis Factors

In 1891, a surgeon, William Coley, working at The Memorial Hospital in New York City observed the disappearance of a neck tumor in a patient who had contracted erysipelas, a streptococcal infection (*1*). Thirty eight additional cases dating back to 1868 were also documented by Coley, who then decided to treat other cancer patients with live streptococci. Because this was not "acceptable" medical practice at the time, however, heat-killed organisms were used instead. This approach failed.

Studies performed at the same time in France, indicated that the virulence of certain bacteria was sometimes increased if the bacteria were grown in the presence of *Serratia marcescens*. Coley tried mixtures of these bacterial cultures prepared for him at the New York College of Physicians and Surgeons. These and at least 15 other preparations of "Coley's mixed toxins," one of which was marketed by Parke Davis and Company (from 1899 until 1907) and another by the Lister Institute for Preventative Medicine in London (from the 1890s until the 1930s), were tested on over 500 cases with inconclusive results. A monograph written by Coley's daughter, Helen Coley Nauts, describing his investigations in detail has recently been published (*2*).

At the Fourth International Lymphokine Meeting Workshop in West Germany in 1984, the molecular cloning of two factor(s) that are possibly the mediators of the antitumor effects of "Coley's mixed toxins" was reported (*3,4*). Critical scientific developments during the intervening 92 years, which led to the isolation of these factors, now termed tumor necrosis

Table 1
History of TNF Developments

| 1891 | Coley: Attempted to treat cancers with mixtures of *Streptococcus pyrogenes* and *Serratia marcescens*. |
|------|------|
| 1931 | Gratia and Linz: Demonstrated the hemorrhagic necrosis of experimental cancer after injection of bacterial filtrates. |
| 1943 | Shear and colleagues: Identified the active agent from bacteria that induced hemorrhagic necrosis of experimental cancer as a polysaccharide subsequently shown to be a component of endotoxin. |
| 1951 | Algire: Postulated that hemorrhagic necrosis was the result of endotoxin-induced hypotension leading to vascular collapse and resulting tumor necrosis. |
| 1960/61 | Govaerts; Rosenau and Moon: Demonstrated that lymphocytes from sensitized animals lysed allogeneic targets. |
| 1968 | Ruddle and Waxman; Granger and Williams; Rosenau: Demonstrated that lymphocyte cytotoxic factor (later termed lymphotoxin and, more recently, TNF-$\beta$) produced by antigen- or mitogen-stimulated lymphocytes caused target cell lysis. |
| 1975 | Carswell and colleagues: Utilized mice infected with *Bacillus Calmette-Guerin* and endotoxin to produce a serum factor capable of inducing tumor necrosis. |
| 1983 | Williams and colleagues: Described a human B-lymphoblastoid cell derived factor (TNF-LUKII) with tumor necrosis activities. |
| 1984 | Gray and colleagues: Cloned cDNA for human tumor necrosis factor-$\beta$. |
| 1984 | Pennica and colleagues: Cloned cDNA for human tumor necrosis factor-$\alpha$. |
| 1985 | Pennica and colleagues: Cloned cDNA for murine tumor necrosis factor-$\alpha$. |

factors (TNF), are outlined in Table 1 (5–14). In this chapter, we discuss (1) the similarities of the in vivo tumor necrosis activities of a predominantly macrophage-derived cytokine termed TNF-$\alpha$, also called cachectin, and a B-lymphoblastoid cell-derived lymphokine termed TNF-$\beta$ (also called lymphotoxin) and (2) the techniques in protein biochemistry and molecular biology that succeeded in producing recombinant human tumor necrosis factor-alpha (rHuTNF-$\alpha$) and tumor necrosis factor-beta (rHuTNF-$\beta$). The studies support the conclusion that these proteins are a family of inter-related molecules with tumor necrosis activities.

## 2. Nomenclature: In Vivo Necrosis Activities

The term tumor necrosis factor describes the in vivo antitumor activities of two distinct cytokines, i.e., classical macrophage-derived TNF

(TNF-α) and B-lymphoblastoid cell-derived TNF-β (3,4). Both cytokines induce hemorrhagic necrosis of the BALB/c chemically induced sarcoma Meth A (3,4). The classical in vivo TNF (13) assay visually measures the hemorrhagic necrosis of a 7–10-d-old intradermal Meth A sarcoma implant measuring approximately 0.5–0.75 cm in diameter in syngeneic (BALB/c) or semisyngeneic (BALB/c × C57BL/6) $F_1$ mice. The scoring is defined as follows:

Hemorrhagic Necrosis Scoring

| | |
|---|---|
| 3+ | Denotes 50–75% hemorrhagic necrosis |
| 2+ | Denotes 25–50% hemorrhagic necrosis |
| 1+ | Denotes <25% hemorrhagic necrosis |
| − | Denotes no visible necrosis |

A comparison of the tumor necrosis activities of both rHuTNF-α and rHuTNF-β is presented in Table 2. Additional studies have been reported previously (3,4). The results clearly show that both rHuTNF-α and rHuTNF-β induce a similar degree of hemorrhagic necrosis of Meth A A sarcoma after intravenous injection and support that these molecules belong to a family of cytokines with similar biologic activities.

Table 2
In Vivo Tumor Necrosis Activities of rHuTNF-α and rHuTNF-β
in Meth A Sarcoma Bearing CB6F₁ Mice

| Intravenous treatment | Hemorrhagic necrosis score[a] |
|---|---|
| PBS[b] | 0.1 ± 0.31 |
| 5 μg rHuTNF-α | 2.6 ± 0.77 |
| 5 μg rHuTNF-β | 2.3 ± 1.0 |

[a]There were 19 animals per group for rHuTNF-α and 20 for rHuTNF-β and PBS controls. Hemorrhagic necrosis score (means ± SD) was determined as described in section 2.
[b]Phosphate buffered saline.

The term TNF (LukII) has been used recently (14) to describe a B-lymphoblastoid cell-derived cytokine that appears to be lymphotoxin-like by virtue of cellular source in vitro and in vivo bioactivities. The term lymphotoxin fails to reflect one of the most important properties of this molecule; namely its tumor necrosis activity. The term TNF-β describes this activity, indicates certain homologies to TNF-α that we will detail in this chapter, and retains the uniqueness of the two molecules. The situation with the TNFs is analogous to that of the interferons (α, β, and γ) and more recently with the interleukin-1s ($\alpha$ and $\beta$) (15,16). In this and the following chapter, we will use the designation TNF-$\alpha$ for classical tumor necrosis factor, and TNF-$\beta$ for lymphotoxin. The term TNF-like will be used in reference to literature reviews in which the exact identity of the factor to recombinant TNF-$\alpha$ or TNF-$\beta$ cannot be determined.

# 3. HuTNF-$\alpha$ and HuTNF-$\beta$:
## Biochemistry and Molecular Biology

The molecular cloning of recombinant HuTNF-$\alpha$ (rHuTNF-$\alpha$) and recombinant HuTNF-$\beta$ (rHuTNF-$\beta$) required two prerequisites: (1) sensitive rapid bioassays for protein detection and (2) a source of RNA to prepare cDNA clones. Of great help in the molecular cloning of both TNF molecules was the availability of ample natural protein for purification to obtain sequence data to biosynthesize HuTNF-$\alpha$ and HuTNF-$\beta$ probes. Each issue will be addressed in detail.

## 3.1. Bioassays

A cytotoxic cell assay utilizing murine L-929 fibroblast cells was used to measure HuTNF-$\alpha$ and HuTNF-$\beta$ bioactivity. Assay sensitivity was enhanced and assay duration time decreased by treatment of the L-929 cells with actinomycin D (17,18). After 18 h of incubation, 96-well, flat-bottom microtiter plates were washed in phosphate buffered saline and stained with a solution of crystal violet in methanol-water. Cytotoxic activity was determined in an automated microelisa plate reader set for absorbance at 450 nm and transmission at 570 nm. One unit of HuTNF-$\alpha$ or HuTNF-$\beta$ was defined as the dilution required for 50% lysis of actinomycin D-treated L-929 fibroblast cells. Recently a more sensitive assay utilizing actinomycin D-treated L-M cells (ATCC no. CCL1.2), a subclone of L-929, was adapted to measure HuTNF-$\alpha$ and HuTNF-$\beta$ bioactivity (19). In addition, the adaptation of a rapid colorimeter assay for the quantitation of cytotoxic and cytostatic lymphokines has been reported (20). The assay utilizes a tetrazolium dye that is reduced to a blue formazan in living, but not dead, cells. The concentration of dye produced can also be quantitated in a microelisa reader similar to the crystal violet assay described above.

## 3.2. HuTNF-$\alpha$ and HuTNF-$\beta$ Induction Schemes

The isolation of continuous cell lines capable of producing significant quantities of the specific protein greatly aided in the molecular cloning of these two molecules. Optimal methods have been described for the induction of HuTNF-α and HuTNF-β from human peripheral blood mononuclear cell cultures (3,21,22). The induction procedures resulting in optimal activation required the addition of 4β-phorbol-12-β-myristate-13α-acetate (PMA), thymosin-$α_1$, and staphylococcus enterotoxin B (SEB). These and other procedures also stimulated the production of both TNFs as well as gamma interferon (IFNγ), and were therefore not considered the method of choice for protein purification and cloning (21,22).

Two human cell lines of hematopoietic origin, HL-60 and U937, were found to produce HuTNF-α after stimulation with PMA (3,21). HL-60 consistently produced the highest levels of HuTNF-α and was therefore used for the protein purification and molecular cloning (Table 3). The B-lymphoblastoid cell lines RPMI 1788, RPMI 8226, and RPMI 8866 were found to produce varying levels of HuTNF-β after stimulation with PMA (Table 3) (14,18). Other B-lymphoblastoid cell lines have also been shown to produce TNF-like proteins (14). The relationship of these factors to rHuTNF-α or rHuTNF-β is not known at present.

Table 3
Production of HuTNF-α and HuTNF-β by Human Transformed Cell Lines

| Cell line[a] | Histological type | HuTNF-α | HuTNF-β |
|---|---|---|---|
| RPMI 1788 | B-Lymphoblastoid | − | + + + + |
| RPMI 8226 | | − | + + + |
| RPMI 8866 | | − | + |
| HL-60 | Monocytic | + + + + | − |
| U937 | | + | − |

[a]Stimulated with PMA (10 ng/mL).
[b](−), <4 units/mL; (+), 4–99 units/mL; (+ +), 100–199 units/mL; (+ + +), 200–399 units/mL; (+ + + +), >400 units/mL.

### 3.3. HuTNF-α

TNF was originally described as an activity present in sera of mice following injection with *Bacillus Calmette-Guerin* (BCG) or other immuno-stimulating agents and subsequently injected with lipopolysaccharide (LPS) (13). Intralesional or intravenous injection of serum from these animals induced hemorrhagic necrosis of certain transplantable tumors 24 h following administration and could also be assayed in vitro on L-929 cells (13,23–27).

HL-60-derived HuTNF-α was purified to apparent homogeneity by controlled pore glass, DEAE cellulose chromatograhy, Mono Q-fast protein liquid chromatography, and reverse phase high-performance chromatography (28). A synthetic 42-base-long gene was constructed from the amino acid sequence data obtained from one of the nine tryptic peptides analyzed (TD-6). RNA from HL-60 cells were used to prepare a cDNA library in vector λgt10. A detailed discussion of the cloning procedure has been previously reported and therefore will not be described in this chapter (3). The $NH_2$ terminal amino acid sequence of natural HuTNF-α showed that the mature polypeptide of 157 amino acids was preceded by a sequence of 76 residues that is probably involved in TNF secretion, since it is not observed on mature HuTNF-α (3). Table 4 lists some of the important characteristics of the natural and recombinant HuTNF-α molecules.

Table 4
Characteristics of Natural and Recombinant Human TNF-α

|  | Natural | Recombinant |
|---|---|---|
| Molecular weight | 17,000 | 17,000 |
| Number of amino acids | 157 | 157 |
| Cysteine residues | 2 | 2 |
| Glycosylated[a] | No | No |
| Specific L-929 bioactivity (U/mg) | $4 \times 10^7$ | $4 \times 10^7$ |
| In vivo tumor necrosis activity | Yes | Yes |

[a]Natural murine TNF-α has been shown to be glycosylated (23). This is in agreement with our data describing a glycosylation site on the recombinant murine TNF-α molecule.

The availability of a cDNA probe for rHuTNF-α resulted in the isolation of the cDNA for murine TNF-α (MuTNF-α) (3,29). Six macrophage cell lines (obtained from the American Type Culture Collection, Rockville, MD) were screened for TNF production. As shown in Table 5, the PU5-1.8 cell line produced the highest levels of TNF at 4 h and was therefore chosen for cDNA cloning. Other macrophage cell lines have also been shown to produce a cytotoxic factor(s) (29–31). The exact relationship between these molecules and MuTNF-α is not known. However, Northern blot analysis determined that the MuTNF was in fact MuTNF-α and not MuTNF-β or a previously uncharacterized cytotoxic factor. The cloning of the cDNA for MuTNF-α has been reported and will also not be discussed in this chapter (29). In comparison to the rHuTNF-α, the isolated MuTNF-α cDNA encoded a polypeptide consisting of a 79-amino-acid presequence region followed by the sequence for mature MuTNF-α of 156 amino acids.

Recombinant MuTNF-α contains two cysteine residues at position 69 and 101, like rHuTNF-α, but does contain one potential N-glycosylation site at amino acid 7 (asparagine), unlike rHuTNF-α. This agrees with previous reports describing the glycoprotein nature of partially purified native murine TNF (23).

Table 5
Production of MuTNF by Murine Macrophage Cell Lines

| Cell line[a] | MuTNF units/mL at 4 h[b] |
|---|---|
| Wehi-3 | − |
| J774A.1 | − |
| P388D$_1$ | − |
| WR19M.1 | + |
| RAW264.7 | + + + |
| PU5-1.8 | + + + + |

[a]Stimulated with 500 ng/mL PMA.
[b]See Table 3 for details of scoring system.

### 3.4. HuTNF-β

HuTNF-β (originally termed lymphotoxin in 1968) was defined as a factor(s) present in supernatants of mitogen- or antigen-stimulated mononuclear cell cultures that could inhibit the growth of neoplastic cell li nes, but had little or no anticellular activities on normal cells (10–12). Human TNF-β was purified recently to homogeneity from serum-free cultures of PMA-stimulated RPMI 1788 cells (18). Purification consisted of DEAE-cellulose chromatograhy, preparative isoelectric focusing, lentil-lectin Sepharose chromatography, and preparative polyacrylamide gel electrophoresis. The purified HuTNF-β glycoprotein was homogeneous, as determined by high-pressure liquid chromatography and polyacrylamide gel electrophoresis. A continuous sequence of 155 residues was determined by biochemical analyses. The exact carboxy terminal region was difficult to determine, however, because of the hydrophobic nature of this region and the limited amount of purified protein available (18).

A synthetic gene was biosynthesized for the 155 residues of the $M_r$ 20,000 form that was determined by microsequencing (4). This gene was constructed assuming that the missing carboxy-terminal amino acids were not necessary for bioactivity. Extracts of Escherichia coli transformed with the synthetic gene were inactive in the L-929 bioassay. Therefore another approach was undertaken to produce rHuTNF-β. RNA was isolated from a culture of nonadherent human peripheral blood mononuclear cells induced with PMA, SEB, and thymosin-$\alpha_1$ and used to prepare a cDNA library. The detailed procedures for the cloning have been previously reported and therefore will not be described (4). Sixteen additional residues were found at the carboxy-terminal end encoded by the cDNA that had not been identified by protein sequencing. These 16 residues were not present in the synthetic inactive gene, and therefore a hybrid expression plasmid was constructed by splicing the coding sequences for the 16 residues onto the carboxy terminal end. *E. coli* cultures containing the hybrid expression plasmid contained significant L-929 bioactivity. Some of the important characteristics of the natural and recombinant HuTNF-$\beta$ molecules are outlined in Table 6.

Table 6
Characteristics of Natural and Recombinant HuTNF-$\beta$

|  | Natural | Recombinant |
|---|---|---|
| Molecular weight[a] | 20,000, 25,000 | 16,000, 18,000 |
| Number of amino acids | 148, 171 | 149, 172 |
| Cysteine residues | 0 | 0 |
| Glycosylated | Yes | No |
| Peptides after tryptic digestion | 2 | ND[b] |
| Specific L-929 bioactivity (U/mg)[c] | $4 \times 10^7$ | $4 \times 10^7$ |
| In vivo tumor necrosis activity | Yes | Yes |

[a]Ninety-five percent of the purified natural HuTNF-$\beta$ material consisted of the $M_r$ 20,000 form, and 5% was the $M_r$ ~25,000 species.

[b]ND, not done.

[c]As determined by the L-929 assay. Utilizing a recently developed bioassay that relies on L-M cells (*19*), rHuTNF-$\beta$ has a specific activity of approximately 1–2 × 10[8] U/mg.

## 3.5. Amino Acid Homologies

An amino acid sequence comparison between rHuTNF-$\alpha$ and rHuTNF-$\beta$ indicated 28% shared identity, and if conservative substitutions are taken into consideration, 51% (*3,4*). Optimal homology requires placing two insertions in the sequences of rHuTNF-$\beta$ at amino acid numbers 110–113 and 148–150. Two particularly conserved regions were detected at amino acids numbers 35–66 and 110–133 (rHuTNF-$\alpha$ numbering). Fifty percent of the amino acids (28 of 56) are identical in these regions. In addition, the carboxyterminal region of the two proteins are also significantly conserved. The fact that the HuTNF-$\beta$ molecule that was expressed minus the last 16 carboxyterminal amino acids was inactive, suggests that this region is involved in certain in vitro biological activities. Whether particular domains of the molecule are important for the function of different activities is not known.

## 4. Summary

We have briefly reviewed the history, nomenclature issues, protein biochemistry, and molecular biology related to HuTNF-$\alpha$ and HuTNF-$\beta$

known at the time this review was written in the spring of 1986. The data presented indicate that macrophage-derived HuTNF-$\alpha$, and $\beta$-lympho-blastoid-derived HuTNF-$\beta$ belong to a family of proteins with tumor necrosis activities. The following chapter will describe some of the previously defined and newly defined in vivo biological activities of this family of interrelated proteins.

NOTE: Since writing this article, numerous advances in our understanding of the biological significance of the Tumor Necrosis Factors have been made. For the latest information on Tumor Necrosis Factor, the reader is requested to examine the abstract book for a recent meeting on Tumor Necrosis Factor held in Heidelberg, West Germany in September 1987. Immunobiology 175, No. 1/2, 1987.

## References

1. Coley, W. B. *Ann. Surg.* **14**, 199 (1891).
2. Nauts, H. C. *Cancer Res. Inst. Monogr.* No. 8 (2nd ed.) (1980).
3. Pennica, D., Nedwin, G. E., Hayflick, J. S., Seeburg, P. H., Derynck, R., Palladino, M. A., Kohn, W. J., Aggarwal, B. B., and Goeddel, D. V. *Nature* **312**, 724 (1984).
4. Gray, P. W., Aggarwal, B. B., Benton, C. V., Bringman, T. S., Henzel, W. J., Jarrett, J. A., Leung, D. W., Moffat, B., Ng, P., Svedersky, L. P., Palladino, M. A., and Nedwin, G. W. *Nature* **312**, 721 (1984).
5. Gratia, A. and Linz, R. *Scramces Soc. Biol. Ses. Fil.* **108**, 427 (1931).
6. Shear, M. J., Turner, F. C., Perrault, A., and Shovelton, T. *J. Natl. Cancer Inst.* **4**, 81 (1943).
7. Algire, G. H., Legallais, F. Y., and Anderson, B. F. *J. Natl. Cancer Inst.* **12**, 1279 (1952).
8. Govaerts, A. *J. Immunol.* **85**, 516 (1960).
9. Rosenau, W. and Moon, H. D. *J. Natl. Cancer Inst.* **27**, 471 (1961).
10. Ruddle, N. H. and Waksman, B. H. *J. Exp. Med.* **128**, 1267 (1968).
11. Granger, G. A. and Williams, T. W. *Nature* **218**, 1253 (1968).
12. Rosenau, W. *Fed. Proc.* **27**, 34 (1968).
13. Carswell, E. A., Old, L. J., Cassel, R. L., Green, S., Fiore, N., and Williamson, B. *Proc. Natl. Acad. Sci. USA* **72**, 3666 (1983).
14. Williamson, B. D., Carswell, E. A., Rubin, B. Y., Prendergast, J. S., and Old, L. J. *Proc. Natl. Acad. Sci. USA* **80**, 5397 (1983).
15. March, C. J., Mosley, B., Larsen, A., Cerretti, D. P., Braedt, G., Price, V., Gillis, S., Henney, C. S., Kronheim, S. R., Grabstein, K., Conlon, P. J., Hopp, T. P., and Cosman, D. *Nature* **315**, 641 (1985).
16. Auron, P. E., Webb, A. C., Rosenwasser, L. J., Mucci, S. F., Rich, A., Wolff, S. M. and Dinarello, C. A. *Proc. Natl. Acad. Sci. USA* **81**, 7907 (1984).

17. Spofford, B., Daynes, R. A., and Granger, G. A. *J. Immunol.* **112**, 2111 (1974).
18. Aggarwal, B. B., Moffat, B., and Harkins, R. N. *J. Biol. Chem.* **259**, 686 (1984).
19. Kramer, S. M. and Carver, M. E. *J. Immunolog. Meth.* **93**, 201 (1986).
20. Green, L. M., Reade, J. L., and Ware, C. F. *J. Immunol. Meth.* **70**, 257 (1984).
21. Nedwin, G. E., Svedersky, L. P., Bringman, T. S., Palladino, M. A., and Goeddel, D. V. *J. Immunol.* **135**, 2492 (1985).
22. Svedersky, L. P., Nedwin, G. E., Goeddel, D. V., and Palladino, M. A. *J. Immunol.* **134**, 1604 (1985).
23. Green, S., Dobrjansky, A., Carswell, E. A., Kassel, R. L., Old, L. J., Fiore, N., and Schwartz, M. K. *Proc. Natl. Acad. Sci. USA* **73**, 381 (1976).
24. Helson, L., Green, S., Carswell, E. A., and Old, L. J. *Nature* **258**, 731 (1975).
25. Matthews, N. and Walkins, J. F. *Br. J. Cancer* **38**, 302 (1978).
26. Matthews, N. *Immunology* **44**, 135 (1981).
27. Ruff, M. R. and Gifford, G. E., in *Lymphokines* (Pick, E., ed.) Academic, New York (1981).
28. Aggarwal, B. B., Kohn, W. J., Hass, D. E., Moffat, B., Spencer, S. A., Henzel, W. J., Bringman, T. S., Nedwin, G. E., Goeddel, D. V., and Harkins, R. N. *J. Biol. Chem.* **260**, 2345 (1985b).
29. Pennica, D., Hayflick, J. S., Bringman, T. S., Palladino, M. A., and Goeddel, D. V. *Proc. Natl. Acad. Sci. USA* **82**, 6060 (1985).
30. Aksamit, R. R. and Kim, K. J. *J. Immunol.* **122**, 1785 (1979).
31. Kull, F. C. J. and Cuatrecasas, P. *Proc. Natl. Acad. Sci. USA* **81**, 7932 (1984).

# Part 2
# CLINICAL APPLICATIONS

## Interferons

# Clinical Aspects of Interferon Therapy in Human Cancer

MARK S. ROTH and KENNETH A. FOON

## 1. Introduction

Over the past decade improved production methods have made feasible large controlled trials with the interferons (IFNs) (Tables 1, 2, and 3). The type of IFN almost exclusively tested until 1981 was crude IFNα obtained from Sendai virus-stimulated buffy coat leukocytes and represented 1% purity ($10^6$ U/mg protein) (*1,2*) (One unit of IFN is roughly the amount that reduces viral replication in tissue culture by half). Refinement in purification methods and the use of recombinant DNA techniques with *Escherichia coli* has allowed for large-scale production and purification to homogeneity ($10^8$ U/mg protein) of all three types of IFN (*3–6*). Clinical trials with pure IFNα began in 1981. Cloning and purification of IFNβ and IFNγ were more difficult, and clinical trials with these proteins began only in the latter part of 1983. A review of these results and proposed mechanisms of antitumor activity are presented.

## 2. Human Trials

A summary of clinical trials for IFNα is presented in Tables 2 and 3. Some reported trials have used highly purified IFN ($10^8$ U/mg protein), whereas others have used crude preparations ($10^6$ U/mg protein). Impurities in the latter preparations include albumin, transferrin, and additional lymphokines. Despite these contaminants, toxicities and antitumor responses seen with both preparations have been similar. Phase I trials establishing toxicities and pharmacokinetics with recombinant IFNα, β, and γ have been reported (*7–8, 10–12*). The major side effects have been

Table 1
Interferons in Clinical Use

| Type | Subtype[a] (new nomenclature) | Source | Purity, % | Amino acid differences |
|---|---|---|---|---|
| α | Leukocyte [IFNα (LE)] | Leukocytes from normal blood | < 1[b] | |
| | Lymphoblastoid (IFN-alfa-N1) | Lymphoblastoid (Namalva) cells in culture | < 1[b] | |
| | Recombinant α2 (IFN-alfa-2b) | Transformed E. coli | >95 | Arginine at position 23. Deletion at position 44 when compared to other α subtypes. |
| | Recombinant αA (IFN-alfa-2a) | Transformed E. coli | >95 | Lysine at position 23. Deletion at position 44. |
| | Recombinant αD (IFNαD) | Transformed E. coli | >95 | 29 variations from αA |
| | Recombinant α-2arg (IFN-alfa-2c) | Transformed E. coli | >95 | Arginine at position 23. Arginine at position 34. |
| β | Fibroblast (IFNβ) | Fetal foreskin fibroblast in culture | < 1[b] | |
| | Recombinant βcys (rIFNβcys) | Transformed E. coli | >95 | Cysteine at position 17. |
| | Recombinant βser (rIFNβser) | Transformed E. coli | >95 | Serine at position 17. |
| γ | Immune (IFNγ) | T-lymphocytes from normal blood | < 1[b] | |
| | Recombinant γ (rIFNγ) | Transformed E. coli | >95 | |

[a]New nomenclature was proposed at a joint meeting of the WHO and USAN council in May, 1985.
[b]These crude preparations can be purified to near homogeneity (see text).

those of a flu-like illness (fever, chills, muscle aches, headache, GI upset, and fatigue). Interferon-α is well absorbed following im or sc injection, and repeated administration results in tachyphylaxis to fever, whereas fatigue and anorexia increase with dosage and duration of treatment. Other reported side effects include dose-related myelosuppression, elevated transaminases, paresthesias, anosmia, somnolence, confusion, impotence in males, and reported cases of interstitial nephritis (7–9). In contrast, initial phase I trials with IFNβ and IFNγ gave no detectable serum levels of IFN following im injection, although enhancement of immune response was reported (10–12). With the more sensitive ELISA testing, however, recombinant IFNγ has been detected in serum following the im route of administration at doses previously reported to show no biological serum activity (12). Additionally, tachyphylaxis as reported following repetitive administration of IFNα does not occur with IFNβ (10). Other toxicities are similar, although rare hepatotoxicity with IFNγ has been reported. In clinical trials the usual dose-limiting toxicity with all three types of IFN is fatigue.

## 3. Solid Malignancies

### 3.1. Osteosarcoma and Soft Tissue Sarcoma

Osteosarcoma is a high-grade malignant spindle cell tumor arising within bone that typically occurs during childhood and adolescence. There is a 1.3:1 male to female predominance. Patients typically present with pain at the site of tumor involvement. When localized, this tumor is likely curable with surgery and chemotherapy. Relapsing or metastatic osteosarcoma has no cure. Interferonα has shown antitumor activity both in vitro and in vivo against murine osteogenic sarcoma (14). In human trials, however, crude IFNα has shown minimal activity in patients with metastatic osteosarcoma treated at doses from 3 to 10 × $10^6$ U im daily, with one partial response among 13 patients reported (15,16). Crude IFNα has been used in an adjuvant trial (17), in which 48 patients with osteosarcoma received 3 × $10^6$ U/d im for 28 d, followed by the same dose every 2 d for 17 mo after surgery. Five year survival of treated patients is 58%, compared to 33% in 30 patients followed in a nonrandomized simultaneous control group. A prospective randomized trial using pure IFN is needed to define the role of IFNα.

Twenty patients with metastatic soft tissue sarcomas have been treated with fibroblast IFNβ at an initial dose of 5 × $10^6$ U iv over 10 min, then 5 × $10^6$ U iv over 3 h daily for 10 d (18). There was only one partial response lasting 10 wk. The authors concluded that IFNβ in this dose and schedule had minimal activity in soft tissue sarcoma.

Table 2
Clinical Trials with Interferon[a]

| Tumor | Number of evaluable patients | Response rates | | | Total response,[a] % | Reference |
|---|---|---|---|---|---|---|
| | | Complete | Partial | Minor | | |
| *Solid malignancies* | | | | | | |
| Osteogenic sarcoma | 15 | 0 | 1 | | 7 | *15,16* |
| Melanoma | 167 | 6 | 13 | 2 | 11 | *19–24* |
| Breast cancer | 187 | 0 | 14 | 10 | 7 | *28–35* |
| Renal cell | 252 | 6 | 37 | 28 | 17 | *37–46* |
| Kaposi's sarcoma (AIDS related) | 44 | 9 | 12 | | 48 | *49–51* |
| Colorectal carcinoma | 65 | 0 | 2 | | 3 | *53–56* |
| Carcinoid | 9 | 0 | 6 | | 67 | *58* |
| Lung | | | | | | |
| Small cell | 10 | 0 | 0 | | 0 | *63* |
| Non-small cell | 70 | 0 | 1 | 1 | 1 | *59–62* |
| Ovarian cancer | 42 | 5 | 3 | | 19 | *64–66* |
| Bladder cancer (papillomatosis or superficial) | 20 | 10 | 8 | | 90 | *67–69* |
| Head and neck (squamous) | 11 | 4 | 6 | | 91 | *70,71* |
| Nasopharyngeal | 13 | 0 | 2 | 2 | 15 | *72* |
| Cervical cancer | 14 | 3 | 3 | | 43 | *73* |

| *Hematologic malignancies* | | | | | | |
|---|---|---|---|---|---|---|
| Hairy cell leukemia[b] | 121 | 14 | 69 | 35 | 97 | 75–83 |
| Non-Hodgkin's lymphoma | | | | | | |
| Low-grade | 92 | 9 | 30 | 6 | 42 | 85–90 |
| Intermediate- and high-grade | 36 | 1 | 4 | 2 | 14 | 28,85,87,89,91 |
| Hodgkin's disease | 8 | 0 | 0 | 2 | 0 | 89 |
| Cutaneous T-cell lymphoma | 20 | 2 | 7 | 2 | 45 | 92 |
| Chronic lymphocytic leukemia | 67 | 0 | 12 | | 18 | 28,89,90,94–97,133 |
| Multiple myeloma | 177 | 3 | 18[c] | | 17 | 28,99–105 |
| Chronic myelogenous leukemia | 68 | 2 | 46 | 7 | 81 | 108–110 |
| Essential thrombocythemia | 4 | 3 | 0 | | 75 | 111 |
| Acute leukemia | 62 | 0 | 19[d] | | 31 | 112–116 |

[a] % Total response = complete + partial/number evaluable patients.

[b] Complete response means absence of hairy cells in the bone marrow and normalization of peripheral blood white cells, platelets, and erythrocytes. Partial response means a normalization of peripheral blood white cells, platelets, and erythrocyte counts and >50% reduction in hairy cells in the bone marrow. Minor response generally means improvement in hemoglobin to more than 10 g/dL or improvement in platelets to more than 100,000 cells/$\mu$L or improvement in neutrophils to more than 1000 cells/$\mu$L. % total response for hairy cell leukemia includes minor responses.

[c] Complete response and partial response not available from all trials, % total response includes all responses.

[d] Most responses were of short duration.

Table 3
Immunomodulatory Activities of the Interferons

| |
|---|
| Enhance (low dose) or suppress (high dose) natural killer activity |
| Augment antibody dependent cellular cytotoxicity (ADCC) |
| Enhance tumoricidal activity of macrophages |
| Regulate antibody production in B-cells |
| Enhance cytotoxic phase of mixed lymphocyte culture (MLC) |
| Depress lymphoproliferative phase of mixed lymphocyte culture |
| Increase expression of cell surface antigens, HLA-A, B, C, DR, and $B_2$ microglobulin[a] |

[a]Only IFNγ has consistently increased expression of HLA-DR (131), and IFNγ unlike α or β, is able to increase expression of HLA-A, B, and C proteins on the cell surface at concentrations that are considerably lower than those necessary to induce an antiviral effect.

## 3.2. Melanoma

Melanoma is a malignant neoplasm arising from melanocytes and accounting for approximately 1% of cancers in the United States. There is no overall sex predilection, and the majority of patients are between 30 and 60 yr old when they present with primary lesions. Cutaneous melanoma is usually curable if it is less than 0.76 mm thick and does not extend beyond the papillary dermis. Unfortunately, metastatic melanoma is generally refractory to standard chemotherapy. A multicenter trial using crude IFNα was initiated by the American Cancer Society in 1978. Forty-four patients with no prior treatment and advanced melanoma (22 with lung metastases and 22 with cutaneous, subcutaneous, or lymph node metastases) received crude IFNα at 1, 3, or 9 × 10⁶ U im daily for 42 d. Partial response was noted in one patient and two had minor responses (19). In another study using partially purified lymphoblastoid IFNα at a dose of 2.5 × 10⁶ U/m² daily for 30 d, one partial response lasting 6 mo among 17 previously treated patients was reported (20). In another study using low-dose 0.5 × 10⁶ U/m² highly purified lymphoblastoid IFN, one complete response (lasting 15 mo and one partial response among 14 patients treated was reported (21). In this study, higher doses (15 × 10⁶ U/m²) were given to 25 patients and only one complete response was seen (lasting 10 mo) (21).

Recombinant IFNα has been given in three trials. Thirty patients with disseminated melanoma received im recombinant IFNα, 12 × 10⁶ U/m², three times weekly for 3 mo. Six responses were observed (one complete response, five partial responses). Responding lesions were limited to soft tissue metastases except for one partial response of a lung nodule. Response durations varied from 2 mo to 13+ mo (22). Using much higher doses (50 × 10⁶ U/m² im of IFNαA), the same investigators found similar results,

23% response rate in 31 patients (*23*). In another study using 3–100 × 10⁶ U/d for up to 4 wk, two of seven partial responses in an im-treated group and two of 16 complete responses in an iv-treated group were reported. The two complete responders, both with metastases to lymph nodes only, are of more than 2.5 yr duration (*24*).

With the aim of potentiating the antitumor effect of IFN, oral cimetidine was used concomitantly in another study. The rationale for these studies is based on the fact that IFN alone has had limited success, perhaps because of induced activation of suppressor cells, and histamine-2 antagonists have been shown to inhibit a variety of regulatory functions mediated by suppressor cells. Using combination treatment two complete and one partial response among six patients failing prior crude IFNα alone were reported (*25*). This observation was expanded in a phase II trial in which 35 patients with disseminated melanoma received im rIFN-αA 50 × 10⁶ U/m² three times a week for 12 wk concomitant with daily oral cimetidine 1200 mg/day. Eight partial regressions were observed, a response similar to previous studies without cimetidine (*26*).

Interferonα has limited, but definite antitumor activity against melanoma. Further phase II and III trials are needed to establish its therapeutic role.

Interferonγ has been used at doses of 3–3000 μg/m²/d for 14 d by iv infusion in 30 patients with advanced melanoma (*27*). Of 24 evaluable patients, one complete and one partial response has been seen. The complete response occurred in a patient with lung and hilar disease.

### 3.3. Breast Cancer

Human breast cancer is a heterogeneous tumor with highly variable patterns of growth and metastatic spread. Each year in the United States about 100,000 cases are diagnosed and 30,000 deaths attributed to the disease. Early detection and diagnosis remain the cornerstone of treatment. Metastatic breast cancers are not curable. Although beneficial palliative responses can be obtained with hormonal or chemotherapy in about 40% of patients, these responses rarely last longer than 1–2 yr. Patients with metastatic breast cancer who have failed hormonal or chemotherapy have a very poor short-term prognosis.

Crude IFNα was given to 17 patients with advanced metastatic disease who had failed chemotherapy or hormonal therapy at daily doses of 3 or 9 × 10⁶ U im (*28*). Six patients achieved a partial remission and one minor tumor response. Duration of response ranged from 8 to 60+ wk (median, 27 wk). Using an identical treatment program, the American Cancer Society phase II trial reported five partial responses among 23 patients with relapsing breast cancer who had not received prior cytotoxic therapy (29). Duration of partial response ranged from 14–176 d with a median range of 59 d. Recombinant and highly purified lymphoblastoid IFNα has been given in six trials (30–35). Doses have ranged from 0.5 × $10^6$ U im three times/wk to 50 × $10^6$ U/m² iv for 5 consecutive d. Of 120 evaluable patients, only two partial and seven minor responses have been reported.

From these studies it is apparent that purified IFNα has minimal activity in breast cancer, whereas in a smaller number of patients treated thus far, crude IFNα preparations may have some antitumor activity. This discordance may be caused by additional substances in the crude preparation. The issue remains unresolved.

Partially pure IFNβ was given at 3 and 6 × $10^6$ U/d im to six patients (36). Three responses (one partial, two minor) were reported.

## 3.4. Renal Cell Carcinoma

Renal cell carcinoma (RCC) comprises 1% of all human cancer. It occurs most often in the fifth decade of life, but is observed in all age groups. There is a 3:1 male to female predominance. If localized, the cancer is curable following nephrectomy. When metastatic, renal cell carcinoma is among the most unresponsive tumors to conventional chemotherapy or hormonal treatment (best responses about 10%). A variety of immune therapies have been attempted with slightly better results in some trials, but no confirmed antitumor responses over 20% reported.

Crude IFNα preparations have shown some activity in this disease. Fifty patients (21 without prior treatment) with advanced RCC have been treated at initial doses of 3 million U/day im and followed for more than 2 yr (37). A 26% response rate was reported (three complete responses and 10 partial responses). The time from initiation of IFNα to response ranged from 1 to 6 mo and duration of response from 2 to 16 mo (median, 6 mo). The survival advantage was not significant. The American Cancer Society sponsored a trial comparing two doses (1 × $10^6$ U/d versus 10 × $10^6$ U/d) of crude IFNα. Three of 30 patients responded (one complete response and two partial responses), all in the group receiving the higher dose (38).

Recombinant IFNα or highly purified lymphoblastoid IFN has been administered to 129 patients, with one patient having a complete response and 19 patients a partial response (39–46). As with the ACS study, it appears that higher doses produced better responses. Thirty patients were randomized between doses of 2 × $10^6$ U/m² and 20 × $10^6$ U/m² daily (39). No complete or partial responses were achieved in 15 patients receiving the low dose. In contrast, 27% receiving the high dose achieved complete or partial response. Other studies (40–46) show variable results dependent upon frequency and route of administration. From these studies it appears that IFNα has antitumor activity in renal cell cancer, although limited, with only six of 252 complete responses reported (2.4%).

Recombinant IFNβ has been given to 11 patients with metastatic RCC in a phase I trial (47). Three patients achieved partial remissions. In vitro synergy has been shown between IFNα and IFNγ for both antiviral and antiproliferative activity (48). Trials combining these two IFNs in the treatment of RCC are currently underway.

### 3.5. Kaposi's Sarcoma

Kaposi's sarcoma is a pigmented sarcoma of the skin that was once rare, but is now occurring in an epidemic-like fashion in patients with the acquired immunodeficiency syndrome (AIDS). Kaposi's sarcoma unassociated with AIDS typically follows an indolent course, whereas Kaposi's sarcoma associated with AIDS can be extremely virulent. Interferonα has produced regression of Kaposi's sarcoma in AIDS patients and offers advantages over standard chemotherapy that might further immunosuppress an already compromised host. Forty-four patients have received recombinant IFN or highly purified lymphoblastoid IFNα at doses from 20 × $10^6$ U/m²/d im to 50 × $10^6$ U/m²/d (49–52). An overall response rate of 48% was reported with nine complete and 12 partial responses. There does not appear to be a correlation between augmentation of natural killer-cell activity or other changes in immunologic variables and tumor regression. Interestingly, however, some remissions have been unmaintained for over 6 mo.

Although these studies are exciting, the numbers are small, and further confirmation is needed as is overall impact on survival in the AIDS population.

### 3.6. Colorectal Adenocarcinoma

Colorectal carcinoma represents the second leading cause of cancer mortality in the United States. Current therapies for metastatic disease produce responses in only a minority of patients (<20%). Four clinical trials with IFNα have been reported (53–56). Nineteen patients were treated with crude IFNα at a dose of 3 × $10^6$ U/d 5 d/wk im (53). Of 18 evaluable patients, there were no objective responses. Purified lymphoblastoid or recombinant IFNα has been administered to 47 evaluable patients at doses from 3 × $10^6$ U/d im to 50 × $10^6$ U/m² 3× weekly im (54–56). Only two partial responses were reported. It appears that IFNα has a minimal effect on this disease.

In vitro IFNγ has a much more potent inhibitory effect against human adenocarcinoma cell lines. Clinical trials have yet to be reported (57).

### 3.7. Carcinoid

Crude IFNα was given to nine patients with midintestinal carcinoid, six with the carcinoid syndrome (58). Treatment with $3 \times 10^6$ U/d im for 1 mo followed by $6 \times 10^6$ U/d for another 2 mo resulted in prompt reduction in symptoms and polypeptide tumor markers in six of nine patients. No patient, however, demonstrated objective decrease in tumor size during therapy.

### 3.8. Lung Cancer

As with colorectal cancer, results with chemotherapy for metastatic non-small cell lung cancer are very poor. By the end of 1986, death from lung cancer will be the leading cause of cancer-related mortality for both men and women. Unfortunately, thus far, trials with IFN have proven unsuccessful. Crude IFNα has been administered to 50 patients with only a single partial response reported (59,60). Recombinant IFNα has been administered to 20 patients with only one minimal response reported (61,62). Ten patients with advanced chemotherapy-resistant small cell lung cancer have been treated with IFNα without any objective responses (63).

### 3.9 Ovarian Carcinoma

Ovarian cancer is the fourth most frequent cause of cancer death in women and is the leading cause of gynecologic cancer death in the United States. Early detected ovarian cancer is curable with surgery. Unfortunately, however, more than two-thirds of the cases initially present as advanced disease and cannot be cured. Although ovarian carcinoma responds to cytotoxic chemotherapy and radiation treatment, disease-free 5-yr survival is uncommon. Both crude and recombinant IFNα have been given systemically to patients with advanced recurrent ovarian cancer with only two of 28 patients achieving a partial response (64,65). More recently rIFN-alfa-2b was administered intraperitoneally (ip) at doses of $5-50 \times 10^6$ U weekly for 16 wk to 14 patients with persistent intraperitoneally ovarian cancer documented at second-look laparotomy after combination chemotherapy (66). Six responses were reported (five complete and one partial response). Five responses were documented by surgical reevaluation, and all responses occurred in patients with residual tumor nodules that were <5 mm prior to rIFN therapy (six of eight). Interestingly, natural killer cell activity from ip lavage fluid was augmented by IFN in both responding and nonresponding patients. Further studies using ip IFNα given to patients with a negative second-look laparotomy are currently underway to assess its role as adjuvant treatment.

### 3.10. Bladder Carcinoma

Bladder carcinoma is the most frequent malignant tumor of the urinary tract. Although localized at the time of diagnosis as either a superficial carcinoma or papilloma in 90% of patients, as many as 80% will subsequently develop recurrent tumors. No well-designed IFN trials have been performed. In an early European trial, $2 \times 10^6$ U of crude IFNα was administered to eight patients with recurrent malignant papillomatosis of the bladder, intralesionally, locally, or systemically daily for 21 d (67). Treatment was repeated at monthly intervals until tumor regression. The authors reported complete regression in all patients with a follow-up period of 4–46 mo. Only one patient had a recurrence after remission. A similar excellent response rate has been reported following im administration in 12 patients (two complete, eight partial responses) (68,69). Controlled trials comparing intravesical chemotherapy with systemic IFNα are required to define the optimal treatment.

### 3.11. Head and Neck Carcinoma

Head and neck carcinoma is an epithelial malignancy associated with pronounced functional and cosmetic deformity that is made worse by conventional treatment. Two reports from Yugoslavia have reported the efficacy of crude IFNα (70,71). Thirty patients with a variety of head and neck tumors, including 11 with squamous cell carcinoma, were treated. Patients received intralesional, topical, or systemic crude IFNα for 1–6 mo. A complete clinical remission was reported in four cases and partial remission in six. Additional trials are required to confirm this data.

Crude IFNα has been given at a dose of $10 \times 10^6$ U im daily to 13 patients with advanced nasopharyngeal carcinoma, which is commonly associated with the Epstein-Barr virus (72). Two partial responses were obtained, suggesting further study is needed to assess response to IFNα in this neoplasm.

### 3.12. Cervical Cancer

Approximately 16,000 new cases of invasive cervical cancer occur annually in the United States. This neoplasm is strongly linked to herpes virus type-II. Early studies on 15 patients with invasive cervical cancer receiving crude IFNα have been reported from Yugoslavia (73). Nine patients were given $2 \times 10^6$ U/daily topically and intramuscularly and six topically only for 3 wk followed by surgical removal of the cervix. Of 14 evaluable patients, three had total regression of tumor and three had regression to *in situ* or microinvasive histology. Additional studies are needed to confirm these early reports.

## 4. Hematologic Malignancies

### 4.1. Hairy Cell Leukemia

Hairy cell leukemia is a well-characterized lymphoproliferative disorder in which cells with lymphoid morphology and villous cytoplasmic projections infiltrate the bone marrow, blood, and reticuloendothelial system. It is of B-cell origin and usually presents with cytopenias (*74*). The disease is often indolent, with median age of onset 50 yr, and a 5:1 male to female predominance. Standard initial therapy has been splenectomy that often restores hematologic parameters to normal; however, most of these patients relapse weeks to years postsplenectomy. Treatment of relapses has been generally poor with standard cytotoxic agents. Excellent responses were reported (*75*) in seven patients with hairy cell leukemia (three complete and four partial) treated with crude IFNα. Similar data have been reported by a number of investigators using recombinant IFNα. Response rates have been comparable with recombinant preparations following three times per week therapy or daily therapy with doses ranging from 3 to 6 $\times 10^6$ U im or sc (*75–83*). Although the initial report suggested that complete responses were frequent, this has not been confirmed, with only 14 of 121 complete responses reported (*75–83*). More important, however, is that virtually all of the partially responding patients normalize their peripheral blood counts and maintain this while on IFN therapy, despite evidence of residual hairy cells in the bone marrow. Some of these patients have had no prior therapy including splenectomy. Responding patients have not been reported to become refractory to IFNα. Many patients have been followed for over 3 yr. In addition, improvement in natural killer activity and immunologic surface markers parallels the hematologic recovery (*81*). On-going studies to assess low ($2 \times 10^6$ U/m²) versus ultralow doses ($0.2 \times 10^6$ U/m²) IFNα are currently underway. Phase III trials randomizing newly diagnosed patients with hairy cell leukemia to splenectomy or IFNα are also underway.

### 4.2. Non-Hodgkin's Lymphoma and Hodgkin's Disease

The histologic classification of non-Hodgkin's lymphoma has recently undergone reformulation from the commonly used Rappaport system. Based on prognosis and morphology, the histologic types of malignant lymphoma have been grouped into low- intermediate-, and high-grade malignancy under the working formulation (*84*). Although many chemotherapy agents produce responses, patients with low-grade non-Hodgkin's lymphoma are not curable with currently available treatment. This, in combination with the indolent nature of the disease, leads to multiple episodes of treatment and relapse with the patient eventually dying of unrelated causes, toxicity of therapy, progressive disease, or emergence of a more aggressive histology. The low-grade non-Hodgkin's lymphoma has shown responses to IFNα. Early results with crude IFNα preparations reported responses in four of seven patients (*85,86*). This response has been confirmed using recombinant IFN-alpha (*87,88*). In the largest series reported to date (*87*), previously treated patients received rIFN-alpha-2a at a dose of $50 \times 10^6$ U/m$^2$ of body surface area three times weekly. Thirteen responses were reported (four complete and nine partial responses) among 24 evaluable patients with a median duration of response of 8 mo. The role of IFNα in combination with standard cytotoxic agents is currently under investigation as first-line therapy.

Interferonα has shown to be less effective in the intermediate- and high-grade lymphomas. Thirty-six cases have been treated with both crude and recombinant IFNα and five responses were reported (*28,85,87,90,91*). Further study of IFNα in intermediate- and high-grade non-Hodgkin's lymphoma may be warranted to establish which histologic subgroups might benefit from treatment.

Eight patients with advanced refractory Hodgkin's disease have been treated with crude IFNα (*89*). Only two brief minor responses were reported.

## 4.3. Cutaneous T-Cell Lymphoma

Cutaneous T-cell lymphoma (mycosis fungoides and the Sezary syndrome), is a non-Hodgkin's lymphoma characterized by a malignant proliferation of mature helper T-lymphocytes that presents with skin infiltration and an indolent clinical course. Effective therapies include topical mechlorethamine, psoralen plus ultraviolet light (PUVA), total skin electron beam irradiation, and systemic chemotherapy. Unfortunately, prolonged disease-free survival has been reported only rarely with these modalities and the best response rates for advanced disease are reported to be about 25% with short duration of response (*92a*). Responses in nine of 20 patients (two complete, seven partial) with advanced stages of disease refractory to prior therapy were observed (*92,92a*) using recombinant IFNα at a dose of $50 \times 10^6$ U/m$^2$ body surface area intramuscularly three times weekly. Responses defined as at least 50% reduction in the sum of perpendicular measurements of malignant lesions lasting at least 1 mo occurred within 4 wk of therapy and lasted 3 mo to more than 25 mo. These results suggest IFNα is perhaps the most effective single agent for cutaneous T-cell lymphoma.

## 4.4. Chronic Lymphocytic Leukemia

Chronic lymphocytic leukemia (CLL) is a hematologic malignancy characterized by proliferation and accumulation of relatively mature-appearing lymphocytes. Most cases involve a clonal proliferation of B-lymphocytes (93). CLL typically occurs in persons over 50 yr (median age, 60 yr) and affects males more than females at a ratio of 2:1 (93). The disease is usually stable over months to years, but transformation to a more aggressive disease state does occur. Alkylating agents, radiation therapy, and corticosteroids are commonly used to treat patients, although few data show that survival is substantially improved. In a number of early studies, crude IFNα preparations were reported to be active in patients with advanced CLL (nine partial responses of 20 treated patients) (28,94,95). In a phase II trial of rIFN-alfa-2a, 18 patients were treated with both high (50 × 10⁶ U/m² intramuscularly) and low dose (5 × 10⁶ U/m² intramuscularly) recombinant IFNα three times weekly (97) with only two partial responses reported. Five patients appeared to have an acceleration of disease while receiving recombinant IFNα. This low response is confirmed by a number of investigators (89,90,94–96,133). This finding is in marked contrast to responses in patients with chemotherapy-refractory low-grade non-Hodgkin's lymphoma and hairy cell leukemia as described above.

## 4.5. Multiple Myeloma

Multiple myeloma is a disease of uncontrolled proliferation of malignant plasma cells in the marrow manifested clinically by tumor formation, osteolysis, hemopoiesis, hypogammaglobulinemia with a paraprotein monoclonal spike, and renal disease. The mean age at the time of diagnosis is 62 yr. Patients with multiple myeloma respond initially to a variety of chemotherapeutic agents; once patients become refractory to first line therapy, however, further responses become difficult (98). In a pilot study, four previously untreated patients were treated with crude IFNα 3 × 10⁶ U im daily. All patients obtained durable responses (two complete and two partial responses) lasting 3–19 mo (99). Disease regression was observed among three patients in 11 additional patients evaluated at the same dose (100). These studies were extended into a prospective randomized trial comparing IFNα (crude) 3 × 10⁶ U im daily with melphalan/prednisone on a 6-wk schedule. Fifty-three patients were allotted to melphalan/prednisone and 62 patients to IFNα. Total response rate was higher in the melphalan/prednisone group (41%) than in the IFNα group (14%) ($p < 0.05$) (response defined as >50% reduction in paraprotein) (101).

Recombinant IFNα has been administered in four trials (102–105). Doses ranged from $2 \times 10^6$ U/m² to $100 \times 10^6$ U/m² daily. Only 14 of 83 previously treated patients responded, whereas 5 of 11 untreated patients responded. Of note is a recent observation of synergy between IFNα and high-dose chlorambucil in refractory myeloma (106). Further trials of combination alkylating agent and IFN are ongoing.

## 4.6. Chronic Myelogenous Leukemia

Chronic myelogenous leukemia (CML) is a neoplastic disease characterized by clonal proliferation of a myeloid stem cell. A unique chromosomal translocation, the Philadelphia (Ph¹) chromosome, is present in about 90% of patients. The peak age of onset is 40 yr. The clinical manifestation of the disease relates to accumulation in the blood and abdominal viscera of large numbers of immature and mature granulocytic cells. In most cases, the proliferation of the hematopoietic cells can be suppressed for 1–4 yr with cytotoxic agents, but transformation to an acute leukemia or blast phase occurs in virtually all patients (median 3 yr) (107). In the blast phase, therapeutic agents, including those useful in the treatment of acute leukemia, are ineffective.

Fifty-one patients in the benign phase of their disease were treated with $3–9 \times 10^6$ U/daily im of crude ($10^6$ U/mg protein) IFNα (108). Forty-one of the patients responded to therapy achieving complete (36 patients) or partial response (five patients) in the peripheral blood. Responding patients showed a gradual decrease in their spleen size and a decrease in bone marrow cellularity. Suppression of the Ph¹ chromosome occurred to varying degrees in 20 of 51 patients and was no longer identified in two patients. Recombinant IFNα seems to be equally efficacious, with 14 of 17 patients responding in early trials (109). Successful lowering of platelet counts in nine patients (all previously treated) with severe symptomatic thrombocytosis has also been demonstrated (110) with crude IFNα. This preliminary evidence for activity of IFNα is encouraging, and phase II trials to assess impact on survival are underway.

## 4.7. Essential Thrombocythemia

Essential thrombocythemia is a myeloproliferative disease defined by a platelet count generally in excess of $1 \times 10^9$ per l, megakaryocyte hyperplasia in the bone marrow, and the absence of another associated disease cause (i.e., Ph[1] chromosome, increased red cell mass, infection or iron deficiency). Essential thrombocythemia usually appears between the ages of 50 and 70 yr. The major morbidity of the disease is bleeding and thrombosis with a 50% 5-yr survival. A number of agents have been effective ($^{32}$P, L-phenylalanine mustard, busalfan, uracil mustard, and hydroxyurea) in lowering platelet counts. Recombinant IFNα has been administered to four previously untreated patients with essential thrombocythemia at a dose of 5–10 × 10$^6$ U/d im for 30 d (111). Platelet counts returned to normal in three of the four patients. Maintenance IFNα twice weekly was given after 30 d, and patients were followed up to 80 d without relapse. Since no known leukemogenic potential exists for IFNα, it may become a useful initial treatment for essential thrombocythemia.

### 4.8 Acute Leukemia

Acute leukemia is a malignant stem cell disorder characterized by uncontrolled growth of poorly differentiated lymphoblasts or myeloblasts. Early studies with crude IFNα were reported to produce responses in six of seven patients with refractory acute lymphoblastic leukemia (ALL) and two of three with acute myelogenous leukemia (AML) at doses of 0.5–5 million U/kg iv daily. Recovery of normal marrow cellularity was not observed, and duration of response not described (112,113). In phase I and II trials (114,115), 53 patients were treated with partially pure lymphoblastoid IFNα (5–200 × 10$^6$ U/m$^2$ daily × 10 d). Five of 33 patients with AML and three of five with ALL experienced significant (80–90%) drops in circulating blast counts, but bone marrow pathology revealed only three patients with any degree of improvement in bone marrow infiltration (two transiently and 1 for 3 mo). Recombinant IFNα (25–100 × 10$^6$ U/d × 7 d) was administered to 13 heavily pretreated patients with only two minimal responses (116). Interferonα in the high doses used above has had limited effectiveness in the management of acute leukemia. The potential role of lower-dose IFNα has yet to be determined.

### 5. Mode of Action

The mechanism of antitumor activity for the IFNs is complex and has not yet been defined. The IFNs have direct in vitro antiproliferative activity in a wide variety of tumors (57,117–121). Interestingly, in comparative antiproliferative studies IFNα has shown a greater inhibitory effect in cells of hematopoietic origin than either IFNβ or IFNγ using both crude and recombinant IFNs (*57,118,119,121*). Of note, noncycling tumor cells (G0-G1) appear to be a more sensitive target for the antiproliferative activity of human IFN (*122,123*).

Further studies in support of a direct antiproliferative effect are studies of transplanted human tumors in immunodeficient nude mice, in which immunomodulatory effects of administered human IFN are minimal (*124,125*). In these models dose-dependent growth inhibition is observed and persists only for the duration of treatment. Evidence for direct antiproliferative effects in human trials is suggested in cutaneous T-cell lymphoma. Four of 10 patients who had relapsed while receiving a 10% maintenance dose, responded after reescalation to a 100% dose (*92*). Renal cell cancer also appears to respond better when higher doses of IFNα are given, again suggesting a direct antiproliferatie effect (*38,39*).

## 5.1. Oncogene Expression

Neoplastic transformation of normal cells to malignant cells may be regulated by expression of cellular oncogenes. Rat fibroblast cells when exposed to the Rous sarcoma virus undergo malignant transformation resulting from the expression of the viral src oncogene. The product of this gene has been shown to be a tyrosine phosphokinase (pp60$^{src}$) (*126*) that is capable of inducing this transformation. Treatment of Rous sarcoma virus-transformed rat cells with crude rat IFNα resulted in a 50% reduction in intracellular pp60$^{src}$ associated protein kinase activity and a more normal growth pattern (*127*). Moreover [$^{3}$H]-leucine pulse labeling experiments showed that IFN worked by selectively reducing the synthesis of the src gene product (*127*).

Purified human IFNα has been shown to decrease accumulation of the cellular myc oncogene messenger RNA in the Daudi cell line (Burkitt's lymphoma) (*128*). The effect is dose dependent and occurs before any inhibition of cell growth can be detected. Interestingly, in studying the mechanism by which c-myc mRNA is decreased, no effect was seen on c-myc transcription rates, but rather an accelerated degradation of c-myc mRNA was noted (67–80% reduction in c-myc mRNA half-life as compared to control cells) (*128*).

Effect of IFNα (crude) on oncogene expression of peripheral blood cells in two patients with CML has also been studied (*129*). Although the expression of several oncogenes (*sis, ras*-Harvey, *ras*-Kirsten, and *myc*) remained unchanged during IFN therapy, a significant reduction in abl oncogene expression was detected within a few days after initiating treatment in both patients. The results of these three studies suggest another mechanism by which IFN may inhibit tumor growth.

## 6. Immunomodulatory Activity

Immunomodulatory activities of IFN are also of considerable interest and possibly play a role in the antitumor effect (*130–132*). The first evidence of this indirect effect of IFN was demonstrated when mice were inoculated with L1210 cells derived from an IFN-resistant clone, but were still protected by daily IFN treatment (*130*). Since the resistant cells did not revert to IFN-sensitive ones in vivo, these experiments were interpreted as suggesting an antitumor effect was mediated by the host, rather than a direct effect on cell multiplication. Subsequently it has been shown that IFN$\alpha$ can enhance as well as suppress cell-mediated and humoral immune responses that are believed to play an active role in tumor surveillance (Table 3). The relative importance in inducing tumor regression by immunomodulatory mechanism versus a direct inhibitory effect remains an important unanswered question.

## 7. Conclusion

The past decade has resulted in remarkable improvements in technology allowing for large-scale production of the IFNs. Although it is clear that the IFNs will not be effective treatment for the majority of cancers by themselves, we have reviewed herein the effectiveness it can have in managing some of the malignancies. Even in diseases in which IFN is effective, we don't know the optimal dose of IFN to use. Although high doses may have greater direct antiproliferative activity, they may in fact suppress the immune system, whereas low doses may be more effective in enhancing the immune system. IFN's role as a first-line treatment or in combination with standard cytotoxic drugs or other biological response modifiers, are areas of on-going research. It is known that IFN$\gamma$ and IFN$\alpha$ bind to different surface receptors (*132*), and combinations of these two IFNs in treating malignancy are being actively studied as well. Regardless of the eventual role of the IFNs in the treatment of cancer, they are an important first member of a family of biological response modifiers used in treating human malignancies.

## Acknowledgments

The authors wish to thank Ms. Anne Brancheau for her excellent secretarial assistance in preparation of this manuscript.

# References

1. Cantell, K. and Hirvonen, S. *Texas Rep. Biol. Med.* **35**, 138-144 (1977).
2. Cantell, K., Hirvonen, S., Kauppinen, H. -L., and Myllyla, G. *Meth. Enzymol.* **78**, 29-38 (1981).
3. Pestka, S. *Sci. Am.* **249**, 37-43 (1983).
4. Lin. L. S. and Stewart, W. E. II. *Meth. Enzymol.* **78**, 481 (1981).
5. Berg, K. and Heron, I. *Meth. Enzymol.* **78**, 487 (1981).
6. Gray, P. W. and Goeddel, D. V. *Nature* **289**, 859-863 (1982).
7. Sherwin, S. A., Knost, J. A., Fein, S., Abrams, P. G., Foon, K. A., Ochs, J. J., Schoenberger, C., Maluish, A. E., and Oldham, RK. *J. Am. Med. Assoc.* **248**, 2461-2466 (1982).
8. Gutterman, J. U., Fine, S., Quesada, J., Horning, S. J., Levine, J. F., Alexanian, R., Bernhardt, L., Kramer, M., Spiegel, H., Colburn, W., Trown, P., Merigan, T., and Dziewanowski, Z. *Ann. Intern. Med.* **96**, 549-556 (1982).
9. Averbuch, S. D., Austin, H. A., Sherwin, S. A., Antonovych, T., Bunn, P. A., and Longo, D. *N. Engl. J. Med.* **301**, 32-35 (1984).
10. Hawkins, M. J., Krown, S. E., Borden, E. C., Krim, S. E., Real, F. X., Edwards, B. S., Anderson, S. A., Cunninningham-Rundles, S., and Oettgen, H. F. *Cancer Res.* **44**, 5934-5938 (1984).
11. Gutterman, J. U., Rosenblum, M. G., Rios, A., Fritsche, H. A., and Quesada, J. R. *Cancer Res.* **44**, 4164-4171 (1984).
12. Vadhan-Rij, S., Al-Katib, A., Bhalla, R., Pelus, L., Nathan, C. F., Sherwin, S. A., Oettgen H. F., and Krown, S. E. *J. Clin. Oncol.* **4**, 137-146 (1986).
13. Foon, K. A., Sherwin, S. A., Abrams, P. G., Stevenson, H. C., Holmes, P., Maluish, A. E., Oldham, R. K., and Heberman, R. B. *Cancer Immunol. Immunother.* **19**, 193-197 (1985).
14. Glasgow, L. A., Crane, J. L., Kern, E. R., and Youngner, J. S. *Cancer Treat. Rep.* **62**, 1881-1887 (1978).
15. Ito, H., Murakami, K., Yanagawa, T., Shinjiro, B., Sawamura, H., Sakakida, K., Matsuo, A., Imanishi,, J., and Kishida, T. *Cancer* **46**, 1562-1565 (1980).
16. Caparros, B., Rosen, G., and Cunningham-Rundles, S. *Proc. Am. Assoc. Cancer Res.* **23**, 121 (abstr.) (1982).
17. Nilsonne, U. *Sem. Hop. Paris* **58**, 1764-1766 (1982).
18. Harris, J. E., Das Gupta, T., and Vogelzang, N. *Proc. Am. Soc. Clin. Oncol.* **4**, 222 (abstr.) (1985).
19. Krown, S. E., Burk, M. W., Kirkwood, J. M., Kerr, D., Morton, D. L., and Oettgen H. F. *Cancer Treat. Rep.* **68**, 723-726 (1984).
20. Retsas, S., Priestman, T. J., Newton, K. A., and Westbury, G. *Cancer* **51**, 273-276 (1983).
21. Goldberg, R. M., Ayoob, M., Silgals, R., Ahlgren, J. D., and Neefe, J. R. *Cancer Treat. Rep.* **69**, 813-816 (1985).

22. Creagan, E. T., Ahmann, D. L., Green S. J., Long, H. J., Frytak, S., O'Fallon, J. R., and Itri, L. M. *J. Clin. Oncol.* **2**, 1002–1005 (1984).

23. Creagan, E. T., Ahmann, D. L., Green, S. J., Long, H. J., Rubin, J., Schutt, A. J., and Dziewanowski, Z. E. *Cancer* **54**, 2844–2849 (1984).

24. Kirkwood, J. M., Ernstoff, M. S., Davis, C. A., Reiss, M., Ferraresi, R., and Rudnick, S. A. *Ann. Intern, Med.* **103**, 32–36 (1985).

25. Borgstrom, S., von Eyben, F. E., Flodgren, P., Atelsson, B., and Sjogren, H. O. *N. Engl. J. Med.* **307**, 1080–1081 (Letter) (1982).

26. Creagan, E. T., Ahmann, D. L., Green, S. J., Long, H. J., Frytak, S., and Itri, L. M. *J. Clin. Oncol.* **3**, 977–981 (1985).

27. Trautman, T., Kirkwood, J. M., Ernstoff, M. S., Davis, C., Coval, S., Reich, S., Rudnick, S., and Fischer, D. *Proc. Am. Soc. Clin. Oncol.* **5**, 232 (abstr.) (1985).

28. Gutterman, J. U., Blumenschein, G. R., Alexanian, R., Yap, H. -Y., Buzdar, A. U., Cabanillas, F., Hortobagyi, G. N., Hersh, E. M., Rasmjssen, S. L., Harmon, M., Kramer, M., and Petska, S. *Ann. Intern. Med.* **93**, 399–406 (1980).

29. Borden, E. C., Holland, J. F., Dao, T. L., Gutterman, J.U., Weiner, L., Chang, Y.-C., and Jashbhaik, P. *Ann. Intern. Med.* **97**, 1–6 (1982).

30. Muss, H. B., Kempf, R. A., Martino, S., Rudnick, S. A., Greiner, J., Cooper, M. R., Decker, D/., Grunberg, S. M., Jackson, D. V., Richards, F., Samal, B., Singhakowinta, A., Spur, C. L., Stuart, J. J., White, D. R., Caponera, M., and Mitchell, M. S. *J. Clin. Oncol.* **2**, 1012–1016 (1984).

31. Sherwin, S. A., Mayer, D., Ochs, J. J., Abrams, P. G., Kinost, J. A., Foon, K. A., Fein, S., and Oldham, R. K. *Ann. Intern. Med.* **98**, 598–602 (1983).

32. Sarna, G.P. and Figlin, R. A. *Cancer Treat. Rep.* **69**, 547–549 (1985).

33. Nethersell, A., Smedley, H., Katrak, M., Wheller, T., and Sikora, K. *Br. J. Cancer* **49**, 615–620 (1984)

34. Quesada, J. R., Hawkins, M., Horning, S., Alexanian, R., Borden, E., Merigan, T., Adams, F., and Gutterman, J. U. *Am. J. Med.* **77**, 427–432 (1984).

35. Goodwin, M. G., Brenckman, W.,m Moore, J., Hood, L., Tso, C. Y., Koren, H., and Laszlo, J. *Proc. Am. Soc. Clin. Oncol.* **3**, 60 (1984).

36. Quesada, J. R., Gutterman, J. U., and Hersh, E. M. *J. Interferson Res.* **2**, 593–599 (1982).

37. Quesada, J. R., Swanson, D. A., and Gutterman, J. U. *J. Clin. Oncol.* **3**, 1086–1092 (1985).

38. Kirkwood, J. M., Harris, H. E., Vera, R., Sandler, S., Fischer, D. S., Khandekar, J., Ernstoff, M. S., Gordon, L., Lutes, R., Bonomi, P., Lytton, B., Cobleigh, M., and Taylor, S. J. *Cancer Res.* **45**, 863–871 (1985).

39. Quesada, J. R., Rios, A., Swanson, D., Trown, P., and Gutterman, J. U. *J. Clin. Oncol.* **3**, 1522–1528 (1985).

40. Vugrin, D., Hood, L., Taylor, W., and Laszlo, J. *Cancer Treat. Rep.* **69**, 817 (1985).

41. Neidhart, J. A., Gagen, M. M., Young, D., Tuttle, R., Melink, T. J., Ziccarrelli, A., and Kisner, D. *Cancer Res.* **44**, 4140–4143 (1984).
42. Krown, S. E., Einzig, A. I., Abramson, J. D., and Oettgen, H. F. *Proc. Am. Soc. Clin. Oncol.* **2**, 58 (abstr.) (1983).
43. Vugrin, D., Hood, L., Taylor, W., and Laszlo, J.*Proc. Am. Soc. Clin. Oncol.* **3**, 153 (abstr.) (1984).
44. Trump, D. Harris, J., Tuttle, R., Oken, M., Bennett, J., Magers, C., and Davis, T. *Proc. Am. Soc. Clin. Oncol.* **3**, 153 (abstr.) (1984).
45. Neidhart,. H. A., Gagen, M. M, Kisner, D., Tuttle, R., and Whisnant, J. *Proc. Am. Soc. Clin. Oncol.* **3**, 60 (abstr.) (1984).
46. de Kernion, J. B., Sarna, G., Figlin, R., Lindner, A., and Smith, R. B. *J. Urol.* **130**, 1063–1066 (1983).
47. Rinehart, J., Neidhart, J., Meyer, M., Hiner, C., and Young, D. *Proc. Am. Soc. Clin. Onkcol.* **4**, 224 (abstr.) (1985).
48. Czarniecki, C. E., Fennie, C. W., and Powers, D. B. *J. Virol.* **49**, 490–496 (1983).
49. Krown, S. E., Real, F. X., Cunningham-Rundles, S., Myskowski, P. L., Koziner, B., Fein, S., Mittelman, A., Oettgen, H. F., and Safai, B. *Med. Intell.* **308**, 1071–1076 (1983).
50. Rios, A., Mansell, P., Newell, G. R., Reuben, J. M., Hersh, E. M., and Gutterman, J. U.*J. Clin. Oncol.* **3**, 506–512 (1985)
51. Groopman, J. E., Gottlieb, M. S., Goodman, J., Mitsuyasu, R. T., Conant, M. A., Prince, H., Fahey, J. L., Derezin, M., Weinstein, W. M., Casavante, C., Rothman, J., Rudnick, S. A., and Volberding, P. A.*Ann. Intern. Med.* **100**, 671–676 (1984).
52. Volberding, P., Gottlieb, M., Rothman, J., Rudnick, S., Conant, M., Derezin, M., Weinstein, W., and Groopman, J.*Proc. Am. Soc. Clin. Oncol.* **2**, 3 (abstr.) (1983).
53. Figlin, R. A., Callaghan, M., and Sarna, G. *Cancer Treat. Rep.* **67**, 493–494 (1983).
54. Chaplinski, T., Laszlo, J., Moore, J., and Silverman, P. *Cancer Treat. Rep.* **67**, 1009–1012 (1983).
55. Neefe, J. R., Silgals, R., Ayoob, M., and Schein, P. S. *J. Biol. Res. Mod.* **3**, 366–370 (1984).
56. Eggermont, A. M., Weimar, W., Marquet, R. L., Lameirs, J. D., and Jeeke, J. *Cancer Treat. Rep.* **69**, 185–187 (1985).
57. Denz, H., Lechleitner, M., Marth, C., Daxenbichler, G., Gastl, G., and Braunsteiner, H. *J. Interferon Res.* **5**, 147–157 (1985).
58. Oberg, K., Funa, K., and Alm, G. *N. Engl. J. Med.* **309**, 129–133 (1983).
59. Figlin, R. A., and Sarna, G. P. *Proc. Am. Soc. Clin. Oncol.* **2**, 45 (abstr.) (1983).
60. Krown, S.E., Stoopler, M. B., Gralla, R. J., Cunningham-Rundles, S., Stewart, W. E., Pollack, M. S., and Oettgen, H. F. in *Immunotherapy of Human Cancer* (Terry W. D. and Rosenberg S. A., eds.) Elsevier-North Holland, New York (1982).

61. Grunberg, S. M., Kempf, R. A., Itri, L.M., Venturi, C. L., Boswell, W. D., and Mitchell, M. S. *Cancer Treat. Rep.* **69**, 1031-1032 (1985).
62. Leavitt, R. D., Duffey, P., and Aisner, J. *Proc. Am. Soc. Clin. Oncol.* **3**, 52 (abstr.) (1984).
63. Jones, D. H., Bleechan, N. M., Slater, A. J., George, P. J., Walker, J. R., and Dixon, A. K. *Br. J. Cancer* **47**, 361-366 (1983).
64. Einhorn, N., Cantell, K., Einhorn, S., and Strander, H.*Am. J. Clin. Oncol.* **5**, 167-172 (1982).
65. Niloff, J. M., Knapp, R. C., Jones, G., Schaetzl, E.M., and Bast, R. C. *Cancer Treat. Rep.* **69**, 895-896 (1985).
66. Berek, J. S., Hacker, N. F., Lichtenstein, A., Jung, T., Spina, C., Knox, R.M., Brady, J., Greene, T., Ettinger, L. M., Lagasse, L. D., Bonnem, E. M., Spiegel, R. J., and Zighelboim, J. *Cancer Res.* **45**, 4447-4453 (1985).
67. Ikic, D., Maricic, A., Oresic, V., Rode, B., Nola, P., Smudj, K., Knezevic, M., and Jusic, D. *Lancet* **1**, 1022-1023 (1981).
68. Scorticatti, C. H., de-de-laPena, N. C., Bellora, O. G., Mariotto, R.A., Casabe, A. R., and Comolli, R. *J. Interferon Res.* **2**, 339-343 (1982).
69. Hill, H. O., Pardue, A., Khan, A., Aleman, C., Hilario, R., and Hill, J. M. *Tex. Rep. Biol. Med.* **41**, 634-640 (1981).
70. Ikic, D., Brodarec, I., Padovan, I., Knezevic, M., and Soos, E. *Lancet* **1**, 1025-1027 (1981).
71. Padovan, I., Brodarec, I., Ikic, D., Knezevic, M., and Soos, E. *J. Cancer Res. Clin. Oncol.* **100**, 295-310 (1981).
72. Connors, J. M., Andimann, W. A., Howarth, C.B., Liu, E., Merigan, T. C., Avage, M. E., and Jacobs, C. *J. Clin. Oncol.* **3**, 813-817 (1985).
73. Ikic, D., Kirhmajer, V., Maricic, Z., Jusic, D., Krusic, J., Knezevic, M., Rode, B., Soos, E. *Lancet* **1**, 1027-1030 (1981).
74. Golomb, J. M. *Cancer* **42**, 946-956 (1978).
75. Quesada, J. R., Reuben, J., Manning, J. T., Hersch, E. M., and Gutterman, J. U., *N. Engl. J. Med.* **310**, 15-18 (1984).
76. Quesada, J. R., Hersch, E. M., and Gutterman, J. U. *Proc. Am. Soc. Clin. Oncol.* **3**, 207 (abstr.) (1984).
77. Quesada, J. R., Hersh, E. M., Reuben, J., and Gutterman, J. U. *Blood* (suppl. 1) **64**, 172 (abstr.) (1984).
78. Ratain, M. J., Golomb, H. M., Vardiman, J. W., Vokes, E. E., Jacobs, R. H., and Daly, K. *Blood* **65**, 644-648 (1985).
79. Jacobs, A. D., Champlin, R. E., and Golde, D. W. *Blood* **65**, 1017-1020 (1985).
80. Thompson, J. A., Brady, J., Kidd, P., and Fefer, A. *Cancer Treat. Rep.* **69**, 791-793 (1985).
81. Foon, K. A., Maluish, A. E., Abrams, P. G., Wrightington, S., Stevenson, H. C., Alarif, A., Fer, M. F., Overton, W. R., Poole, M., Schnipper, E. F., Jaffe, E. ⸱., and Herberman, R. B. *Am. J. Med.* **80**, 351-356 (1986).

82. Worman, C. P., Catovsky, D., Bevan, P. C., Camba, L., Joyner, M., Green P. J., Williams, H. J. H., Bottomley, J. M., Gordon-Smith, E. C., and Cawley, J. C. *Br. J. Haem.* **60**, 759–763 (1985).

83. Habermann, T., Hoagland, H., Chang, M., and Phylidy, R. *Blood* (suppl. 1) **66**, 2009 (abstr.) (1985).

84. The non-Hodgkin's lymphoma pathologic classification project: National Cancer Institute sponsored study of classifications of non-Hodgkin's lymphomas. Summary and description of a working formulation for clinical use. *Cancer* **49**, 2112–2135 (1982).

85. Merigan, T. C., Sikora, K., Bredden, J. H., Levy, R., and Rosenberg, S. A. *N. Engl. J. Med.* **299**, 1449–1453 (1978).

86. Louie, A. C., Gallagher, J. G., Sikora, K., Levy, R., Rosenberg, S. A., and Merigan, T. C. *Blood* **58**, 712–718 (1981).

87. Foon, K. A., Sherwin, S. A., and Abrams, P. G. *N. Engl. J. Med.* **311**, 1148–1152 (1984).

88. Leavitt, R. D., Kaplan, R., and Ozer, H. *Blood* (suppl. 1) **64**, 182 (abstr.) (1984).

89. Horning, S. J., Merigan, T. C., Krown, S. E., Gutterman, J. U., Louie, A., Gallagher, J., McCravey, J., Abramson, J., Cabanillas, F., Oettgem, J., and Rosemberg, S. A. *Cancer* **56**, 1305–1310 (1985).

90. O'Connell, M. J., Colgan, J. P., Oken, M. M., Ritts, R. E., Kay, N. E., and Itri, L. M. *J. Clin. Oncol.* **4**, 128–136 (1986).

91. Leavitt, R. D., Ratanatharathorn, V., Ozer, H., Rudnick, S., and Feraresi, R. *Proc. Am. Soc. Clin. Oncol.* **2**, 54 (abstr.) (1983).

92. Bunn, P. A., Idhe, D. C., and Foon, K. A. *Cancer* **57**, 1315–1321 (1986).

92a. Bunn, P. A., Foon, K. A., and Ihde, D. C. *Ann. Intern. Med.* **101**, 484–487 (1984).

93. Gale, R. P. and Foon, K. A. *Ann. Intern. Med.* **103**, 101–120 (1985).

94. Misset, J. L., Mythe, G., Gastiaburu, J., Goutner, A., Dorval, T., Schwarqenberg, L., Machover, D., Ribaud, P., and de Vassal, F. *Biomed. Pharmacother.* **36**, 112–116 (1982).

95. Huang, A., Laszlo, J., and Brenckman, W. *Proc. Am. Assoc. Cancer Res.* **23**, 113 (1982).

96. Ozer, H., Leavitt, R., and Ratanatharathorn, V. *Am. Soc. Hematol.* **62**, 211 (abstr.) (1983).

97. Foon, K. A., Bottino, G., and Abrams, P. G. *Am. J. Med.* **78**, 216–220 (1985).

98. Bergsagel, D. in *Hematology* (Williams, W., Beutler, E., Ersleu, A., and Lichtman, M., eds.) McGraw Hill, New York (1983).

99. Mellstedt, H., Bjorkholm, M., Hohansson, B., Ahre, A., Holm, G., and Strander, H. *Lancet* **1**, 245–248 (1979).

100. Osserman, E. F., Sherman, W. H., Alexanian, R., and Gutterman, J. *Am. Assoc. Cancer Res.* **21**, 161 (abstr.) (1980).

101. Bjorkholm, M. *Proc. Am. Soc. Clin. Oncol.* **2**, 242 (abstr.) (1983).

*102.* Costanzi, J. J., Cooper, M. R., Scarffe, J. H., Ozer, H., Grubbs, S. S., Ferraresi, R. W., Pollard, R. B., and Spiegel. R. J. J. *Clin. Oncol.* **3**, 654-659 (1985).

*103.* Quesada, J. R., Alexanian, R., and Gutterman, J. U. *Blood* (supple. I) **64**, 183 (abstr.) (1984).

*104.* Wagstaff, J., Loynds, P., and Scarffe, J. H. *Cancer Treat. Rep.* **69**, 495-498 (1985).

*105.* Case, D. C., Sonneborn, H. L., Paul, S. O., Hiegel, J., Boyd, M. A., Shepp, M. A., Dorsk, B. M., and Bonnem, E. *Blood* (suppl. 1) **66**, 213 (abstr.) (1985).

*106.* Clark, R. H., Dimitrov, N. V., Axelson, J. A., and Charamella, L . J. *J. Biol. Resp. Modif.* **3**, 613-619, (1984).

*107.* Champlin, R. E. and Golde, D. W. *Blood* **65**, 1034-1047, (1985).

*108.* Talpaz, M., Kantarjuan, H., McCredie, M. J., Keating, J., Trujillo, J., and Gutterman, J. U. *Blood* (suppl. 1) **66**, 209 (abstr.) (1985).

*109.* Talpaz, M., Kantarjian, H., McCredie, K. B., Keating, M. J., and Gutterman, J. U. *Blood* (suppl. 1) **66**, 209 (abstr.) (1985).

*110.* Talpaz, M., Mavligit, G., Keating, M., Walters, R. S., and Gutterman, J. U. *Ann. Intern. Med.* **99**, 789-792 (1983).

*111.* Velu, T., Delwiche, F., Flument, J., Monsieur, R., Stryckmans, P., and Wybran, U., *Blood* (suppl. 1) **64**, 176 (abstr.) (1984).

*112.* Hill, N. O., Pardue, A., Khan, A., Aleman, C., Hilario, R., and Hill, J. M. *Texas Rep. Biol. Mod.* **41**, 634-638 (1982).

*113.* Hill, N. O., Pardue, A., Khan, A., Aleman, C., Dorn, G., and Hill, J. M. *J. Clin. Hematol. Oncol.* **11**, 23-35 (1981).

*114.* Rohatiner, A. Z. S., Balkwill, F. R., Griffin, D. B., Malpas, J. S., and Lister, T. A. *Cancer Chemother. Pharmacol.* **9**, 97-102 (1982).

*115.* Rohatiner, A. Z. S., Balkwill, F. R., Malpas, J. S., and Lister, T. A. *Cancer Chemother. Pharmacol.* **11**, 56-58 (1983).

*116.* Leavitt, R. D., Duffey, P., and Wiernik, P. H. *Am. Soc. Hematol.* **62**, 205 (abstr.) (1983).

*117.* Balkwill, F. R. and Oliver, R. T. D. *Int. J. Cancer* **20**, 500-505 (1977).

*118.* Borden, E. C., Hogan, T. F., and Voelkel, J. G. *Cancer Res.* **42**, 4948-4953 (1982).

*119.* Chadha, K. C. and Srivastava, B. I. *J. Clin. Hematol. Oncol.* **11**, 55-60 (1981).

*120.* Salmon, S. E., Durie, B. G. M., Young, L., Liu, R. M., Trown, P., and Stebbing, N. *J. Clin. Oncol.* **1**, 217-225 (1983).

*121.* Blalock, J., Georgiades, J. E., Longford, M. P., and Johnson, H. M. *Cell Immunol.* **49**, 390-394 (1980).

*122.* Horoszewicz, J. S., Leong, S. S., and Carter, W. S. *Science* **206**, 1091-1093 (1979).

*123.* Creasey, A. A., Bartholomew, J. C., and Merigan, T. C. *Proc. Natl. Acad. Sci. USA* **77**, 1471-1475 (1980).

*124.* Yoshitake, Y., Kishida, T., Esaki, K., and Kawamata, J. *Giken J.* **1**, 125-127 (1976).

125. Balkwill, F. R., Moodie, E. M., Freedman, V., and Fantes K. H. *Int. J. Cancer.* **30**, 231–235 (1982).
126. Erikson, R. L., Purchio, A. F., Erikson, E., Collet, M. S., and Brugge, J. S. *J. Cell Biol.* **87**, 319–325 (1980).
127. Lin, S. L., Garber, E. A., Wang, E., Caliguiri, L. A., Schellekens, H., Goldberg, A. R., and Tamm, I. *Mol. Cell. Biol.* **3**, 1656–1664 (1983).
128. Dani, C. H., Mechti, N., Piechaczyk, M., Lebleu, B., Jeanteur, P. H., and Blanchard, J. M. *Proc. Natl. Acad. Sci. USA* **82**, 4891–4899 (1985).
129. Strayer, D. R., Gillespie, D. H., Bressuer, J., and Brodsky, I. **Blood** (suppl. 1) **64**, 175 (abstr.) (1984).
130. Gresser. I. in *Advances in Cancer Research* (Klein, G. and Weinhouse, S., eds.) Academic, New York and London, (1972).
131. Kelley, V. E., Fier, W., and Strom, T. B. *J. Immunol.* **132**, 240 (1984).
132. Williams, B. R. G. in *Interferon and Cancer* (Sikora, K., ed.) Plenum, New York (1983).
133. Schulof, R. S., Lloyd, M. J., Stallings, J. J., Mai, D., Phillips, T. M., Jones, G. J., and Schechter, G. P. *J. Biol. Resp. Mod.* **4**, 310–323 (1985).

# Antiproliferative and Clinical Antitumor Effects of Interferons

## JOAN H. SCHILLER and ERNEST C. BORDEN

## 1. Introduction

Interferons (IFN) are a family of proteins produced and secreted by cells in response to virus infection, double-stranded RNA, antigens, or other low molecular weight agents (1). Three major classes, which have significant differences in primary amino acid sequence, have now been defined. Human IFNs α and β (type I IFNs) are 165 or 166 amino acids in length, with an additional 20-amino-acid secretory peptide present on the amino terminal end. A comparison of the sequences of IFNα and IFNβ demonstrates a 29% homology of amino acids (2). IFNγ (type II IFN) is 143 amino acids in length, also with an additional 20-amino-acid secretory peptide present on the amino terminal end. It has approximately a 12% amino acid sequence homology with IFNα (3).

IFNα is a family of more than 20 proteins, differing by 15–25% in amino acid sequence (4). These proteins have been produced from eukaryotic cells by Sendai virus stimulation of human buffy coat leukocytes. Two species of IFNβ have been identified; these have been produced from foreskin fibroblasts after induction by synthetic polynucleotides. IFNγ is produced by T-lymphocytes in response to specific antigenic or mitogenic stimuli. Only one naturally produced protein species has been identified.

Although the initial clinical trials in Scandinavia and the US utilized leukocyte IFNα that was approximately 1% pure, improvements have occurred in the large-scale production and purification of these proteins. Preparations of IFNα from a Burkitt lymphoblastoid line (Namalva) that are over 70% pure are now available (lymphoblastoid IFN). In addition, IFNα, β, and γ produced by recombinant DNA technology and purified to homogeneity are now available on an industrial scale for clinical and laboratory use. These bacterially synthesized IFNs are not glycosylated.

IFNs have aroused a great deal of interest in the recent scientific and lay literature because of their antiviral and antineoplastic effects. Although the mechanism responsible for clinical antitumor activity has not yet been dissected, IFNs have both direct antiproliferative and immunomodulatory activity. The immunoregulatory effects of IFN, reviewed elsewhere (5,6), include stimulation of immune effector cells, such as T-cells and macrophages, enhanced expression of tumor-associated antigens, modulation of class I (HLA-A,B,C) and II (HLA-DR and the noncovalently linked $\beta$-2 microglobulin) major histocompatibility complex antigens, and the regulation of oncogene expression. This review will focus on the clinical antitumor aspects of IFN, with an emphasis on the experimental evidence demonstrating a direct antiproliferative effect.

## 2. Direct Antiproliferative Activity of Interferons

Antiproliferative activity of IFN has been demonstrated both in vitro and in vivo. A direct action of IFN on tumor cells, as opposed to an augmentation of immunological activity, has been supported by studies in athymic nude mice. Human tumors have been inhibited in their growth in the nude mouse by human IFN$\alpha$ and IFN$\beta$, but not mouse IFN (7–9). Human lymphoblastoid IFN inhibited the growth of human breast carcinoma xenografts in nude mice and stimulated 2-5 A synthetase levels in the tumor cells, but did not affect 2-5 A synthetase levels in mouse spleen cells and did not influence mouse NK activity (10). Although human lymphoblastoid IFN did not affect hepatic levels of drug metabolizing enzymes, whereas mouse IFN caused significant and differential changes in the isozymic forms of these enzymes, the addition of mouse IFN to human lymphoblastoid IFN and cyclophosphamide did not alter the antitumor effect on human breast cells grown as xenografts (11). Treatment of HeLa tumor-bearing mice with human IFN$\beta$ resulted in enhanced levels of 2-5 A synthetase and protein kinase activities in the HeLa tumor cells, whereas treatment with mouse interferon ($\alpha$ and $\beta$) had no apparent effects on the HeLa cells, but increased activity of 2-5 A synthetase and protein kinase in the mouse spleen and lung (12). These results suggest that the activity of the IFN is caused by direct effects on the tumor rather than the host.

A direct antiproliferative effect on tumor cells is further supported by in vitro studies, in which modulation of immunological parameters would not be expected to play a role. The human tumor colony-forming assay (HTCFA) is an assay that has been used as an "in vitro phase II test" of a variety of new anticancer drugs (13,14). Although limited by technical considerations inherent in the assay methodology (15), it has a 60–65% true positive and 85–95% true negative rate for predicting response or lack of response to standard cytotoxic agents in prospective trials (16,17). This assay has been used to determine the antitumor effects of both natural and recombinant produced interferons. For example, eight of 25 solid tumor specimens (four of 10 ovarians, two of five melanomas, one of two osteogenic sarcomas, and one of one chondrosarcoma) were inhibited by 70% or more in the HTCFA (18). Five of nine evaluable hematological tumors (one of three chronic myelogenous leukemias, three of five acute myelogenous leukemias, one of one myeloma) had at least a 70% inhibition of colony formation.

Other investigators testing human leukocyte IFN against 62 patients' tumors, however, representing 14 tumor types, in the HTCFA, noted an antiproliferative effect, as evidenced by a ⩾70% decrease in tumor colony-forming units (TCFUs) in five tumors: one lymphosarcoma cell leukemia, one small cell lung cancer, one adenocarcinoma of the lung, one breast cancer, and one pancreatic cancer (19). One patient with lymphosarcoma cell leukemia who was treated clinically with IFN and had his tumor tested in vitro had a clinical response to IFN.

Two highly purified recombinant leukocyte IFNs (IFNαA and IFNαD) were tested against 273 and 71 tumors, respectively (20). Sixteen tumor types were encompassed. Thirty-eight percent of tumors tested against IFNαA and 16% tested against IFNαD had TCFUs reduced to 50% of control or less. Fifty-one percent of melanoma tumors tested against IFNαA exhibited at least 50% inhibition of tumor colony formation, as did 50% of the lung cancer tumors tested, 33.9% of the ovarian cancer tumors, 33.4% of myeloma, 33.3% of sarcoma, 30.4% of adenocarcinomas of unknown primary, 28% of breast cancers, 30.8% of acute leukemias, and 23.1% of renal carcinomas. IFNαD was slightly less active than IFNαA when compared on a weight basis.

Although the antitumor effect of IFN in the HTSCA could potentially be related to host immunoreactive or stromal cells present in the agar, IFN has also been shown to be active against a number of tumor cell lines (18). The absence of immune competent cells when tumor cell lines are cultivated in the HTCFA or when grown in suspension or as a monolayer makes immune enhancement as a mechanism of antiproliferation unlikely. These in vitro studies have allowed comparisons between IFN types to be made. For example, we compared the relative antiproliferative activity of natural IFNα and IFNβ in 43 in vitro assays of 25 human cell lines or strains (21). IFNβ produced >20% growth inhibition in 22 cells (88%), and IFNα produced growth inhibition in nine cells (36%). Only Daudi cells (Burkitt's lymphoma) were consistently more inhibited by IFNα. In the other 24 human cells, the effect of IFNβ was greater than or equal to IFNα.

We also evaluated the antiproliferative activity of five IFNs against 22 ovarian cancer cells grown in the HTCFA (22). Two naturally produced IFNαs (human lymphoblastoid IFN and buffy coat leukocyte-derived IFN); two recombinant human leukocyte IFNs (IFNαA and IFNαD); and a naturally produced IFNβ were studied. The native IFNαs were equivalent in their antiproliferative potency when compared in 22 tumors. The antiproliferative effect of IFNαA was greater than IFNαD in the 14 tumors tested. When compared to the naturally produced IFNβ in 13 tumors, both native IFNαs were more potent.

These in vitro assays may provide useful data for clinical trial design. They may be helpful in identifying IFN-sensitive and IFN-resistant tumors, as well as in determining differences in potency and specificity for tumors of differing histologic origin, thus allowing for maximum utilization of clinical resources. They also raise interesting biological questions. For example, these in vitro tests have demonstrated a dose–response relationship, with increasing concentrations of IFN causing increasing inhibition of cell growth (18,22). The optimal biologic dose for producing the maximal immunologic effect may differ, however, from the maximal tolerated clinical dose. In two separate trials, we demonstrated greater stimulation of NK cell activity at lower than at higher doses of IFNα$_2$ (23,24). In both trials, $3 \times 10^6$ unit of IFNα given intramuscularly provided maximal NK cell stimulation. This dose is 10 to 50 times less than the maximally tolerated single dose of IFNα. Other studies have failed to demonstrate any correlation between IFN-induced enhancement of natural killer activity and clinical response of multiple myeloma patients to leukocyte interferon (25). Thus the relative importance of immunoregulatory and antiproliferative properties of IFNs in achieving an antitumor effect remains to be determined.

# 3. Clinical Antitumor Activity

## 3.1. Solid Tumors (Table 1)

### 3.1.1. Breast Cancer

Preclinical studies demonstrating an antitumor effect against breast carcinoma cells in nude mice (9) and human cancer cell lines (26) were undertaken in conjunction with clinical trials in human breast cancer patients. Initial clinical studies evaluated the antitumor effects of naturally produced, partially purified IFNα. Six responses were reported in 17 patients with advanced metastatic disease who had failed chemotherapy (16 of 17) or hormonal therapy (1 of 17) and were subsequently treated with $3 \times 10^6$ or $9 \times 10^6$ unit of partially purified Cantell leukocyte IFN (27). An American Cancer Society trial using the same dosage and schedule noted five partial responses in 23 patients (28). No relationship was found between response and menopause, estrogen receptor status, prior hormonal therapy, or disease-free interval. Patients who responded were significantly older than nonresponders.

More recently, however, studies utilizing highly purified preparations of IFNα have been less successful. No responses were observed in 17 patients treated with $50 \times 10^6$ unit/m$^2$ of recombinant IFNαA im three times a week (29). Limited therapeutic efficacy has been observed by other investigators using similar doses, routes, and schedules of IFNαA (30–32). No responses were seen in 15 patients treated with lymphoblastoid IFN (33) or 14 patients treated with IFNα$_2$ (34). The lack of efficiency of purified alpha IFNαs in these studies may be because of the absence of contaminants such as other IFNs or lymphokines contained in the partially purified Cantell preparation that accounted for its antitumor activity. Alternatively, differences in patient populations studied, such as tumor estrogen receptor content, previous therapy, and sites of disease, may be important.

### 3.1.2. Renal Cell Carcinoma

We employed cell culture techniques and highly purified recombinant IFNs to confirm the antiproliferative activity seen with impure preparations of IFN (35). Significant dose-dependent inhibition was seen with several recombinant IFNα subtypes and IFNβ$_{ser}$, whereas no significant alteration in growth kinetics was seen with recombinant IFNγ. In addition, the rare observation of spontaneous regressions of metastatic renal cell tumors has suggested that host immune factors may be important in this otherwise unresponsive tumor type, generating interest in the role of IFN in this disease. Original reports described five responses in series of 19 patients treated with leukocyte interferon (36). These studies have subsequently been extended to a total of 50 patients, with a response rate of 26% (37). Similar trials done at UCLA and at Karolinska Hospital in Sweden using the same IFN, dose, and schedule have reported partial and complete response rate of 16.5 and 27%, respectively (38,39). A prospective, randomized collaborative trial of low vs high doses of leukocyte IFN ($1 \times 10^6$ unit/d for 28 d versus $10 \times 10^6$ unit/d for 28 d) was carried out in 30 patients with metastatic disease (40). None of the 14 patients who received the low dose of IFN had a response, whereas three of 16 (19%) of patients treated with the high dose responded (one complete, two partial responses). Although not statistically significant, this result suggested a dose–response relationship.

Table 1
Combined Results of Phase II Trials in Solid Tumors

| Study, ref. number | IFN | Dose and schedule, × 10⁶ unit | Route | No. of responders/no. evaluable |
|---|---|---|---|---|
| *Breast* | | | | |
| Partially purified preparations | | | | |
| Gutterman et al. (27) | Leukocyte | 3 or 9 qd × 28 d | im | 6/17 |
| Borden et al. (28) | Leukocyte | 3 or 9 qd × 28 d | im | 5/23 |
| | | | | Total: 11/40 = 27.5% |
| Purified preparations | | | | |
| Sherwin et al. (29) | rIFNαA | 50/m² tiw | im | 0/17 |
| Nethersell et al. (30) | rIFNαA | 20 or 50/m² tiw | im | 2/12 |
| Muss et al. (31) | rIFNα2 | 30/m² qd × 5 | im | 0/33 |
| | | or | | |
| | | 50/m² qd × 5 | im | 0/15 |
| | | or | | |
| Quesada et al. (32) | rIFNαA | 2/m² tiw | sc | 0/11 |
| Sarna et al. (33) | Lymphoblastoid | 3–50 qd × 8 wk | im | 1/19 |
| Padmanabhan et al. (34) | rIFNα2 | 30/m² q wk | im | 0/15 |
| | | 2/m² tiw | sc | 0/7 |
| | | randomized vs | | |
| | | 50/m² qd × 5 | iv | 0/7 |
| | | | | Total: 3/110 = 3% |
| *Renal cell* | | | | |
| Partially purified preparations | | | | |
| Quesada et al. (37) | Leukocyte | 3 qd | im | 13/50 |
| DeKernion et al. (38) | Leukocyte | 3 qd × 5 | im | 7/43 |

| | | | | |
|---|---|---|---|---|
| Edsmyr et al. (39) | Leukocyte | 3 qd | im | 3/11 |
| Kirkwood et al. (40) | Leukocyte | 1 randomized vs 10 qd × 28 | im | 0/14 |
| | | | | 3/16 |
| | | | Total: 26/134 = 19% | |
| **Purified preparations** | | | | |
| Neidhart et al. (41) | Lymphoblastoid | 5/m² tiw | im | 5/33 |
| Vugrin et al. (42) | Lymphoblastoid | 3/m² tiw × 6 wk | im | 1/21 |
| Quesada et al. (43) | rIFNαA | 2/m² randomized vs | im | 0/15 |
| | | 20/m² qd | im | 4/15 |
| | | 20/m² qd | im | 8/26 |
| | | | Total: 18/110 = 16% | |
| *Melanoma* | | | | |
| **Partially purified preparations** | | | | |
| Krown et al. (48) | Leukocyte | 1 qd × 42 randomized vs | im | 1/16 |
| | | 3 qd × 42 randomized vs | | 0/14 |
| | | 9 qd × 42 | im | 0/14 |
| | | | Total: 1/44 = 2% | |
| **Purified preparations** | | | | |
| Retsas et al. (49) | Lymphoblastoid | 2.5/m² qd | im | 1/15 |
| Creagan et al. (50) | rIFNαA | 12/m² tiw | im | 6/30 |
| Creagan et al. (51) | rIFNαA | 50/m² tiw | im | 7/31 |
| Creagan et al. (52) | rIFNα2 | 50/m² tiw | im | 8/35 |
| Goldberg et al. (53) | Lymphoblastoid | plus cimetidine 15/m² tiw × 2 wk | im | 1/12 |
| | | 5/m² q wk | im | 0/6 |
| Kirkwood et al. (54) | rIFNα2 | 0.5/m² q 5d/wk | im | 2/14 |
| | | 3, 30, or 50 qd | im | 2/7 |
| | | 10, 30, 50, or 100 5 d/wk | iv | 2/16 |
| | | | Total: 29/166 = 17% | |

*(continued)*

Table 1 (*continued*)
Combined Results of Phase II Trials in Solid Tumors

| Study, ref. number | IFN | Dose and schedule, $\times 10^6$ unit | Route | No. of responders/no. evaluable |
|---|---|---|---|---|
| *Ovary* | | | | |
| Niloff et al. (*55*) | rIFNαA | $20/m^2$ tiw $\times$ 8 wk | im | 0/15 |
| Berek et al. (*56*) | rIFNα2 | 5 escalating up to 50 q wk | ip | 5/11 |
| | | | | Total: 5/26 = 19% |
| *Bronchogenic (non-small cell)* | | | | |
| Grunberg et al. (*57*) | rIFNα | $50/m^2$ tiw | im | 0/12 = 0% |
| *Primary hepatocellular carcinoma* | | | | |
| Partially purified preparations | | | | |
| Nair et al. (*60*) | Leukocyte | 3 qd $\times$ 60 | im | 0/4 = 0% |
| Purified preparations | | | | |
| Sachs et al. (*61*) | rIFNA | $12/m^2$ tiw or $50/m^2$ tiw | im | 0/8 |
| | | | im | 0/8 |
| | | | | Total: 0/16 = 0% |
| *Glioblastoma multiforme* | | | | |
| Alpha | | | | |
| Hirakawa et al. (*64*) | Leukocyte | $5 \times 10^4$ units q wk or | im | 1/3 |
| Boethius et al. (*65*) | Leukocyte | 1 or 3 q od 3 or 9 qd | im | 0/2 |
| Mahaley et al. (*66*) | Lymphoblastoid | 10 to $30/m^2$ 3x/wk to 5x/wk | im | 1/12 |
| | | | iv or im | 7/17 |
| | | | | Total: 9/34 = 26% |

| | | | | |
|---|---|---|---|---|
| **Beta** | | | | |
| Duff et al. (67) | β (Fibroblast) | 10 qd and 1 q od | iv Intratumor | 0/12 = 0% |
| *Carcinoid* | | | | |
| Oberg et al. (68) | Leukocyte | 3–6 qd | im | 6/9 = 67% |
| *Colon* | | | | |
| Partially purified preparations | | | | |
| Figlin et al. (69) | Leukocyte | 3 q 5d/wk | im | 0/18 = 0% |
| Purified preparations | | | | |
| Chaplinski et al. (70) | Lymphoblastoid rIFNαA | 3/m² tiw | im | 0/19 |
| Neefe et al. (71) | rIFNα2 | 50/m² tiw | im | 1/19 |
| Eggermont et al. (72) | | 20/m² biw | im | 1/10 |
| | | | | Total: 2/66 = 3% |
| *Bladder papillomatosis* | | | | |
| Ikic et al. (73) | Leukocyte | 2 qd × 21 | Trans-urethral | 8/8 |
| Scorticatti et al. (74) | Leukocyte | 1 qod | im | 2/4 |
| | | | | Total: 10/12 = 83% |
| *Nasopharyngeal* | | | | |
| Connors et al. (75) | Leukocyte | 10 qd × 30 | im | 2/13 = 15% |
| *Cervical* | | | | |
| Ikic et al. (76) | Leukocyte | 2 qd × 21 or 2 qd × 21 + 1 qd × 21 | Topically Topically im | 6/15 = 40% |
| | | | | Total: 6/15 = 40% |

*(continued)*

Table 1 (*continued*)
Combined Results of Phase II Trials in Solid Tumors

| Study, ref. number | IFN | Dose and schedule, $\times 10^6$ unit | Route | No. of responders/no. evaluable |
|---|---|---|---|---|
| *Kaposi's sarcoma* | | | | |
| Alpha | | | | |
| Krown et al. (*77*) | rIFNαA | 36 or 54 qd × 28 | im | 5/12 |
| Groopman et al. (*78*) | rIFNα2 | 1/m² 5 d/wk, qo wk, randomized vs 50/m² 5 d/wk, qo wk | sc | 2/10 |
| Rios et al. (*79*) | Lymphoblastoid | 20/m² qd × 2 mo | iv | 4/10 |
| Gelmann et al. (*80*) | Lymphoblastoid | 7.5/m² qd × 28 or 15/m² qd × 10 or 25/m² qd × 28 | im | 8/12 |
| | | | im | 1/10 |
| | | | im | 0/10 |
| | | | im | 3/10 |
| Real et al. (*81*) | rIFNαA | 3 qd × 28 | im | 1/36 |
| | | 36 or 54 qd × 28 | im | 13/34 |
| | | | | Total: 37/144 = 26% |
| Gamma | | | | |
| Krigel et al. (*82*) | γ | 0.5 qd × 10; repeated 2 wk later | im | 0/7 = 0% |

The effects of purified preparations of IFNαs are also currently being evaluated. Recent clinical trials of human lymphoblastoid IFN have demonstrated response rates of 15 and 5% (41,42). A trial initiated to determine the dose–response relationships with rIFNαA given at 2 × 10⁶ unit/m² or 20 × 10⁶ unit/m² im every day showed no responses in 15 patients treated with the low dose, but 11 responses in 41 patients treated with high dose (43).

These data support the clinical activity of IFNα in renal cell carcinoma and suggest its effect may be dose related. Although further studies will be necessary to define the exact role of IFN in this disease, IFNα would appear to be a promising treatment for this tumor.

### 3.1.3. Melanoma

Malignant melanoma is a disorder that is traditionally refractory to standard chemotherapeutic agents, and against which in vitro data have demonstrated an IFN antitumor effect. For example, in the B16 murine melanoma model, partially purified mouse interferon achieved a statistically significant antitumor effect in vivo and in vitro compared with controls (44). HMV-1 human melanoma cells were highly sensitive to human fibroblast interferon in vitro and were inhibited over 85% by the intratumor injection of 6 × 10⁵ unit in nude mice (45). We have evaluated the effects of seven different human IFNs on 30 fresh human melanomas using the HTCFA (46). Fourteen of 19 evaluable tumors were sensitive to at least one IFN, although none of the IFNs differed significantly in their antiproliferative effect. These data and others have supported the clinical evaluation of IFN against melanoma (20,47).

Initial trials of partially purified leukocyte IFN demonstrated minimal and mixed responses in patients treated with 1, 3, or 9 × 10⁶ unit/d, with no clear dose–response relationships (48). A similar trial design using lymphoblastoid IFN produced only one partial response in 15 patients, raising questions regarding optimum dose (49). A series of trials undertaken at the Mayo Clinic demonstrated similar response rates in patients given 12 × 10⁶ unit/m² TIW (20%), 50 × 10⁶ unit/m² TIW (23%), or 50 × 10⁶ unit/m² plus cimetidine (23%) (50–52). No advantage was seen, however, in patients given three different dosages and schedules of lymphoblastoid IFN (53). Similarly, no advantage was seen in patients who received different doses of rIFNα₂ by either the iv or im route (54). Clearly further studies are needed to determine the optimal dose and schedule in this resistant tumor type.

### 3.1.4. Ovarian Carcinoma

Ovarian cancer is a tumor type particularly suited to in vitro studies because of the relative ease of access to tumor cells in the peritoneum, as well as the high percentage of tumors capable of growing in the HTCFA. We evaluated the antiproliferative potency of five IFNs in 22 evaluable ovarian tumors (*22*). Fourteen (64%) were sensitive to at least one IFN. Other investigators have demonstrated sensitivity to IFNαA in 33.9% of tumors studied (*20*). Although a recent study that utilized rIFNαA intramuscularly in 15 patients with recurrent or persistent ovarian cancer demonstrated no antitumor effect (*55*), five of 11 patients who received intraperitoneal rIFNα$_2$ responded (*56*). Three complete responses and one partial response were documented by repeat laparatomy, and all took place in patients whose residual tumor had been less than five mm, suggesting that ip rIFNα$_2$ may be effective in patients with minimal disease.

### 3.1.5. Non-Small Cell Bronchogenic Carcinoma

Non-small cell lung cancer is a tumor type against which no effective chemotherapy is available. A recent study performed at the University of Southern California was unable to document any antitumor effect in 12 patients treated with rIFNα (*57*). A similar refractoriness to therapy has been observed in previous trials with partially purified IFNα (*58,59*).

### 3.1.6. Primary Hepatocellular Carcinoma

Primary hepatocellular carcinoma (PHC) is another tumor for which new modalities of treatment are currently being sought. Five patients, four of whom were evaluable for response, were treated with partially purified IFNα (*60*). Three patients had progressive disease and one remained stable. None of 16 patients treated with IFNαA responded (*61*).

### 3.1.7. Glioblastoma Multiforme

The effect of interferons against malignant glioma has been examined in both in vitro and in vivo studies. Interferons inhibit the growth of glioblastoma cells maintained in tissue culture (*62*), as well as transplanted into nude mice (*63*). Intramuscular injection of leukocyte interferon brought about a partial response in two of 17 patients with glioblastoma (*64,65*). Nineteen patients with recurrent gliomas who had previously undergone surgery and radiation therapy were treated with escalating doses of lymphoblastoid IFN (*66*). Seven of 17 evaluable patients responded. Twelve patients with recurrent glioblastoma multiforme were entered on a phase II study of IFNβ, in which treatment consisted of combined intravenous (10 × 10⁶ unit/d) and intratumor (1 × 10⁶ qod) administration of IFNβ$_{ser}$ over three 10-d cycles (*67*). No responses were seen.

### 3.1.8. Carcinoid

Nine patients with midgut carcinoid tumors were treated with daily intramuscular doses of leukocyte interferon (*68*). All six patients with liver metastases had a prompt reduction in urinary levels of 5-hydroxyindolacetic acid and serum levels of human chorionic gonadotropin subunits and pancreatic polypeptides. None of the three patients with lymph node involvement responded. Although no dimunition in tumor size was observed, interferon may be of benefit in treating patients with the carcinoid syndrome.

### 3.1.9. Colon

Clinical activity of either partially purified (69) or purified preparations (70–72) of IFNα against human colorectal tumors has not been observed. Phase II studies involving different schedules and dosages have failed to demonstrate any significant response rates. The lack of activity in vivo of this tumor type to IFN may play a useful role in studying mechanisms of in vitro IFN resistance.

### 3.1.10. Bladder Papillomatosis

Recurrent bladder papillomatosis is an attractive tumor type in which to study IFN activity because of the relatively easy accessibility of the tumor for monitoring as well as controlled intravesical exposure to IFN. Complete regressions in eight of eight patients, lasting from 4 to 46 mo, were reported when the tumor bases or surrounding tissue was injected with leukocyte IFN transurethrally (73). Another trial, using systemic IFNa treatment of multiple bladder papilloma grade I or II patients, observed complete and partial tumor regressions, decreases in the recurrence of frequency rates, and recurrences with smaller papillomas (74).

### 3.1.11. Nasopharyngeal Carcinoma

Nasopharyngeal carcinoma (NPC) is a malignancy associated with Epstein-Barr virus that carries a relatively poor prognosis in patients with advanced disease. The association of this tumor with virus provides an additional rationale for the evaluation of this disease. Two partial responses were seen in 13 patients with recurrent NPC treated with leukocyte IFN (75), suggesting that IFN had sufficient activity in advanced NPC to justify further investigation.

### 3.1.12. Cervical Carcinoma

Cervical carcinoma is another tumor associated with viruses that allows for topical treatment. Investigators from Yugoslavia treated 15 patients with invasive squamous cell carcinoma of the uterine cervix with topical leukocyte IFN plus or minus im IFN (46). Three patients had total regression of their disease, two had regression to in situ histology, and one had regression to microinvasive disease.

### 3.1.13. Kaposi's Sarcoma

The association of Kaposi's sarcoma with the acquired immune deficiency syndrome (AIDS) has provided the unique opportunity to study the antitumor and immunomodulatory effects of a virus-associated tumor. Initial trials reported response rates of 42%, with modest increases in OKT4$^+$ ratios (77). Although subsequent trials have confirmed the activity of IFNα in this disease (78,79), no consistent or sustained changes have been seen in immunological variables during or after treatment. A moderate to marked suppression of host defense parameters has been observed that appears within 7 d of the start of interferon and occasionally is improved by d 28 (79). Therapy has not eradicated cytomegalovirus carriage or prevented opportunistic infections related to cytomegalovirus (78). Different response rates reported by other investigators may be the result of differences in the severity of the underlying AIDS between patient populations as assessed by OKT4$^+$/OKT8$^+$ ratios and total lymphocyte counts (80), tumor burden, and patient performance status (79). Low doses of rIFNαA (81) or IFNγ have been ineffective in this disease (82).

## 3.2. Hematological Malignancies (Table 2)

### 3.2.1. Multiple Myeloma

Preclinical studies documenting the antiproliferative activity of natural and recombinant interferons against myeloma cell lines provided rationale for continuing investigation into the clinical usefulness of these agents (83,84). Early studies with partially purified preparations of leukocyte interferon have confirmed activity in this disease (27,85–87). Optimal doses, schedules, and patient populations have yet to be identified, however. For example, response rates of only 8 and 11% were observed when patients with advanced disease were treated with 3–50 × 10$^6$ unit/d of rIFNαA im (32) or 2 × 10$^6$ unit/m$^2$ of rIFNα2 by sc injection 3 d/wk (88). Seven of 38 patients (18%) who received one of three different schedules of iv or sc rIFNα2 had an objective response (89), as did 10 of 47 (21%) evaluable patients treated with escalating doses of im rIFNαA (90). When 27 patients who received 12 × 10$^6$ unit/m$^2$ of rIFNαA im daily were analyzed according to prior therapy, however, seven of 14 (50%) of previously untreated patients had a documented response (91). Only two of 13 (15%) of patients who had relapsed or failed prior chemotherapy had objective tumor regression. In all patients who had tumor response, there was restoration from subnormal levels of serum immunoglobulins, an effect infrequently seen with chemotherapy. Thus, interferon may have a role in the treatment of early stages of multiple myeloma.

## 3.2.2. Hairy Cell Leukemia

Hairy cell leukemia (HCL) is a B-cell malignancy characterized by massive splenomegaly, pancytopenia, characteristic "hairy cells" in the peripheral blood, and an increased incidence of fatal bacterial or fungal infections. Although splenectomy can result in hematological improvement, the disease usually progresses, requiring further therapy. Recently, seven patients with progressive hairy cell leukemia were treated with partially purified leukocyte interferon (92). Three complete responses and four partial responses were observed and maintained for over 6 to over 10 mo. Similar results have subsequently been reported with rIFNα2 (93,94), as evidenced by significant improvements in hemoglobin, granulocyte, and platelet counts. Bone marrow biopsies in six of 14 patients after 6 mo of therapy showed a >50% decrease in the infiltration of leukemic cells (95). Natural killer activity returned and immunological surface markers normalized in responding patients treated with IFNαA (96). Although the optimal dose and schedule are unknown, IFN may be the treatment of choice for patients with progressive disease.

## 3.2.3. Lymphomas

Lymphomas represent a group of hematological malignancies consisting of a variety of histological types that differ in their natural history, treatment, and prognosis.

*3.2.3.1. Cutaneous T-Cell Lymphoma.* High-dose rIFNαA has been effective in patients with advanced cutaneous T-cell lymphoma (97). Nine objective partial remissions lasting 3 to more than 25 mo (median, 5 mo) were documented among 20 evaluable patients. IFN may prove to be more effective for advanced refractory cutaneous T-cell lymphomas than any other reported agent.

*3.2.3.2. Hodgkin's Disease.* Eight patients with Hodgkin's disease were entered into a multi-institutional phase II trial to evaluate the antitumor activity of leukocyte IFN (98). Two brief, minimal responses were observed and not believed to be clinically significant.

*3.2.3.3. Non-Hodgkin's Lymphoma—Favorable Histologies.* More encouraging results have been seen in patients with the more indolent lymphomas. Initial reports described three partial responses in three patients with nodular lymphoma poorly differentiated (NLPD) (99). This experience has subsequently been updated, with one complete response and two partial responses observed in seven evaluable patients with NLPD and nodular mixed lymphoma (NML) (100). One patient had a second partial response on retreatment with interferon, in spite of having received chemotherapy in the interval between IFN treatments. Response rates of 50, 11, and 20%

Table 2
Combined Results of Phase II Trials in Hematological Malignancies

| Study | IFN | Dose and schedule, $\times 10^6$ unit | Route | No. of responders/no. evaluable |
|---|---|---|---|---|
| *Multiple myeloma* | | | | |
| Partially purified preparations | | | | |
| Gutterman et al. (27) | Leukocyte | 3–9 qd | im | 1/3 Previously untreated |
| | | | | 2/7 Previously treated |
| Osserman et al. (85) | Leukocyte | 3 qd | im | 3/18 Previously untreated |
| | | | | 1/3 Previously treated |
| Alexanian et al. (86) | Leukocyte | 3–9 qd | im | 3/12 Previously untreated |
| | | | | 2/9 Previously treated |
| Ahre et al. (87) | Leukocyte | 3 or 6 qd | im | 10/74 Previously treated |
| | | | | Total: 22/126 = 17% |
| | | | | Previously untreated: |
| | | | | 17/107 = 16% |
| | | | | Previously treated: |
| | | | | 5/19 = 26% |
| Purified preparations | | | | |
| Quesada et al. (32) | rIFNαA | 3–50 qd × 8 wk | im | 1/12ᵃ |
| Wagstaff et al. (88) | rIFNα2 | 2–10/m² tiw × 3 mo | sc | 2/18 Previously treated |
| Costanzi et al. (89) | rIFNα2 | 3–100/m²/d tiw × 2 wk, then 10/m² tiw or | iv | 3/18 Previously treated |
| | | | sc | |
| | | 30–50/m²/d for 5 d every 14 d × 4, then 10/m² tiw or | iv | 2/7 Previously treated |
| | | | sc | |
| | | 2/m²/d tiw × 3 mo, then 10/m² tiw | sc | 2/13 Previously treated |
| | | | sc | |

| | | | | |
|---|---|---|---|---|
| Ohno et al. (90) | rIFNαA | 3–50 qd | im | 10/47ᵃ |
| Quesada et al. (91) | rIFNαA | 12/m² qd | im | 7/14 Previously untreated 2/13 Previously treated Total: 29/142 = 20% Previously untreated: 7/14 = 50% Previously treated: 11/69 = 16% |
| *Hairy cell leukemia* Partially purified preparations | | | | |
| Quesada et al. (92) | Leukocyte | 3 qd | im | 7/7 = 100% |
| Purified preparations | | | | |
| Thompson et al. (93) | rIFNα2 | 2/m² tiw | sc | 13/13 |
| Ratain et al. (94) | rIFNα2 | 2–10/m² tiw | sc | 7/8 |
| Jacobs et al. (95) | rIFNα2 | 2/m² tiw | sc | 6/14 |
| Foon et al. (96) | rIFNαA | 3 qd | im | 13/14 Total: 39/49 = 80% |
| *Cutaneous T-cell lymphoma* | | | | |
| Bunn et al. (97) | rIFNαA | 50/m² tiw | im | 9/20 = 45% |
| *Lymphoma* Hodgkin's | | | | |
| Horning et al. (98) | Leukocyte | 1, 3, or 9 qd × 30 | im | 0/8 = 0% |

*(continued)*

Table 2 (*continued*)
Combined Results of Phase II Trials in Hematological Malignancies

| Study | IFN | Dose and schedule, $\times 10^6$ unit | Route | No. of responders/no. evaluable |
|---|---|---|---|---|
| Non-Hodgkin's | | | | |
| Favorable histology | | | | |
| Partially purified alpha | | | | |
| Gutterman et al. (*27*) | Leukocyte | 3–9 qd | im | 3/6 |
| Horning et al. (*98*) | Leukocyte | 1, 3, or 9 qd × 30 | im | 3/28 |
| Louie et al. (*100*) | Leukocyte | 5 bid × 60 | im | 3/7 |
| | | | | Total: 9/41 = 22% |
| Purified alpha | | | | |
| Quesada et al. (*32*) | rIFNαA | 3–50 qd | im | 6/17 |
| Foon et al. (*102*) | rIFNαA | 50/m² tiw | im | 13/24 |
| | | | | Total: 19/41 = 46% |
| Partially purified beta | | | | |
| Siegert et al. (*101*) | β | 4.5 qd × 4 wk, then 9.0 qd × 2 wk | iv | 2/10 = 20% |
| Unfavorable histology | | | | |
| Partially purified preparations | | | | |
| Gutterman et al. (*27*) | Leukocyte | 3–9 qd | im | 0/1 |
| Horning et al. (*98*) | Leukocyte | 1, 3, or 9 qd × 30 | im | 0/8 |
| Louie et al. (*100*) | Leukocyte | 5 bid × 60 | im | 0/3 |
| | | | | Total: 0/12 = 0% |
| Purified preparations | | | | |
| Foon et al. (*102*) | rIFNαA | 50/m² tiw | im | 1/7 |
| | | | | Total: 1/7 = 14% |

| | Preparation | Dose | Route | Response |
|---|---|---|---|---|
| **Chronic lymphocytic leukemia** | | | | |
| Partially purified preparations | | | | |
| Misset et al. (103) | Leukocyte | 1.5–6 qd | sc | 3/9 |
| Gutterman et al. (27) | Leukocyte | 3–9 qd | im | 1/4 |
| | | | | Total: 4/13 = 31% |
| Purified preparations | | | | |
| Foon et al. (104) | rIFNαA | 50/m² tiw or | im | 2/12 |
| | | 5/m² tiw | im | 0/6 |
| | | | | Total: 2/18 = 11% |
| **Chronic myelogenous leukemia** | | | | |
| Talpaz et al. (107) | Leukocyte | 9–15 qd | im | 5/7 |
| Talpaz et al. (108) | rIFNαA | 5/m² qd | im | 14/17 |
| Talpaz et al. (109) | Leukocyte | 9 qd | im | 8/9[b] |
| | | | | Total: 19/33 = 56% |
| **Acute lymphocytic leukemia** | | | | |
| Hill et al. (110) | Leukocyte | 0.5–5/kg qd | iv | 5/5 = 100% |
| **Acute myelogenous leukemia** | | | | |
| Hill et al. (110) | Leukocyte | 0.5–5/kg qd | iv | 2/4 |
| Rohatimer et al. (111) | Lymphoblastoid | 100/m² ad × 7 | iv | 1/10 |
| | | | | Total: 3/14 = 21% |

[a]Details regarding previous therapy not given.
[b]Reduction in thrombocytosis only.

have been reported by other investigators to partially purified preparations of IFN$\alpha$ (27,98) or IFN$\beta$ (101), and of 35% to rIFN$\alpha$A (32). The most encouraging results occurred in a trial of 24 evaluable patients in which 13 responses occurred (102). All responding patients had been heavily pretreated with combination chemotherapy. Relapses occurred within 2–7 mo of cessation of therapy. Three patients who had relapsed after the course of IFN subsequently responded to a second course.

*3.2.3.4. Non-Hodgkin's Lymphoma—Unfavorable Histologies.* Several clinical trials have evaluated the effect of IFN on patients with non-Hodgkin's lymphomas, unfavorable histologies with disappointing results. Despite different doses, schedules, and preparations of IFN, few responses have been seen (27,98,99,102).

### 3.2.4. Chronic Lymphocytic Leukemia

Treatment of chronic lymphocytic leukemia has been reported by several groups. One of four patients (27) and three of nine (103) receiving 3–9 × 10⁶ unit of leukocyte IFN im a day or 1.5 to 6 × 10⁶ unit sc a day, respectively, had partial responses. A good correlation between NK cell activity and clinical response was noted in this latter study. Eighteen evaluable, previously treated patients received either 50 × 10⁶ unit/m² or 5 × 10⁶ unit/m² of rIFN$\alpha$A im three times a week, depending on their pretreatment platelet count (104). Two of 12 patients treated at the higher dose and none of six treated at the lower dose responded. Five patients with progressive disease had an acceleration of their disease while receiving IFN.

### 3.2.5. Chronic Myelogenous Leukemia

Human leukocyte IFN has significant antiproliferative activity against normal myeloid (105) and chronic myelogenous leukemia (CML) progenetor cells (106) in vitro, prompting clinical evaluation. Seven patients with CML, five of whom were untreated and two of whom had single-agent chemotherapy, were treated with leukocyte IFN (107). Hematological remission was obtained in five patients to daily im injections of 9–15 × 10⁶ unit. Among the responding patients, the mean white blood count decreased from 97.4 × 10³/cu mm to 4.2 × 10³/cu mm. Fourteen of 17 patients with "benign-phase" disease responded to 5 × 10⁶ unit/m²/d of IFN$\alpha$A (108). In another study of nine patients with refractory chronic CML and severe thrombocytosis, however, none had a significant cytoreduction of the peripheral leukocyte count (109). A significant decline in platelet counts, from a mean of 1.71 × 10⁶/mm³ to a mean of 0.52 × 10⁶/mm³, was seen in all patients, indicating that leukocyte IFN may be helpful in alleviating progressive thrombocytosis in advanced CML. It is unclear why there is a discrepancy in the control of myeloid cells in patients with advanced, progressive disease and patients who were previously untreated or had benign phase disease.

### 3.2.6. Acute Leukemia

The role of IFN in the treatment of acute leukemias has not been as extensively studied. Objective benefit occurred in two of three patients with acute myelogenous leukemia (AML) and five of five with acute lymphocytic leukemia (ALL) treated with intravenous leukocyte IFN at 0.5–5 × 10⁶ unit/kg/d (*110*). Only one partial response occurred in 10 patients with AML who received lymphoblastoid IFN, however (*111*).

## 4. Toxicities

Phase I trials have defined both subjective and objective side effects that occur with IFNα, IFNβ, and IFNγ (*112–115*). Similar toxicities, both quantitatively and qualitatively, have been described with partially purified and purified preparations. Acute side effects include an influenza-like syndrome of fever, chills, myalgias, arthralgias, headache, and occasional nausea and vomiting. A tachyphylaxis to these acute symptoms has been noted in patients treated on repetitive dosing schedules. Chronic side effects include anorexia and fatigue, which may be dose limiting. Mild to moderate neutropenia is common and rapidly reversible upon cessation of therapy. Hepatotoxicity (elevation of serum glutamic-oxalacetic transaminase), neurologic toxicity (changes in sensorium, diffuse slowing of γ waves on EEG), and cardiac toxicity (tachyarrhythmias) are infrequent and rarely require dose modification.

## 5. Perspective

Interferons are prototype biologic response modifiers that have clinical activity against a broad range of human neoplasms as documented by emerging results from current phase II trials. Optimal doses, schedules, routes, and species of IFNs remain to be defined in upcoming phase III studies. In addition, the role of IFNs in combination with other modalities of cancer treatment, such as chemotherapy and other biological response modifiers, has just begun to be defined.

## 5.1. IFN and Other Lymphokines

Lymphokine interactions is currently an area of exciting research. For example, the in vitro antiproliferative effect of IFN has been enhanced when given with tumor necrosis factor (*116*). IFNs have been shown to enhance the expression of tumor-associated antigens, and thus may have a role in combination treatment with monoclonal antibodies (*117–119*). Combinations of types I and II IFN have resulted in an enhanced antiproliferative effect in vitro and in vivo in both the mouse (*120–122*) and human systems (*123*). Our investigations into the effects of combinations of types I and II IFN have demonstrated a synergistic antiproliferative effect in nine of 10 human cell lines of various histogenesis, including cells that differed in their sensitivities to each IFN (*124*). For example, despite only 10% inhibition in colony formation by 4.0 ng/mL of IFNα54 or 8.0 ng/mL of IFNγ, the T24 human bladder carcinoma cell line was inhibited over 90% by combining these two doses.

## 5.2. IFN and Hyperthermia

In studying the effects of combined IFN and hyperthermia, we demonstrated enhanced antiproliferative effects of interferons at elevated temperatures against human bladder carcinoma cell lines (*125*). For example, T24 human bladder carcinoma cells grown at 37°C and treated with 200 unit of naturally produced IFNα or IFNβ per mL for 7 d were inhibited 50–60%. No change in cell proliferation occurred in untreated T24 cells grown at 39.5°C. Treatment with 200 unit of IFNα or IFNβ per mL at 39.5°C inhibited these cells 80–90%.

## 5.3. IFN and Cytotoxic Agents

In vitro and in vivo evidence suggests that in many systems, IFN may be more effective when given with standard chemotherapeutic agents. The interaction of human leukocyte interferon with vinca alkaloids and other chemotherapeutic agents against human tumors has been studied in the clonogenic assay (*83*). Synergistic activity against colony formation was observed with the combination of vinblastine and IFNαA. An additive or subadditive effect was observed with the other cytotoxic agents tested. IFNβ was capable of synergistically potentiating the cytotoxic effects of 5FU on three human neoplastic cell lines, whereas in two others the combination was additive and in an additional two neither synergistic nor additive effects were observed (*126*). In vivo, human lymphoblastoid interferon enhanced the antitumor activity of suboptimal doses of cyclophosphamide and adriamycin on a human breast tumor xenograft growing in nude mice (*127*).

## 6. Conclusion

Interferons have a level of therapeutic activity in neoplastic disease that is comparable to many cytotoxic drugs currently in clinical practice. Although it is difficult to rank drugs as to level of activity because of their selectivity for specific neoplasms, as a single agent interferons compare favorably. Although IFNα does not have broad spectrum activity, its level of activity in hematologic malignancies and selected solid tumors makes it probable that it will be licensed and marketed for additional applications. Although the side effects of fatigue and anorexia are troublesome, compared to cytotoxic agents, no residual toxicities for vital organs occur. Thus as a biological agent it is meeting expectations of lesser side effects. With improved preclinical models and better understanding of the mechanism of antitumor action, it can be anticipated that the therapeutic index of interferons may improve.

Regardless of how successful interferons are as broadly applicable antineoplastics, it is clear that their introduction into clinical trials has pioneered a new approach to cancer treatment. The development and application of recombinant DNA technology to produce large quantities of highly purified human cytokines has been a major advance. As we better understand protein conformation and the interaction of cytokines with cells, it can be envisioned that the optimal interferon for a specific biological effect could be constructed. Site-specific mutagenesis for alteration of nucleotide sequences has already been applied to specifically engineer an interferon with desirable effects (*128*). New methods in protein synthesis together with protein modeling studies should enable construct of shorter protein sequences or even entirely synthetic organics. There seems little doubt that interferons will be the prototype of biological therapeutics for treatment of neoplastic diseases.

## Acknowledgments

JHS is an American Cancer Society Fellow and a recipient of a Stetler Research Fund for Women Physicians. ECB is an American Cancer Society Professor of Clinical Oncology. Work in ECB's laboratory is supported by the Eastern Cooperative Oncology Group, CA 21076, NCI-CM-07343, NCI-CM-07434, and a grant from Triton Biosciences.

# References

*1.* Stewart, W. E., II, in *The Interferon System* Springer-Verlag, Vienna and New York (1979).

*2.* Taniguchi, T., Ohno, S., Fujii-Kuriyama, Y., and Muramatusu, M. *Gene* **10**, 11 (1980).

*3.* Epstein, L. B. *Nature* **295**, 453–454 (1982).

*4.* Goeddell, D. V., Yelverton, E., Ullrich, A., Heyneker, H. L., Miozzari, G., Holmes, W., Seeburg, P. H., Dull, T., May, L., Stebbing, N., Crea, R., Maeda, S., McCandliss, R., Sloma, A., Tabor, J. M., Gross, M., Familletti, P. C., and Pestka, S. *Nature* **287**, 411–416 (1980).

*5.* Stiehm, E. R., Kronenberg, L. H., Rosenblatt, H. M., Bryson, Y., and Merigan, T. C. *Ann. Intern. Med.* **96**, 80–93 (1982).

*6.* Borden, E. C., Edwards, B. S., Hawkins, M. J., and Merritt, J. A., in *Biological Response in Cancer: Progress Toward Potential Applications* (Michich, E., ed.) Plenum, New York (1982).

*7.* Horoszewicz, J. S., Leong, S. S., Ito, M., Buffett, R. F., Karakousis, C., Holyoke, E., Job, L., Dolen, J. G., and Carter, W. A. *Cancer Treat. Rep.* **62**, 1899–1906 (1978).

*8.* Balkwill, F. Taylor-Papadimitriou, J., Fantes, K. H., and Sebesteny, A. *Eur. J. Cancer* **16**, 569–573 (1980)

*9.* Balkwill, F. R., Moodie, E. M., Freedman, V., and Fantes, K. H. *Int. J. Cancer* **30**, 231–235 (1982).

*10.* Balkwill, F. R., Moodie, E. M., Freedman, V., Lane, E. B. and Fantes, K. H. *J. Interferon Res.* **3**, 319–326 (1983).

*11.* Balkwill, F. R., Mowshowitz, S., Seilman, S. S., Moodie, E. M., Griffin, D. B., Fantes, K. H., and Wolf, C. R. *Cancer Res.* **44**, 5249–5255 (1984).

*12.* Riviere, Y. and Hovanessian, A. G. *Cancer Res.* **43**, 4596–4599 (1983).

*13.* Salmon, S. E., in *Cloning of Human Tumor Stem Cells* (Salmon, ed.) Liss, New York (1980).

*14.* Salmon, S. E., in *Cancer Achievements, Challenges, and Prospects for the 1980's* (Burchenal, J. H. and Oettgen, H. F., eds.) Grune and Stratton, New York (1980).

*15.* Selby, P., Buick, R. N., and Tannock, I. *N. Engl. J. Med.* **308**, 129–134 (1983).

*16.* Von Hoff, D. D., Clark, G. M., Stogdill, B. J., Sarosdy, M. F., O'Brien, M. T., Casper, J. T., Mattox, D. E., Page, C. P., Cruz, A. B., and Sandbach, J. F. *Cancer Res.* **43**, 1926–1931 (1983).

*17.* Alonso, K. *Cancer* **54**, 2475–2479 (1984).

*18.* Bradley, E. C. and Ruscetti, F. W. *Cancer Res.* **41**, 244–249 (1981).

*19.* Von Hoff, D. D., Gutterman, J., Portnoy, B., and Coltman, C. A. *Cancer Chemother. Pharmacol.* **8**, 99–103 (1982).

*20.* Salmon, S. E., Durie, B. G. M., Young, L., Liu, R. M., Trown, P. W., and Stebbing, N. *J. Clin. Oncol.* **1**, 217–225 (1983).

21. Borden, E. C., Hogan, T. F., and Voelkel, J. G. *Cancer Res.* **42**, 4948-4953 (1982).
22. Willson, J. K. V., Bittner, G., and Borden, E. C. *J. Interferon Res.* **4**, 441-447 (1984).
23. Edwards, B. S., Hawkins, M. J. and Borden, E. C. *J. Biol. Resp. Mod.* **2**, 409-417 (1983).
24. Edwards, B. S., Hawkins, M. J., and Borden, E. C. *Cancer Res.* **44**, 3135-3139 (1984).
25. Einhorn, S., Ahre, A., Blomgren, H., Johansson, B., Mellstedt, H., and Strander, H. *Int. J. Cancer* **30**, 167-172 (1982).
26. Shibata, H. and Taylor-Papadimitriou, J. *Int. J. Cancer* **28**, 447-453 (1981).
27. Gutterman, J. U., Blumenschein, G. R., Alexanian, R., Yap, H-Y., Buzdar, A. U., Cabanillas, F., Hortobagyi, G. N., Hersh, E. M., Rasmussen, S. L., Harmon, M., Kramer, M., and Pestka, S. *Ann. Int. Med.* **93**, 399-406 (1980).
28. Borden, E. C., Holland, J. F., Dao, T. L., Gutterman, J. U., Wiener, L., Chang, Y-C., and Patel, J. *Ann. Int. Med.* **97** 1-6 (1982).
29. Sherwin, S. A., Mayer, D., Ochs, J. J., Abrams, P. G., Knost, J. A., Foon, K. A., Fein, S., and Oldham, R. K. *Ann. Int. Med.* **98**, 598-602 (1983).
30. Nethersell, A., Smedley, H., Katrak, M., Wheeler, T., and Sikora, K. *Br. J. Cancer* **49**, 615-620 (1984).
31. Muss, H. B., Kempf, R. A., Martino, S., Rudnick, S. A., Greiner, J., Cooper, M. R., Decker, D., Grunberg, S. M., Jackson, D. V., Richards, F., II, Samal, B., Singhakowinta, A., Spurr, L. C., Stuart, J. J., White, D. R., Caponera, M., and Mitchell, M. S. *J. Clin. Oncol.* **2**, 1012-1016 (1984).
32. Quesada, J. R., Hawkins, M., Horning, S., Alexanian, R., Borden, E., Merigan, T., Adams, F., and Gutterman, J. U. *Am. J. Med.* **77**, 427-432 (1984).
33. Sarna, G. P. and Figlin, R. A. *Cancer Treat. Rep.* **69**, 547-549 (1985).
34. Padmanabhan, N., Balkwill, F. R., Bodmer, J. G., and Rubens, R. D. *Br. J. Cancer* **51**, 55-60 (1985).
35. Schmid, S. M., Borden, E. C., Bryan, G. T., Trump, D. L., and Cummings, K. B. *Surg. Forum* **35**, 655-657 (1984).
36. Quesada, J. R., Swanson, D. A., Trindale, A., and Gutterman, J. U. *Cancer Res.* **43**, 940-947 (1983).
37. Quesada, J. R., Swanson, D. A., and Gutterman, J. U. *J. Clin. Oncol.* **3**, 1086-1092 (1985).
38. deKernion, J. B., Sarna, G., Figlin, R., Lindner, A., and Smith, R. B. *J. Urol.* **130**, 1063-1066 (1983).
39. Edsmyr, R., Esposti, P. L., Andersson, L., Steineck, G., Lagergren, C., and Strander, H. *Radiother. Oncol.* **4**, 21-26 (1985).
40. Kirkwood, J. M., Harris, J. E., Vera, R., Sandler, S., Fischer, D. S., Khandekar, J., Ernstoff, M. S., Gordon, L., Lutes, R., Bonomi, P., Lytton, B., Cobleigh, M., and Taylor, S. J., IV *Cancer Res.* **45**, 863-871 (1985).

41. Neidhart, J. A., Gagen, M. M., Young, D., Tuttle, R., Melink, T. J., Ziccarrelli, A., and Kisner, D. *Cancer Res.* **44**, 4140–4143 (1984).

42. Vugrin, D., Hood, L., Taylor, W., and Laszlo, J. *Cancer Treat. Rep.* **69**, 817–820 (1985).

43. Quesada, J. R., Rios, A., Swanson, D., Trown, P., and Gutterman, J. U. *J. Clin. Oncol.* **3**, 1522–1528 (1985).

44. Bart, R. S., Porzio, N. R., Kopf, A. W., Vilcek, J. T., Cheng, E. H., and Farcet, Y. *Cancer Res.* **40**, 614–619 (1980).

45. Ida, N., Uenishi, N., Kajita, A., and Satoh, Y. *Gann* **73**, 952–960 (1982).

46. Schiller, J. H., Willson, J. K. V., Bittner, G., Wolberg, W., Hawkins, M. J., and Borden, E. C. *J. Interferon Res.* **6**, 615–625 (1986).

47. Salmon, S. E., Meyskens, F. L., Jr., Alberts, D. S., Soehnlen, B., and Young, L. *Cancer Treat. Rep.* **65**, 1–12 (1981).

48. Krown, S.E., Burk, M., Kirkwood, J. M., Kerr, D., Morton, D. L., and Oettgen, H. F. *Cancer Treat. Rep.* **68**, 723–726 (1984).

49. Retsas, S., Priestman, T. J., Newton, K. A., and Westbury, G. *Cancer* **51**, 273–276 (1983).

50. Creagan, E. T., Ahmann, D. L., Green S. J., Long, H. J., Frytak, S., O'Fallon, J. R., and Itri, L. M. *J. Clin. Oncol.* **2**, 1002–1005 (1984).

51. Creagan, E. T., Ahmann, D. L. Green, S. J., Long, H. J., Rubin, J., Schutt, A. J., and Dziewanowski, Z. E. *Cancer* **54**, 2844–2849 (1984).

52. Creagan, E. T., Ahmann, D. L., Green, S. J., Long, H. J., Frytak, S., and Itri, L. M. *J. Clin. Oncol.* **3**, 977–981 (1985).

53. Goldberg, R. M., Ayoob, M., Silgals, R., Ahlgren, J. D., and Neefe, J. R. *Cancer Treat. Rep.* **69**, 813–816 (1985).

54. Kirkwood, J. M., Ernstoff, M. S., Davis, C. A., Reiss, M., Ferraresi, R., and Rudnick, S. A. *Ann. Int. Med.* **103**, 32–36 (1985).

55. Niloff, J. M., Knapp, R. C., Jones, G., Schaetzl, E. M., and Bast, R. C. *Cancer Treat. Rep.* **69**, 895–896 (1985).

56. Berek, J. S., Hacker, N. F., Lichtenstein, A., Jung, T., Spina, C., Knox, R. M., Brady, J., Greene, T., Ettinger, L. M., Lagasse, L. D., Bonnem, E. M., Spiegel, R. J., and Zighelboim, J. *Cancer Res.* **45**, 4447–4453 (1985).

57. Grunberg, S. M., Kempf, R. A., Itri, L. M., Venturi, C. L., Boswell, W. D., Jr., and Mitchell, M. S. *Cancer Treat. Rep.* **69**, 1031–1032 (1985).

58. Krown, S. E., Stoopler, M. B., Gralla, R. J., Cunningham-Rundles, S., Stewart, W. E., Pollack, M. S., and Oettgen, H., in *Immunotherapy of Human Cancer* Elsevier/North-Holland, New York (1982).

59. Figlin, R. A. and Sarna, G. P. *Proc. Am. Soc. Clin. Oncol.* **2**, 45 (1983).

60. Nair, P. V., Tong, M. J., Kempf, R., Co., R., Lee, S-D, and Venturi, C. L. *Cancer* **56**, 1018–1022 (1985).

61. Sachs, E., DiBisceglie, A. M., Dusheiko, G. M., Song, E., Lyons, S. F., Schoub, B. D., and Kew, M. C. *Br. J. Cancer* **52**, 105–109 (1985).

62. Cook, A., Carter, W., Nidagorski, F., and Akhtar, L. *Science* **219**, 881–883 (1983).

63. Tanaka, N., Nagao, S., Tohgo, A., Sekiguchi, F., Kohno, M., Ogawa, H., Matsui, T., and Matsutani, M. *Gann* **74**, 308–316 (1983).

64. Hirakawa, K., Ueda, S., Nakagawa, Y., Suzuki, K., Fukuma, S., Kita, M., Imanishi, J., and Kishida, T. *Cancer* **51**, 1976–1981 (1983).
65. Boethius, J., Blomgren, H., Collins, V. P., Greitz, T., and Strander, H. *Acta Neurochirurgica* **68**, 239–251 (1983).
66. Mahaley, M. S., Urso, M. B., Whaley, R. A., Blue, M., Williams, T. E., Guaspari, A., and Selker, R. G. *J. Neurosurg.* **63**, 719–725 (1985).
67. Duff, T. A., Borden, E., Bay, J., Peipmeier, J., and Sielaff, K. *J. Neuro. Surg.* **64**, 408–413 (1986).
68. Oberg, K., Funa, K., and Alm, G. *N. Engl. J. Med.* **309**, 129–132 (1983).
69. Figlin, R. A., Callaghan, M., and Sarna, G. *Cancer Treat. Rep.* **67**, 493–494 (1983).
70. Chaplinski, T., Laszlo, J., Moore, J., and Silverman, P. *Cancer Treat. Rep.* **67**, 1009–1012 (1983).
71. Neefe, J. R., Silgals, R., Ayoob, M., and Schein, P. S. *J. Biol. Resp. Modif.* **3**, 366–370 (1984).
72. Eggermont, A. M., Weimar, W., Marquet, R. L., Lameris, J. D., and Jeekel, J. *Cancer Treat. Rep.* **69**, 185–187 (1985).
73. Ikic, D., Maricic, Z., Oresic, V., Rode, B., Nola, P., Smudj, K., Knezevic, M., Jusic, D., and Soos, E. *Lancet* **1**, 1022–1024 (1981).
74. Scorticatti, C. H., De De LaPena, N. C., Bellora, O. G., Mariotto, R. A., Casabe, A. R., and Comolli, R. *J. Interferon Res.* **2**, 339–343 (1982).
75. Connors, J. M., Andiman, W. A., Howarth, C. B., Liu, E., Merigan, T. C., Savage, M. E., and Jacobs, C. *J. Clin. Oncol.* **3**, 813–817 (1985).
76. Ikic, D., Krusic, J., Kirhmajer, V., Knezevic, M., Marcic, Z., Rode, B., Jusic, D., and Soos, E. *Lancet* **1**, 1027–1036 (1981).
77. Krown, S. E., Real, F. X., Cunningham-Rundles, S., Myskowski, P. L., Koziner, B., Fein, S., Mittelman, A., Oettgen, H. F., and Safai, B. *N. Engl. J. Med.* **308**, 1071–1076 (1983).
78. Groopman, J. E., Gottlieb, M. S., Goodman, J., Mitsuyasu, R. T., Conant, M. A., Prince, H., Fahey, J. L., Derezin, M., Weinstein, W. M., Casavante, C., Rothman, J., Rudnick, S. A., and Volberding, P. A. *Ann. Int. Med.* **100**, 671–676 (1984).
79. Rios, A., Mansell, P. W. A., Newell, G. R., Reuben, J. M., Hersh, E. M., and Gutterman, J. U. *J. Clin. Oncol.* **3**, 506–512 (1985).
80. Gelmann, E. P., Preble, O. T., Steis, R., Lane, H. C., Rook, A. H., Wesley, M., Jacob, J., Fauci, A., Masur, H., and Longo, D. *Am. J. Med.* **78**, 737–741 (1985).
81. Real, F. X., Oettgen, H. F., and Krown, S. E. *J. Clin. Oncol.* **4**, 544–551 (1986).
82. Krigel, R. L., Odajynk, C. M., Laubenstein, L. J., Ostreicher, R., Wernz, J., Vilcek, J., Rubenstein, P., and Friedman-Kien, A. E. *J. Biol. Resp. Modif.* **4**, 358–364 (1985).
83. Aapro, M., Alberts, D., and Salmon, S. E. *Cancer Chemother. Pharmacol.* **10**, 161–166 (1983).
84. Salmon, S. E. *Clin. Hematol.* **11**, 47–63 (1982).
85. Osserman, E. F., Sherman, W. H., Alexanian, R., Gutterman, J. U., and Humphrey, R. L. in *The Biology of the Interferon System* (DeMaeyer, E.,

Galasso, G., and Schelekens, H., eds.) Elsevier/North-Holland Biomedical Press, Amsterdam (1981).

86. Alexanian, R., Gutterman, J., and Levy, H. *Clin. Hematol.* **11**, 211–220 (1982).

87. Ahre, A., Bjorkholm, M., Mellstedt, H., Brenning, G., Engstedt, L., Gahrton, G., Gyllenhammar, H., Holm, G., Johannson, B., Jarnmark, M., Karnstrom, L., Killander, A., Lerner, R., Lockner, D., Lohnqvist, B., Nilsson, B., Simonsson, B., Stalfelt, A. -M., Strander, H., Svedmyr, E., Wadman, B., and Wedelin, C. *Cancer Treat. Rep.* **68**, 1331–1338 (1984).

88. Wagstaff, J., Loynds, P., and Scarffe, J. H. *Cancer Treat. Rep.* **69**, 495–498 (1985).

89. Costanzi, J. J., Cooper, M. R., Scarffe, J. H., Ozer, H., Grubbs, S. S., Ferraresi, R. W., Pollard, R. B., and Spiegel, R. J. *J. Clin. Oncol.* **3**, 654–659 (1985).

90. Ohno, R. and Kimura, K. *Cancer* **57**, 1685–1688 (1986).

91. Quesada, J. R., Alexanian, R., Hawkins, M., Barlogie, B., Borden, E., Itri, L., and Gutterman, J. U. *Blood* **67**, 275–278 (1986).

92. Quesada, J. R., Reuben, J., Manning, J. T., Hersh, E. M., and Gutterman, J. U. *N. Engl. J. Med.* **310**, 15–18 (1984).

93. Thompson, J. A., Brady, J., Kidd, P., and Fefer, A. *Cancer Treat. Rep.* **69**, 791–793 (1985).

94. Ratain, M. J., Golomb, H. M., Vardiman, J. W., Vokes, E. E., Jacobs, R. H., and Daly, K. *Blood* **65**, 644–648 (1985).

95. Jacobs, A. D., Champlin, R. E., and Golde, D. W. *Blood* **65**, 1017–1020 (1985).

96. Foon, K. A., Maluish, A. E., Abrams, P. G., Wrightington, S., Stevenson, H. C., Alarif, A., Fer, M. F., Overton, W. R., Poole, M., Schnipper, E. F., Jaffe, E. S., and Herberman, R. B. *Am. J. Med.* **80**, 351–356 (1986).

97. Bunn, P. A., Foon, K. A., Ihde, D. C., Longo, D. L., Eddy, J., Winkler, C. F., Veach, S. R., Zeffren, J., Sherwin, S., and Oldham, R. *Ann. Int. Med.* **101**, 484–487 (1984).

98. Horning, S. J., Merigan, T. C., Krown, S. E., Gutterman, J. U., Louie, A., Gallagher, J., McCravey, J., Abramson, J., Cabanillas, F., Oettgen, H., and Rosenberg, S. A. *Cancer* **56**, 1305–1310 (1985).

99. Merigan, T. C., Sikora, K., Breeden, J. H., Levy, R., and Rosenberg, S. A. *N. Engl. J. Med.* **299**, 1449–1453 (1978).

100. Louie, A. C., Gallagher, J. G., Sikora, K., Levy, R., Rosenberg, S. A., and Merigan, T. C. *Blood* **58**, 712–718 (1981).

101. Siegert, W., Theml, H., Fink, U., Emmerich, B., Kaudewitz, P., Huhn, D., Boning, L., Abb, J., Joester, K. E., Bartl, R., Riethmuller, G., and Wilmanns, W. *Anticancer Res.* **2**, 193–198 (1982).

102. Foon, K. A., Sherwin, S. A., Abrams, P. G., Longo, D. L., Fer, M. F., Stevenson, H. C., Ochs, J. J., Bottino, G. C., Schoenberger, C. S., Zeffren, J., Jaffe, E. S., and Oldham, R. K. *N. Engl. J. Med.* **311**, 1148–1152 (1984).

103. Misset, J. L., Mathe, G., Gastiaburu, J., Goutner, A., Dorval, T., Gouveia, J., Hayat, M., Jasmin, C., Schwarzenberg, L., Machover, D., Ribaud, P., and DeVassal, F. *Anticancer Res.* **2**, 67–69 (1982).
104. Foon, K. A., Bottino, G. C., Abrams, P. G., Fer, M. F., Longo, D. L., Schoenberger, C. S., and Oldham, R. K. *Am. J. Med.* **78**, 216–220 (1985).
105. Verma, D. S., Spitzer, G., Gutterman, J. U., Zander, A. R., McCredie, K. B., and Dicke, K. A. *Blood* **54**, 1423–1427 (1979).
106. Oladipupo-Williams, C. K., Svet-Moldavskaya, I., and Vilcek, J. *Oncology* **38**, 356–360 (1981).
107. Talpaz, M., McCredie, K. B., Mavligit, G. M., and Gutterman, J. U. *Blood* **62**, 689–692 (1983).
108. Talpaz, M., Kantarjian, H. M., McCredie, K., Trujillo, J. M., Keating, M. J., and Gutterman, J. U. *N. Engl. J. Med.* **314**, 1065–1069 (1986).
109. Talpaz, M., Mavligit, G., Keating, M., Walters, R. S., and Gutterman, J. U. *Ann. Int. Med.* **99**, 789–792 (1983).
110. Hill, N. O., Pardue, A., Khan, A., Aleman, C., Dorn, G., and Hill, J. M. *J. Clin. Hematol. Oncol.* **11**, 23–35 (1981).
111. Rohatiner, A. Z. S., Balkwill, F. R., Malpas, J. S., and Lister, T. A. *Cancer Chemother. Pharmacol.* **11**, 56–58 (1983).
112. Laszlo, J., Huang, A. T., Brenckman, W. D., Jeffs, C., Koren, H., Cianciolo, G., Metzgar, R., Cashdollar, W., Cox, E., Buckley, C. E., Tso, C. Y., and Lucas, V. S. *Cancer Res.* **43**, 4458–4466 (1983).
113. Kurzrock, R., Rosenblum, M. G., Sherwin, S. A., Rios, A., Talpaz, M., Quesada, J. R., and Gutterman, J. U. *Cancer Res.* **45**, 2866–2872 (1985).
114. Hawkins, M., Horning, S., Konrad, M., Anderson, S., Sielaff, K., Rosno, S., Schiesel, J., Davis, T., DeMets, D., Merigan, T., and Borden, E. C. *Cancer Res.* **45**, 5914–5920 (1985).
115. Gutterman, J. U., Fine, S., Quesada, J., Horning, S. J., Levine, J. F., Alexanian, R., Bernhardt, L., Kramer, M., Spiegel, H., Colburn, W., Trown, P., Merigan, T., and Dziewanowski, Z. *Ann. Int. Med.* **96**, 549–556 (1982).
116. Sugarman, B. J., Aggarwal, B. B., Hass, P. E., Figari, I. S., Palladino, M. A., and Shephard, H. M. *Science* **230**, 943–945 (1985).
117. Ziai, M. R., Imberti, L., Tongson, A., and Ferrone, S. *Cancer Res.* **45**, 5877–5882 (1985).
118. Liao, S. K., Kwong, P. C., Khosravi, M., and Dent, P. B. *J. Nat. Cancer Inst.* **68**, 19–25 (1982).
119. Greiner, J. W., Hand, P. H, Nogucki, P., Fisher, P. B., Pestka, S., and Schlom, J. *Cancer Res.* **44**, 3208–3214 (1984).
120. Fleischmann, W. R., Georgiades, J. A., Osborne, L. C., and Johnson, H. M. *Infect. Immunol.* **26**, 248–253 (1979).
121. Fleischmann, W. R., Kleyn, K. M., and Baron, S. *J. Natl. Cancer Inst.* **65**, 963–966 (1980).
122. Zerial, A., Hovanessian, A. G., Stefanos, S., Huygen, K., Werner, G. H., and Falcoff, E. *Antiviral Res.* **2**, 227–239 (1982).

123. Czarniecki, C. W., Fennie, C. W., Powers, D. B., and Estell, D. A. *J. Virol.* **49**, 490–496 (1984).
124. Schiller, J. H., Groveman, D. S., Schmid, S. M., Willson, J. K. V., Cummings, K. B., and Borden E. C. *Cancer Res.* **46**, 483–488 (1986).
125. Groveman, D. S., Borden E. C., Merritt, J. A., Robins, H. I., Steeves, R., and Bryan, G. T. *Cancer Res.* **44**, 5517–5521 (1984).
126. Miyoshi, T., Ogawa, S., Kanamori, T., Nobuhara, M., and Namba, M. *Cancer Lett.* **17**, 239–247 (1983).
127. Balkwill, F. R. and Moodie, E. M. *Cancer Res.* **44**, 904–908 (1984).
128. Mark, D. F., Lu, S. D., Creasy, A., Yamamoto, R., and Lin, L. *Proc. Natl. Acad. Sci. USA* **81**, 5662–5666 (1984).

# Biologic Effects of Tumor Necrosis Factors Alpha and Beta

ARTHUR J. AMMANN and MICHAEL A. PALLADINO, JR.

## 1. Introduction

As early as 1891, clinical reports suggested that major components of the cell wall of gram-negative bacteria such as endotoxins were associated with antitumor activities; Bruns (*1*) and Coley (*2*) described the regression of tumors in patients with tumors who were deliberately injected with mixtures of killed bacterial toxins. Gratia and Linz (*3*) and Shear et al. (*4*) subsequently demonstrated that bacterial filtrates or endotoxins were capable of inducing hemorrhagic necrosis of specific transplanted tumors. A significant advance in distinguishing the effects of endotoxin from a specific "tumor necrosis factor" was reported in 1975 by Carswell et al. (*5*). They were impressed with the observations and hypothesis of Algire (*6*), who suggested that hemorrhagic necrosis of tumors might be secondary to endotoxin-induced hypotension resulting in circulatory stasis and ischemia of the tumor. They argued, however, that rather than an indirect action, endotoxin probably caused the host to release a factor that was directly toxic to the tumor. This hypothesis led Carswell et al. (*5*) to the discovery of an endotoxin-induced serum factor, which caused necrosis of tumors and which they termed tumor necrosis factor (TNF-like). [Note: The term tumor necrosis factor-like (TNF-like) will be used in reference to reports in which the exact identity of the factor in relation to recombinant human tumor necrosis factor-alpha (rHu TNF-$\alpha$) or recombinant human tumor necrosis factor-beta (rHu TNF-$\beta$) cannot be determined.] Carswell et al. were the first to demonstrate that an endotoxin-induced serum factor, which was toxic to tumor cells in vitro, also resulted in tumor necrosis in vivo.

## 2. In Vivo Production of TNF

In the original studies of Carswell et al. (*5*), the production of TNF-
like activity in vivo was accomplished by first inoculating animals with
*Bacillus Calmette-Guerin* (BCG) and subsequently treating with endotoxin.
Other agents including *Corynebacterium granulosum*, *Corynebacterium
parvum*, and zymosan were also shown to be effective priming agents.
In these models, optimal TNF-like production occurred 2 h following endotoxin treatment. The authors noted that the animals were usually in shock
at this time. Rats and rabbits were also shown to produce TNF-like factors following similar induction regimens. Based on observations in animals,
Carswell et al. (*5*) suggested that the macrophage was the probable source
of TNF.

More recently, Haranaka et al. investigated TNF-like activity in different strains of mice following the administration of lipopolysaccharide
(LPS) (*7*). Differences in the ability to produce TNF-like activity were
demonstrated in various murine strains with BALB/C nu/nu exhibiting the
lowest levels and ICR nu/nu the highest. Sensitivity to LPS (specifically
the lipid A component) was considered the most important factor in the
ability to stimulate TNF-like production. In subsequent studies performed
by Nitusu et al. (*8*), depressed TNF production in BALB/C nu/nu mice
could be enhanced by reconstitution with T-cells. The authors attributed
this effect to macrophage activation by T-cells. Few studies are available
comparing relative production of cytokines by similar populations of cells.
The amounts of cytokine produced are probably independently variable,
however, suggesting that there are "high" or "low" producers of specific
cytokines. For example, in a study by Neta et al. (*9*), considerable variation was observed among different strains of mice in their ability to produce interferon vs TNF-like activity as well as other cytokines.

Little is known regarding the distribution and metabolism of TNF-
like activity in vivo. Beutler et al. (*10*) performed limited pharmacokinetic
studies in rabbits and mice. A radioreceptor assay was used to determine
TNF-like activity in rabbits, and radioiodinated murine TNF-like material
was utilized to determine the half-life and distribution of TNF-like activity
in mice. Following LPS stimulation of rabbits, nanomolar concentrations
of TNF-like activity were found in rabbit serum. Peak levels were observed
at 2 h following injection. TNF-like material had a plasma half-life of 6
min following intravenous injection of radiolabeled material into mice.
The radiolabel was distributed primarily to the liver, kidneys, skin, and
gastrointestinal tract.

## 3. Effects of TNF on Tumors In Vivo

The first documentation of an endotoxin-induced serum factor causing tumor necrosis was reported by Carswell et al. (5). Several different
tumors, S-180 sarcoma (CD-1 Swiss), BP8 leukemia (C3H), P815 masto-
cytoma (DBA/2), several leukemia cell lines, and meth-A sarcoma were
inoculated subcutaneously into mice, and after 7 d the mice were injected
intravenously with serum containing TNF-like activity. After 24 h, tumor
necrosis was graded on a 0 to 3+ scale based on the degree of visible
necrosis. This assay has become a standard means to assay TNF and related
cytokines (11). Although Carswell et al. (5) demonstrated that their TNF-
like material was most effective in tumors that had been established for
more than 5 d, they argued that the effect was a direct cytotoxic effect
on tumor cells and not an indirect effect on blood vessels supplying the
tumor. Because TNF-like material was less effective in tumor-bearing
BALB/C nu/nu mice, Haranaka et al. (11) suggested that it may have an
effect that is both direct and mediated through the immune response of
the host. Regression of tumor by intralesional injection of a TNF-like
cytokine in other animal models was demonstrated by Kahn et al. (12).
In a dog with malignant melanoma, necrosis and decreased tumor size
occurred within the first 3 d following injection, and complete remission
occurred after 3 wk.

The first contemporary report of the use of a TNF-like factor in humans
was published by Papermaster et al. (13), who described tumor regression in humans following intralesional administration of a lymphoid cell
culture supernatant. The lymphokine was isolated from the human B-
lymphoblast cell line RPMI 1788, partially purified, and subsequently injected intralesionally into the metastatic skin lesions of patients with breast
carcinoma and other malignancies. Of 30 patients thus treated, 16 under-
went greater than 50% regression and nine had complete disappearance
of their tumor confirmed by biopsy. The factor produced delayed type
hypersensitivity skin test reactions when injected into the uninvolved skin
of patients and an inflammatory reaction when injected directly into the
metastatic lesions. Although this factor was not identified, it was probably
closely related to TNF-β (previously termed lymphotoxin).

In addition to a specific necrotic effect on subcutaneously transplanted
tumors following intravenous or intralesional injection, TNF may prevent
the growth of tumors inoculated intravenously or intraperitonally (11,14).
More recently it has been demonstrated that rHu TNF-α and rHu TNF-β
can cause necrosis of meth-A sarcomas established in mice and human

tumors established in nude mice (15,16). Intralesional, intramuscular, or intravenous routes of administration were effective (15,16). Studies of the mechanism of tumor killing indicate that rHu TNF-α is the primary cytokine responsible for macrophage killing of macrophage-sensitive tumors (17,18).

In vitro studies demonstrated synergy between recombinant human interferon-γ (rHuIFN-γ) and rHuTNF-α in tumor cell antiproliferative assays. Sugarman et al. (19) studied a variety of tumor cell lines in vitro and found them to be either insensitive or sensitive to the antiproliferative effects of rHuTNF-α alone. Combined with rIFN-γ, several of the insensitive cell lines became sensitive. Although rHuIFN-γ increased the number of TNF-α receptors, the sensitivity to antiproliferative effects of rHuTNF-α could not be related to receptor number. Studies performed in murine tumor models in vivo confirmed the initial in vitro observations of synergy between rHuTNF-α and rHuIFN-γ and suggested that future approaches to the treatment of human malignancies may include the use of combination cytokine therapy (20).

## 4. Metabolic Effects of TNF In Vivo

Based on the observations that certain infections and malignancies in mammals were associated with the development of cachexia, Kawakami et al. (22) studied the effects of endotoxin on lipid metabolism. They observed that endotoxin decreased lipoprotein lipase (LPL) activity and subsequently reported that an endotoxin-induced factor, termed cachectin, was primarily responsible for this effect (22). Cachetin was capable of decreased LPL activity in endotoxin-sensitive C3H/HeN mice, but not in endotoxin-resistant C3H/HeJ mice. The ability of cachetin to inhibit LPL activity was offered as an explanation for the wasting and hypertriglyceridemia in animals with chronic infection or malignancy. Subsequently, cachectin was shown to be identical to TNF-α (19) and to inhibit LPL activity in cultured 3T3-L1 adipocytes (23). Although the effect of TNF-like material on LPL was postulated to be a major cause of wasting, it is unlikely that TNF plays a singular role since both interleukin-1 and interferon have been shown to affect lipid metabolism in vitro and in vivo (24–26).

Because endotoxin shock results in hypoglycemia, Satomi et al. investigated the relationship of endotoxin-induced TNF-like production and hypoglycemia (27). Glucose administration to mice primed by injection of *Propionibacterium acnes* prior to LPS administration inhibited subsequent TNF-like activity induced by LPS. Insulin prevented the in vitro production of TNF-like activity by peritoneal exudate cells in primed mice. The administration of TNF-like material without concomitant LPS was not associated with hypoglycemia, but did result in specific tumor necrosis. The authors concluded that hypoglycemia does not accompany the action of TNF in vivo. Additional metabolic effects include the ability of both rHuTNF-α and rHuTNF-β to induce bone resorption in vitro. This effect was associated with an increased number of osteoclasts and decreased mineralized bone matrix (27). Both cytokines also inhibited bone collagen synthesis as measured by the incorporation of [³H]-proline into collagenase-digestible protein (27).

In contrast to the antiproliferative effect of rHuTNF-α on tumor cells, normal fibroblasts undergo increased proliferation (19). The mechanism for the differential effect is not known, but is not related to receptor numbers (19).

# 5. Tumor Necrosis Factor: Additional Biological Effects

## 5.1. Endotoxin Shock

Because of the observation that endotoxin results in the production of TNF in vitro and shock in vivo, Beutler et al. (28) postulated that TNF was a mediator of endotoxin shock (28). To test this hypothesis, they passively immunized BALB/C mice with specific polyclonal rabbit anti-murine TNF (TNF-like) and demonstrated that they were partially protected against the lethal effects of LPS. Although a dose response to the antibody was observed in their study, mortality was reduced by only 50%, suggesting that either the antibody failed to completely neutralize TNF, or more likely, that other cytokines and pharmacologic agents were released in vivo following endotoxin injection and were not neutralized by antibody to TNF-like material.

## 5.2. Inflammation

Recent studies suggest that TNF has important biologic functions in inflammation whether mediated by endotoxin, infection, or autoimmune factors. In relation to inflammation, rHuTNF-α in vitro results in increased superoxide production by neutrophils, increased production of interleukin-1, stimulation of the mixed lymphocyte culture response, enhanced antibody-dependent cytotoxicity, enhanced neutrophil phagocytosis, enhanced Class I and II MHC antigen expression, increased adherence of neutrophils to endothelial cells, and release of arachodonic acid metabolites from human synovial cells (29–36). A TNF-like cytokine has also been implicated in kidney transplant rejection in a rat model (37).

## 5.3. Autoimmune Disease

Johnson et al. (*38*) demonstrated that autologous peripheral blood lymphocytes from patients with polymyositis produced a TNF-like cytokine when stimulated by muscle cells. The specific type of TNF was not identified, since they utilized crude supernatants from lymphocyte cultures. In a study of postmyocardial infarction patients, Mirrakhimov et al. demonstrated TNF-like activity in supernatants of lymphocytes stimulated with myoglobin in vitro, suggesting that TNF may have a role in the postmyocardial infarction syndrome (*39*).

## 5.4. Infection

TNF may also have a biologic function in the control of infection. Cells infected with vesicular stomatis virus were found to be susceptible to the cytotoxic effects of lymphotoxin, whereas uninfected cells remained intact (*40*). Interferon-γ potentiated this effect in a manner similar to the synergistic action of rHuTNF-α and rHuIFN-γ on tumor cell proliferation. In another study, rHuTNF-α was found to have a cytotoxic effect on Herpes virus infected, but not uninfected, cells (*41*). IFN-γ had no effect on either cell population. Based on in vitro and in vivo studies in mice, Taverne et al. (*42*) concluded that TNF-like material was cytotoxic to *Plasmodium* and prevented the mortality associated with this parasitic infection. Recently, rHuTNF-α was found to be similar to eosinophil-cytotoxicity-enhancing factor and to mediate identical in vitro eosinophil toxicity to *Schistosoma mansoni* larvae (*43*). Patients with the acquired immunodeficiency syndrome (AIDS) and AIDS-related complex, were found to produce significantly less TNF-α and TNF-β in vitro than controls (*32*). Since these patients are susceptible to both infection and malignancy, TNF-α and TNF-β may play a role in their susceptibility to opportunistic infection and malignancy. In a study of newborns, decreased TNF-like activity was observed following phytohemagglutinin stimulation of cord blood mononuclear cells; the authors postulated that this might be an explanation for the undue susceptibility of newborn infants to certain infections (*44*).

## 6. Summary

The availability of recombinant human tumor necrosis factors-α and TNF-β has resulted in the ability to define the biologic activity of various cytokines and allowed for the identification of the specific cells that produce them. TNF has been associated with a number of important activities including: (1) enhanced immunologic function, (2) tumor necrosis, (3) inflammation, (4) endotoxin shock, (5) autoimmune disease, (6) infection, (7) regulation of lipid metabolism, and (8) bone growth. The effects of TNF on immunologic function include enhanced phagocytosis, superoxide production, antibody-dependent cellular cytotoxicity, mixed lymphocyte culture response, and class I and class II antigen expression. TNF is a potent antitumor agent when administered intralesionally or systemically and acts synergistically with interferon-γ. In relation to inflammation, TNF increases neutrophil adherence to endothelial cells and stimulates the release of arachodonic acid metabolites from synovial cells and fibroblasts. TNF is released during endotoxin shock and may therefore be a mediator of some of the physiologic changes that occur following exposure to endotoxin. Preliminary evidence suggests that TNF may play a role in the inflammation associated with autoimmune disease. Recent studies indicate that TNF may have a role in infection, as evidenced by a cytotoxic effect against virus-infected cells and killing of parasites. Finally, TNF administration results in a number of metabolic effects that include inhibition of lipoprotein lipase activity, hypertriglyceridemia, and regulation of bone resorption.

NOTE: Since writing this article, numerous advances in our understanding of the biological significance of the Tumor Necrosis Factors have been made. For the latest information on Tumor Necrosis Factor, the reader is requested to examine the abstract book for a recent meeting on Tumor Necrosis Factor held in Heidelberg, West Germany in September 1987. Immunobiology 175, No. 1/2, 1987.

## References

1. Bruns, P. *Beitr. Z. Klin. Chir.* **3**, 433 (1888).
2. Coley, W. B. *Ann. Surg.* **14**, 199 (1891).
3. Gratia, A. and Linz, R. *Scamces. Soc. Biol. Ses. Fil.* **108**, 427–428 (1931).
4. Shear, M. J. *J. Natl. Cancer Inst.* **4**, 461–587 (1944).
5. Carswell, E. A., Old, L. J., Kassell, R. L., Green, S., Riore, N., and Williamson, B. *Proc. Natl. Acad. Sci. USA* **72**, 3666–3670 (1975).
6. Algire, G. H., Legallais, F. Y., and Kunii, O. *Tohoku J. Exp. Med.* **144**, 385–396 (1984).
7. Haranaka, K., Satomi, N., and Kunii, O. *Tohoku J. Exp. Med.* **144**, 385–396 (1984).
8. Niitusu, Y., Watanabe, N., Sone, H., Neda, H., and Uruushizakaki, I. *Jpn. J. Cancer Res.* **76**, 395–399 (1985).
9. Neta, R., Salvin, S. B., and Sabaawi, M. *Cell Immunol.* **64**, 203–219 (1981).
10. Beutler, B. A., Milsark, I., and Cerami, A. *J. Immunol.* **135**, 3972–3977 (1985).

11. Haranaka, K., Satomi, N., and Satomi, A. *Int. J. Cancer* **34**, 263–267 (1984).
12. Kahn, A., Martin, E. S., Webb, K., Weldon, D., Hill, N. O., Duvall, J., and Hill, J. M. *Soc. Exp. Biol. Med.* **169**, 291–294 (1982).
13. Papermaster, B. W., Holterman, O. A., Klein, E., Dejerassi, I., Rosner, D., Dao, T., and Constanzi, J. J. *Clin. Immunol. Immunopath.* **5**, 31–47 (1976).
14. Fun, K. P., Leung, S. W., Ha, D. K. K., Ng, S. W., Choy, Y. M., and Lee, C. Y. *Cancer Lett.* **27**, 269–276 (1985).
15. Pennica, D., Nedwin, G. E., Hayflick, J. S., Seeburg, P. H., Derynck, R., Palladino, M. A., Kohr, W. J., and Goeddel, D. V. *Nature* **312**, 724–729 (1984).
16. Talmadge, J. E., Tribble, H. R., Pennington, R. W., and Wiltrout, R. H., submitted (1986).
17. Philips, R. and Epstein, L. B. *Nature* **323**, 86–89.
18. Urban, J. L., Shepard, H. M., Rothstein, J. L., Sugarman, B. J., and Schreiber, H., *Proc. Natl. Acad. Sci. USA* **83**, 5233–5237 (1986).
19. Sugarman, B. J., Aggarwal, B. B., Hass, P. E., Palladino, M. A., and Shepard, H. M. *Science* **230**, 943–945 (1985).
20. Williamson, B. D., Carswell, E. A., Rubin, B. Y., Prendergasdt, J. S., and Old, L. J. *Proc. Natl. Acad. Sci. USA* **80**, 5397–5401 (1983).
21. Kawakami, M., Pekala, M., Lane, D., and Cerami, A. *J. Exp. Med.* **154**, 631–639 (1981).
22. Beutler, B., Mahoney, J., Trang, N. L., Pekla, P., and Cerami, A. *J. Exp. Med.* **161**, 984–995 (1985).
23. Beutler, B. A., Greenwald, D., and Hulmes, J. *Nature* **316**, 552–554 (1985).
24. Beutler, B. A. and Cerami, A. *J. Immunol.* **135**, 3969–3971 (1985).
25. Keay, S. and Grossberg, S. E. *Proc. Natl. Acad. Sci. USA* **70**, 4099–4103 (1980).
26. Dixon, R. M., Bordon, E. C., Kein, H. L., Anderson, S., Spennelta, T. L., Tormey, D. C., and Shrago, E. *Metabolism* **33**, 440–404 (1984).
27. Satomi, N., Sakurai, A., and Haranaki, K. *J. Natl. Cancer Inst.* **74**, 1255–1260 (1985).
28. Beutler, B. A., Milsark, I., and Cerami, A. *Science* **229**, 869–871 (1985).
29. Shalaby, M. R., Aggarwal, B. B., Rinderknecht, E., Svedersky, L. P., Finkle, B. S., and Palladino, M. A. *J. Immunol.* **135**, 2069–2073 (1985).
30. Dayer, J. M., Beutler, B. A., and Cerami, A. *J. Exp. Med.* **162**, 2163–2168 (1985).
31. Gamble, J. R., Harlan, J. M., Klebanoff, S. J., and Vadas, V. A., *Proc. Natl. Acad. Sci. USA* **82**, 8667–8671 (1986).
32. Ammann, A. J., Palladino, M. A., Volberding, P., Abrams, D., Martin, N. L., Wert, R., and Conant, M., *Clin. Lab. Immunol.* (1987).
33. Chang, R. and Lee, S. H. *TNO-ISR Meeting on the Interferon System* **55** (1985).
34. Dayer, J. M., Beutler, B. A., and Cerami, A. *J. Exp. Med.* **162**, 2163–2168 (1985).

35. Collins, T., Lapierre, L. A., Fiers, W., Strominger, J. L., and Pober, J. S. *Proc. Natl. Acad. Sci. USA* **83**(2), 446–450 (1986).
36. Shalaby, M. R., Palladino, M. A., Hirabayashi, S. E., Eessalu, T. E., Lewis, G. D., Shepard, H. M., and Aggarwal, B. B. *J. Immunol.* **137**, 2592–2598 (1986).
37. Lowry, R. P., Marghiesco, O. M., and Blackburn, J. H. *Transplantation* **40**, 183–188 (1985).
38. Johnson, R. L., Fink, C. W., and Ziff, M. *J. Clin. Invest.* **51**, 2435–2449 (1972).
39. Mirrakhimov, M. M., Kitaev, M. I., Imanbaev, A. S., and Markovich, M. O. *Ter Arkh.* **56**, 53–56 (1985).
40. Aderka, D., Novick, D., Hahn, T., Fischer, D. G., and Wallach, D. *Cell Immunol.* **92**, 218–225 (1985).
41. Koff, W. C. and Fann, A. V. *Lymphokin Res.* **5**, 215–221 (1986).
42. Taverne, J., Matthews, N., Depledge, P., and Playfair, H. L. *Clin. Exp. Immunol.* **57**, 293–300 (1984).
43. Silberstein, D. S. and David, J. R. *Proc. Natl. Acad. Sci. USA* **83**, 1055–1059 (1986).
44. Eife, R. F., Eife, G., August, C. S., Kuhre, W. L., and Staehr-Johansen, K. *Cell Immunol.* **14**, 435–442 (1974).

# Leukoregulin
## Potential as a Clinical Cancer Therapeutic Agent

JANET H. RANSOM and LINDA S. CLEVELAND

## 1. Introduction

Leukoregulin has not been introduced into clinical trials yet; it has, however, been evaluated in a three-phase preclinical screen. This screen consisted of evaluation of leukoregulin's growth inhibition of human tumor and normal cell lines, measurement of the inhibition of tumor stem cell colony formation in agar using freshly dissociated human tumor cells, and inhibition of human tumor xenograft growth in athymic nude mice. The data regarding the growth inhibition of human tumor cell lines were presented in the preceeding chapter on leukoregulin. Leukoregulin activity ranging from 1 to 1200 units inhibited human gastrointestinal, bladder, head, and neck carcinomas, glioblastomas, and leukemia cell lines, but not normal cell counterparts. The second phase of the screen, clonogenic growth of tumor cells in semisolid agar medium, has been used as an indicator of patient clinical response with a relatively high degree of correlation (1,2). This type of assay allows for the determination of the types of tumor cells that may respond clinically to a given therapeutic agent. The third phase of the screen, evaluation of growth inhibition of human tumor xenografts, further enables appropriate selection of dosage, route of administration, and length of exposure required for a clinical response.

## 2. In Vitro Preclinical Tests

Fresh surgical specimens of human colon adenocarcinoma and small cell lung tumors were digested with collagenase (3), and single-cell suspensions were cultured in 0.3% agar medium (4) with or without the addition

313

of leukoregulin (Table 1). Some human tumors were established in nude mice either from collagenase-dissociated cell suspensions or from tissue fragments transplanted subcutaneously. These established tumors were dissociated and cultured similarly to the fresh surgical specimens and tested for leukoregulin sensitivity (Table 2). About half of the tumors cultured immediately after surgery developed colonies in agar. Three of the five tumors that grew displayed significant inhibition of colony formation. There was a much higher success rate, 11 out of 15, when human tumor xenografts were tested and 10 of 11 tumors responded with significant inhibition of colony formation. Therefore, the high sensitivity of human colon and lung tumor cell lines to leukoregulin directly compares to the susceptibility of these tumor types in the clonogenic assay when noncultured human tumor cells are evaluated.

Table 1
Susceptibility of Freshly Excised Colon Tumors to Leukoregulin
in an Agar Clonogenic Assay[a]

| Patient number | Control colonies per well ± SE | Percent growth inhibition | Leukoregulin, units/mL |
|---|---|---|---|
| CHN | 22 ± 6 | 98 | 50 |
| 84-1991 | 44 ± 6 | 38 | 4000 |
| 84-2027 | 72 ± 4 | 42 | 4000 |
| 845-1752 | 60 ± 11 | 25 | 400 |
| 61-WHC | 32 ± 2 | 12 | 400 |

[a]$2 \times 10^5$ Tumor cells were plated/mL 35-mm culture dish and assessed for colony formation after 2 wk. Colonies 200 $\mu$m or larger were enumerated.

## 3. In Vivo Preclinical Tests

Our in vivo preclinical test consists of treating athymic nude mice bearing human tumor xenografts with leukoregulin. Tumor cells were implanted intrasplenically, resulting in primary tumor growth in the spleen and formation of metastatic tumor foci in the lung and liver. It was reasoned that this model system would more closely resemble clinical tumor therapy than treating subcutaneously transplanted tumors. Because this was a metastatic model, and metastatic foci can be heterogenous in their response to therapies, we evaluated leukoregulin's growth inhibitory effects on several human tumor cells and in vivo-selected variants with increased metastatic capabilities (Table 3). These tumors were kindly provided by Dr. Jim Kozlowski and were selected for increased metastases formation by repeated subcutaneous tumor implantation, surgical tumor excision, and reimplantation, by trocar, of tumor foci that developed in the lung (5). We found that the metastatic variants did not differ significantly in their susceptibility to leukoregulin from their nonselected counterparts.

Table 2
Susceptibility of Freshly Excised Human Tumor Xenografts to Leukoregulin in an Agar Clonogenic Assay[a]

| Tumor type | Control colonies per well ± SE | Percent growth inhibition[b] |
|---|---|---|
| Colon carcinomas | | |
| THO | 38 ± 4 | 92 |
| ATK | 160 ± 22 | 91 |
| EPP | 86 ± 17 | 91 |
| BLV | 66 ± 15 | 40 |
| Lung carcinomas | | |
| LS-1 | 32 ± 6 | 78 |
| LX-1 | 2742 ± 1160 | 53 |
| LS-16 | 61 ± 18 | 74 |
| LS-13 | 106 ± 14 | 34 |
| Mammary carcinoma | | |
| MX-1 | 12 ± 3 | 29 |
| Sarcoma | | |
| BRT | 8 ± 4 | 94 |

[a]$2 \times 10^5$ tumor cells were plated/mL/35-mm culture dish and assessed for colony formation after 2 wk. Colonies 200 $\mu$m or larger were enumerated.
[b]In the presence of 50 units of leukoregulin.

We therefore injected one of the most leukoregulin-sensitive tumors, HT-29, intrasplenically into mice. To maximize the therapeutic effect, leukoregulin was administered intravenously three times a week for 8 wk starting 4 h after tumor cell inoculation (Table 4). The primary tumor incidence in the spleens of mice treated with leukoregulin was 40% compared to 86% for saline-treated controls. Moreover, those 40% of tumors that did grow in leukoregulin-treated mice were 84% smaller than those in control tumors. The incidence of metastatic tumor formation in control mice was too low to register significant differences; treated mice had fewer metastases, however. There was no difference in mouse weight or other adverse pathologies in control and treated mice. The finding that leukoregulin can inhibit the growth of a human tumor in a mouse suggests possible clinical therapeutic effectiveness.

Table 3
Susceptibility of Human Tumor Cell Lines and Metastatic Variants to Leukoregulin In Vitro

| Cell line | Type | Units causing 50% growth inhibition | Metastatic tumor incidence | | | |
|---|---|---|---|---|---|---|
| | | | Intravenous[a] | Subcutaneous[b] | Intrasplenic[c] | |
| | | | % Lung mets. | % Lung mets. | % Lung mets. | % Liver mets. |
| HT-29 | Colon | 1.7 | 20 | 70 | 80 | 20 |
| HT-29M | Colon metastatic | 1.5 | 50 | 60 | 100 | 70 |
| A375P | Melanoma | 1.8 | 40 | 0 | ND[d] | ND |
| A375M | Melanoma metastatic | 4.2 | 100 | 93 | ND | ND |
| DX-3 | Melanoma | 25 | 40 | 20 | 60 | 100 |
| DU-145 | Prostate | 48 | 7 | 20 | 30 | 0 |
| PC-3 | Prostate | 7.3 | 7 | 15 | 80 | 100 |
| PC-3M | Prostate metastatic | 7.7 | 87 | 55 | ND | ND |

[a] $1 \times 10$ tumor cells were injected iv. Mice were euthanized after 8 wk and microscopic lung tumor burden was assessed (5).

[b] $1 \times 10$ tumor cells were injected sc, and the tumors were allowed to grow for 2 wk, then excised, and microscopic lung tumor burden was assessed at 8 wk (5).

[c] $5 \times 10$ tumor cells were injected is. Mice were euthanized after 8 wk and microscopic lung and liver tumor burden was assessed (5).

[d] ND, not determined.

Table 4
Leukoregulin Therapy of HT-29 Injected Intrasplenically[a]

| Tumor site | Control | Leukoregulin treated | % Inhibition |
|---|---|---|---|
| *Spleen* | | | |
| Incidence | 12/14 | 4/10 | |
| Tumor burden, g | 1.08 | 0.17 | 84 |
| *Liver* | | | |
| Incidence | 2/14 | 0/10 | |
| *Lung* | | | |
| Incidence | 4/14 | 1/10 | |
| Mice weight, g | 22.5 | 22.3 | |

[a]Leukoregulin was injected three times a week for 8 wk until a total of 600 units was administered. Mice were euthanized at 8 wk and microscopic metastatic foci enumerated. Mice were weighed at the end of treatment.

## 4. Conclusions

Leukoregulin inhibits the growth of numerous human tumor cell lines and freshly dissociated noncultured human tumor cells. Leukoregulin also inhibits human tumor cell outgrowth in nude mice, suggesting that leukoregulin may have great clinical therapeutic potential.

## References

*1.* Van Hoff, D. D., Clark, G. M., Stogdill, B. J., Sarosdy, M. F., O'Brien, M. T., Casper, J. T., Mattox, D. E., Page, C. P., Cruz, A. B., and Sandbach, J. F. *Cancer Res.* **43**, 1926–1931 (1983).
2. Alonso, K. *Cancer* **54**, 2475–2479 (1984).
*3.* Peters, L. C., Brandhorst, J. S., and Hanna, M. G., Jr. *Cancer Res.* **39**, 1353–1360 (1979).
*4.* Hamburger, A. W. and Salmon, S. E. *Science* **197**, 461–463 (1977).
*5.* Kozlowski, J. M., Fidler, I. J., Campbell, D., Xu Z-l, Kaign, M. E., and Hart, I. R. *Cancer Res.* **44**, 3522–3529 (1984).

# Index

## A

Actinomycin D, 91, 197
Antibodies
    to cytolysin, 55, 56

## B

Bladder carcinoma, 257, 285
Breast cancer, 253, 254, 276, 277

## C

Calcium
    requirement in cell cytolysis, 53
Cell-mediated cytotoxicity
    formation of ion pores, 10
    mechanisms of, 9, 45
Cervical cancer, 257, 258, 285
Colorectal carcinoma, 255, 256, 285, 313–317
Complement
    C9, 36
    mechanism of cell cytolysis, 36
Cytolysin (*see* perforin)
    antibodies, 55, 56
    biological actions, 5, 53–55, 149
    cell source, 5, 46
    definition of, 7, 53
    mechanism of action, 55–60
    molecular weight, 5, 52
Cytoplasmic granules
    isolation of, 22, 46–48

lesions produced by, 22–27
    molecular contents, 49, 50
    target cell sensitivity, 56
Cytotoxic T-lymphocytes
    mechanism of action, 20–22

## E

Eosinophils
    cationic protein, 34
    granules, 51
    mechanism of cell-mediated cytotoxicity, 32–34

## G

Glioblastoma, 284

## H

Head and neck carcinoma, 257, 285
Hematologic malignancies, 258–262, 286–293
Hepatocellular carcinoma, 284

## I

Inhibitors
    of cytolysin, 57, 58
    of endotoxin, polymyxin B, 78

319

Interferon
   assay, 108
   definition of, 107, 273
   gene structure, 102
   immunomodulation, 264
   mechanism of action, 105–110,
      151, 262, 263, 274–276
   neutralizing antibodies, 112
   protein structure, 102, 273
   receptors, 103
   synergisms, 110, 294
Interferon-α
   biological effects, 4, 5, 89, 91,
      112–114, 262, 275
   cell source, 5, 101
   clinical trials, 247–264, 276–293
   inducing agents, 5
   molecular weight, 5, 102
   specific activity, 5, 247
   toxicity, 5, 249, 293
Interferon-β
   biological effects, 4, 5, 262
   cell source, 5, 101
   clinical trials, 248, 276–293
   inducing agents, 5
   molecular weight, 5, 102
   specific activity, 5, 247
   toxicity, 5, 249, 293
Interferon-gamma
   biological effects, 4, 5, 89, 91,
      262
   cell source, 5, 107
   clinical trials, 248, 276–293
   inducing agents, 5
   molecular weight, 5, 103
   specific activity, 5, 247
   toxicity, 5, 249, 293
Ion channels
   in cytolysin mechanism of action,
      58–60
   in leukoregulin mechanism of ac-
      tion, 198–202
   in NKCF mechanism of action,
      125

K

Kaposi's sarcoma, 255, 286
Kinetics
   of cytolysin-mediated killing, 55
   of macrophage cytolysis, 80, 81

L

Leukolysins
   definition of, 3
Leukoregulin
   assays, 192–194
   biological effects, 5, 172–182,
      208–214, 313–317
   cell source, 5, 169–172
   definition of, 6, 169–189
   inducing agents, 5, 170, 202–204
   mechanism of action, 178–182,
      189–191, 194–202
   molecular weight, 5, 182, 183,
      207
   pI, 5, 183
   relationship to other lymphokines,
      173–178
   species specificity, 178
   toxicity, 315
Lipid A, 74
Lipopolysaccharide (see endotoxin),
      68, 69
   inducer of monocyte cytotoxic
      factor, 89
   role in monocyte cytolysis, 72–76
Lung cancer, 256, 284, 313–315
Lymphotoxin (see TNF-β)
   antibodies, 221, 222
   biological effects, 5, 131, 222–
      229
   cell source, 5, 218, 219
   definition of, 4, 217, 241
   inducing agents, 5, 219, 220, 238,
      239, 241

molecular weight, 5, 218–220,
    241, 242
pI, 5, 220
relationship to TNF, 221–227
Lysomotropic agents, 161


**M**

Macrophage activating factors, 68
Macrophages (*see* mononuclear
    phagocytes)
functions, 67, 69, 72–81, 87
mechanism of action, 87
soluble toxic factors
    complement, 7
    H$_2$O$_2$, 7, 69, 70
    lysozyme, 7, 69
    macrophage cytotoxic factor, 7
    proteases, 7, 70, 71
    thymidine, 7, 69
    tumor necrosis factor, 71
Melanoma, 252, 283
Membranes
    synthetic membranes, 13
Monocyte cytotoxic factor
    biological actions, 95–97
    definition of, 87, 88
    kinetics of lysis, 90
    proteolytic enzyme sensitivity, 93
    source, 88
    temperature sensitivity, 92


**N**

Natural killer cell cytotoxic factor
    antibodies, 142, 143
    biological actions, 5, 125–133,
        156–162
    cell source, 5, 123, 138, 149–151
    definition of, 6, 121, 149

divalent cation requirements, 151
human, 123, 138
inducing agents, 5, 122, 123
inhibitors, 140
kinetics, 125, 138
molecular weight, 5, 130, 139,
    141, 155
murine, 123
receptor, 151, 152
relationship to other cytokines,
    131, 132, 141–144
Natural killer cells
    mechanism of action, 20–22, 121,
        122, 137, 138, 144–146


**O**

Ovarian carcinoma, 256, 257, 283,
    284


**P**

Pore-forming proteins
    from amebae, 10–18
        biophysical properties, 17
        molecular weight, 11
        purification, 14, 15
    from mammalian lymphocyte
        granules
        cytolytic activity, 32
        isolation, 27
        polymerization, 29
    from other protozoan parasites,
        18–20
    in NK mediated cytotoxicity, 58–
        60
Protease inhibitors
    effect on MCF, 94
    effect on NKCF, 124, 158
    effect on TNF, 94

## R

Renal cell carcinoma, 254, 277–283

## T

Tumor necrosis factor
  assays, 238
  biological effects, 5, 131, 303–309
  cell source, 5, 241
  definition of, 5, 71, 235–238, 239
  homology to lymphotoxin, 242
  inducing agents, 5, 71, 238, 239
  mechanism of action, 71, 236–238
  molecular weight, 5, 240
  pI, 5
  toxicity, 5, 307, 308

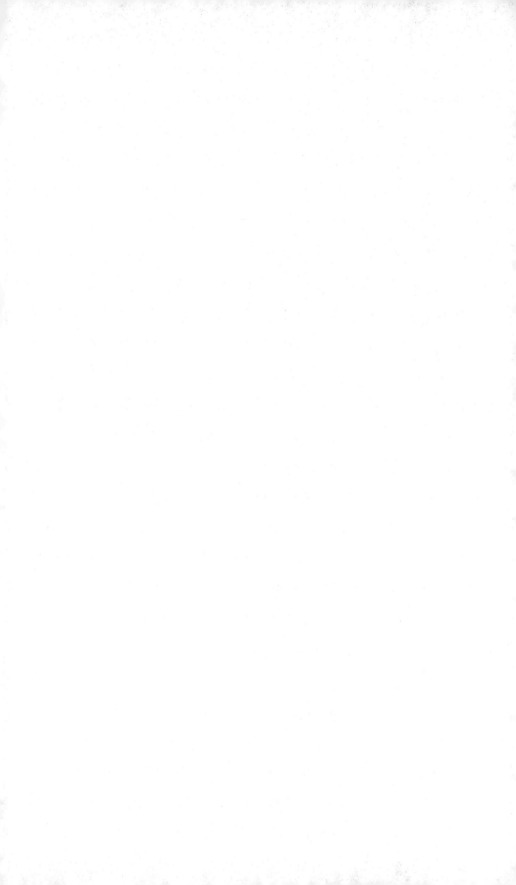